I0754513

technics used in the work, arranged so luminously as to form an admirable guide to every medical student. The whole system is here displayed with a modesty of pretension, and a scrupulosity in statement, well calculated to bespeak candid investigation. This laborious work is indispensable to the students and practitioners of Homœopathy, and highly interesting to medical and scientific men of all classes. Complete Repertory, one volume, bound, $3.

Jahr's New Manual: originally published under the name of Symptomen-Codex. (Digest of Symptoms.) This work is intended to facilitate a comparison of the parallel symptoms of the various Homœopathic agents, thereby enabling the practitioner to discover the characteristic symptoms of each drug, and to determine with ease and correctness what remedy is most Homoeopathic to the existing group of symptoms. Translated, with important and extensive additions from various sources, by Charles Julius Hempel, M. D., assisted by James M. Quin, M. D., with revisions and clinical notes by John F. Gray, M. D.; contributions by Drs. A. Gerald Hull, George W. Cook, and Dr. B. F. Joslin, of New-York; and Drs. C. Hering, J. Jeanes, C. Neidhard, W. Williamson, and J. Kitchen, of Philadelphia; with a Preface by Constantine Hering, M. D. 2 vols., bound, 1848. $11.

Laurie, Dr. J., Homœopathic Domestic Me-dicine, with the Treatment and Diseases of Females, Infants, Children, and Adults. 5th American edition, much enlarged, with additions by A. Gerald Hull, M. D. 1849. Bound, $1 50.

Laurie, Dr. J., Elements of Homœopathic Practice of Physic. An Appendix to Laurie's Domestic, containing also all the Diseases of the URINARY AND GENITAL ORGANS. Bound, 1849. $1 25.

F. Humphrey's, M. D. The Cholera and its Homœopathic Treatment. 1849. 38 cts.

B. F. Joslin, M. D. Homoeopathic Treatment of Diarhœa, Dysentery, Cholera Morbus and Cholera, with repertories. 50 cts.

Jahr's Clinical Guide, or Pocket Repertory. Translated from the German, by Chs. J. Hempel, M. D. Bound, (just published,) $1 50.

Hahnemann's Organon of Homœopathic Medicine, 3d American edition, with improvements and additions from the last German edition, and Dr. C. Hering's introductory remarks, 1848. Bound, $1.

G. L. Rau's Organon of the Specific Healing Art of Homoeopathy. By C. J. Hempel, M.D. $1 25.

Hahnemann, Dr. S., Materia Medica Pura. Translated by C. J. Hempel, M. D. 4 vols. 1846. $6.

E. Stapf's Additions to the Materia Medica Pura. Translated by C. J. Hempel, M. D. $1 50.

Hahnemann, Dr. S., the Chronic Diseases, their Specific Nature and Homoeopathic Treatment. Translated and edited by Charles J. Hempel, M. D., with a Preface by Constantine Hering, M. D., Philadelphia. 8vo. 5 vols. Bound, 1845. $7.

Transactions of the American Institute of Homoeopathy. 1846. Bound. $1 50.

C. Hering's Domestic Physician. Fourth American edition, revised, with additions from the author's manuscript of the sixth German edition. The part relating to the diseases of Females and Children, by Walter Williamson, M. D. 1848. $2.

Homœopathic Cookery. Second edition, with additions, by the Lady of an American Homoeopathic Physician. Designed chiefly for the use of such persons as are under Homoeopathic Treatment. 50 cts.

Rueckert's Therapeutics: or, Successful Homoeopathic Cures, collected from the best Homoeopathic Periodicals, translated and edited by C. J. Hempel. 1 large 8vo. vol., bound. 1846. $3 50.

Hempel's Homœopathic Domestic Physician. Bound. 1850. 50 cts.

Jahr, G. H. G., M. D., Short Elementary Treatise upon Homoeopathia and the Manner of its Practice; with some of the most important effects of ten of the principal Homoeopathic Remedies, for the use of all honest men who desire to convince themselves by experiment of the truth of the doctrine. Second French edition, corrected and enlarged. Translated by Edward Bayard, M. D. Bound. 37 1-2 cts.

J. A. Tarbell, M. D. Sources of Health and the Prevention of Disease. Bound. 1850. 50 cts.

Bœnninghausen's Essay on the Homoeopath-ic Treatment of Intermittent Fevers. Translated and edited by Charles J. Hempel, M. D. 1845. 38 cts.

A Treatise on the Use of Arnica, in cases of Contusions, Wounds, Sprains, Lacerations of the Solids, Concussions, Paralysis, Rheumatism, Soreness of the Nipples, etc., etc., with a number of cases illustrative of the use of that drug. By Charles Julius Hempel, M. D. 1845. 19 cts.

Ruoff's Repertory of Homoeopathic Medi-cine, nosologically arranged. Translated from the German by A. H. Okie, M. D., translator of Hartmann's Remedies. Second American edition, with additions and improvements, by G. Humphrey, M. D., etc. $1 50.

The Family Guide to the Administration of Homoeopathic Remedies. Third edition, after the second London edition, with additions. Price 25 cts.

A Systematic Report of 392 cases Treated Hydropathically at Brattleboro', 1848; with a plan of the walks in the vicinity. Also, Causes and Hydropathic Treatment of the Cholera, by Drs. R. Wesselhoeft and Wm. Grau. 1849. 50 cts.

Ed. C. Chepmell's Domestic Homoeopathy restricted to its legitimate sphere of practice, together with rules for diet and regimen. First American edition, with additions and improvements by Samuel B. Barlow, M. D. 1849. Bound, 50 cts.

Laurie's Homoeopathic Domestic, by A. Gerald Hull, M. D. Small edition, bound. 1849. 75 cts.

Hempel's Boenninghausen, for Homoeopathic Physicians; to be used at the Bedside of the Patient, and in studying the Materia Medica Pura. 1 octavo vol., most complete edition, including the Concordances of Homoeopathic Remedies. Translated and adapted to the use of the American profession, by C. J. Hempel, M. D. 1847. $1 50.

Hartmann's Acute Diseases, and their Homoeopathic Treatment. Third German edition, revised and considerably enlarged by the Author. Translated, with additions, and adapted to the use of the American profession, by C. J. Hempel, M. D. 2 vols. $2 75.

Hartmann's Chronic Diseases. 2 vols. 1849. $3.

Becker, M. D., on Consumption. Translated from the German. 1848. 38 cts.

——— on Diseases of the Eye. Translated from the German. 1848. 38 cts.

——— on Constipation. Translated from the German. 1848. 38 cts.

——— on Dentition. Translated from the German. 1848. 38 cts.

☞ The above four works, bound in one volume, $1.

Hartmann, Dr. F., Practical Observations on some of the chief Homoeopathic Remedies. Translated from the German by A. H. Okie, M. D. First series. Bound, $1.

The second and last series. Bound, $1.

Epps, Dr. J., Domestic Homoeopathy: or, Rules for the Domestic Treatment of the Maladies of Infants, Children, and Adults, etc. Third American from the fourth London edition. Edited and enlarged by George W. Cook, M. D. 1848. Bound, 75 cts.

W. Williamson, M. D., Diseases of Females and Children. 38 cts.

Wm. Henderson, M, D., Homoeopathic Practice. 1846. 50 cts.

Forbes, M. D., Homoeopathy, Allopathy, and Young Physic. 1846. 19 cts.

Wm. Henderson, M. D. Letter to J. Forbes, 1846. 19 cts.

☞ The above three books, bound in one volume, $1.

Quarterly Homoeopathic Journal, Vol. I., complete with Index, for 1849, by Drs. J. Birnstill and B. de Gersdorf. $3.

The Homoeopathic Examiner, by A. Gerald Hull, M. D. The second and third volume, $10. Also, vols. IV. and V., or under the title:

The Homoeopathic Examiner, Vols. I. and II., new series, by Drs. Gray and Hempel, 1845-1847, bound, in two volumes, with an inoptical index over the 2 volumes, can be used as a manual. $6.

This is the most valuable collection of Essays on the treatment of all the more important diseases, such as *croup*, *inflammation*, *typhus*, *measles*, *scarlatina*, etc., etc. The work contains, likewise, many valuable provings, a number of interesting cases from practice, critical discussions, and original articles, and is altogether an indispensable aid to the physician.

The British Journal of Homoeopathy, edited by J. J. Drysdale, M. D., J. R. Russel, M. D., and R. J. Dudgeon, M. D. The four quarterly numbers of 1849 are on hand, at 75 cts. each number. Several volumes of 1846 and 1849 are complete on hand, at $3 each vol. of four quarterly numbers, with title and index.

On Eclecticism in Medicine: or, a Critical Review of the leading Medical Doctrines. An inaugural thesis, presented at the New York University, on the 1st of March, 1845. By C. J. Hempel, M. D. 25 cts.

Joslin, B. F., M. D., Principles of Homoeo-pathia. In a series of Lectures. Price 75 cts.

Reasons why Homoeopathy should receive an Impartial Investigation from the Medical Profession and the Public. By B. F. Bowers, M. D. 18 cts.

Defence of Hahnemann and his Doctrines, including an exposure of Dr. Alex. Wood's "Homoeopathy Unmasked." London, 1844. 50 cts.

F. Vanderburgh, M. D., an Appeal for Homoeopathy; or, Remarks on the Decision of the late Judge Cowan, relative to the legal rights of Homoeopathic Physicians. 1844. 12 cts.

Sherril's Manual of Homoeopathic Prescription, with an improved Repertory; also, an Introduction in which the doctrine and nature of the Homoeopathic system is explained. 1845. 38 cents.

F. A. Guenther's New Manual of Homoeopathic Veterinary Medicine; or, the Homoeopathic Treatment of the Horse, the Ox, the Sheep, the Dog, and other Domestic Animals. $1 25.

Just Published:

E. E. Marcy, M. D., The Homoeopathic Theory and Practice of Medicine. Bound, 1850. $2.

Jahr's and Gruner's New Homoeopathic Pharmacopiæ and Posology of the mode of preparing Homoeopathic Medicine, and the Administration of Doses, compiled and translated from the German works of Buchner, Gruner, and the French work of Jahr, by C. J. Hempel, M. D. Bound, 1850. $2.

Jahr's Diseases of the Skin: or, Alphabetical Repertory of the Skin Symptoms and External Alterations of Substance, together with the morbid phenomena observed in the glandular, osseous, mucous and circulatory systems, arranged with pathological remarks on the Diseases of the Skin. By Dr. A. G. Jahr. Edited by C. J. Hempel, M. D. Price $1.

Just imported: the New Edition.

M. J. Weber, M. D., Large Anatomical Atlas of the Human Body in Natural Size, coloured. Eighty-four plates, also the six newest supplement plates, and a text book or explanation of the Atlas. This is the original and correct edition, and has been always sold for $40 without the six supplement plates. At present, but for an uncertain time only, at $25.

Hydriatics, or Manual of the Water Cure, especially as practised by Vincent Priesnitz, in Græffenberg, compiled and translated from the writings of Charles Munde, Dr. Oertel, Dr. B. Hirschel, and other eye-witnesses and practitioners. Fourth edition, by Francis Græter. Price 50 cts., with one plate or six engravings. 1844.

Rokytansky's Pathological Anatomy. Trans-lated from the German, with additions on Diagnosis, from Schönlein, Skoda, and others, by Dr. John C. Peters. 1844. 75 cts.

Opinions of the Press.—" Dr. Rokytansky's book is no more than it professes to be: it is morbid Anatomy in its densest and most compact form, scarcely ever alleviated by histories, cases or hypotheses. It is just such a work as might be expected from its author, who is said to have written in it the result of his experience gained in the careful examination of over 12,000 bodies, and who is possessed of a truly marvellous power of observing and amassing facts. In the course of our analysis we have said comparatively little of its merits, the best evidence of which is found in the length to which our abstracts have been carried without passing beyond the bounds of what is novel and important. Nor would this fault have been committed though much more had been borrowed, for no modern volume on morbid Anatomy contains half so many genuine facts as this; it is alone sufficient to place its author in the highest rank of European medical observers."—*British and Foreign Medical Review*, January, 1843.

Enchiridion Medicum, or the Practice of Medicine; the result of fifty years' experience, by C. W. Hufeland, counsellor of state, physician in ordinary of the late King of Prussia, Professor in the University of Berlin. From the sixth German edition; translated by C. Bruckhausen, M. D. Revised by R. Nelson, M. D. Second American edition. 1844. Bound, $2 50.

ALPHABETICAL REPERTORY

OF THE

SKIN-SYMPTOMS

AND

External Alterations of Substance,

TOGETHER WITH THE MORBID PHENOMENA OBSERVED IN

THE GLANDULAR, OSSEOUS, MUCOUS AND CIRCULATORY SYSTEMS,

ARRANGED, WITH

PATHOLOGICAL REMARKS ON THE DISEASES OF THE SKIN.

BY DR. G. H. G JAHR.

EDITED BY

CHARLES J. HEMPEL, M. D.

NEW-YORK:

WILLIAM RADDE, 322 BROADWAY.

1850.

H. Ludwig & Co., Printers, 53 Vesey-st. N.Y.

PREFACE

THIS little work contains, beside the skin symptoms, a number of symptoms which do not strictly belong to this class of diseases, such as *sprains* and *pains as if sprained, affections of the bones* and *glands, disorganizations of the mucous membrane* of the inner mouth, fauces, sexual organs, &c. Although, logically speaking, these affections do not strictly belong to the diseases of the skin, yet no practitioner will object to finding these various maladies arranged side by side in this volume; he will even think that I might have taken a wider scope than I have done, though it is but just to say, that I have endeavoured to make this little work as complete as possible.

The plan which I have pursued in this work, will facilitate the comparison of analogous symptoms and the finding the desired information. This facility is afforded not only by the *alphabetic arrangement* of the symptoms, but also by the *twofold indication* of the remedies: first according to the *sensations and symptoms,* and secondly according to the *organs* and *parts of the body,* so that, in the former the parts of the body, and in the latter the symptoms, constitute the subdivisions. In order to afford practitioners the means of instituting comparisons in accordance with their own judgment, I have arranged under every leading or alphabetical word or name all that which belongs to this division, and have not only chosen nouns, but also adjectives, as such leading alphabetical words or names, so that ***red, blue,*** &c. swelling, for example, will not only be found under ***swelling***, but also, in conjunction with other ***red, blue,*** &c. things, under ***red*** and ***blue appearances*** generally, in order to be enabled to compare with each other all the morbid phenomena the characteristic distinction of which is ***red, blue,*** &c. colour. In the divisions by organs and parts, these appearances will be found mentioned again in the adjective form, so that "***red swelling of the face,***" in the article "***face,***" should not be looked for as a subdivision under "***swelling,***" but under "***red,***" (***red*** and ***swollen*** meaning ***red-swollen,***) &c. Upon the same principle we have constantly distinguished ***itching*** and ***itching parts,*** tumours, eruptions, &c., ***inflammations*** and ***inflamed parts,*** tumours, eruptions, &c., the former to be understood in the general sense, as a main division, the latter being mentioned as a secondary symptom characterizing a more general morbid state.

It has been deemed unnecessary, in this work, to copy the text of the symptoms from the Materia Medica, which every one is at liberty to consult at any time, either in the original form or as modified in my "*Symptomen-Codex.*" It should be mentioned, however, that this work has been enriched with a number of additional symptoms and indications, from *unprinted papers* and other sources. The signs which I have used in my Symptomen-Codex, asterisks and ciphers (*°), have likewise been employed in this little work, and have been arranged with as much care as possible; they have only now and then been omitted in the general paragraphs at the commencement of a new article. These omissions have been deemed proper, and, in some cases, even necessary, for this reason, that those general paragraphs, though constituting, for the most part, a résumé of the local symptoms which follow, are, nevertheless, to be considered in many respects as an independent and self-existing whole; it will be for the reader to judge whether a remedy which refers exclusively to a local symptom should have been mentioned in the résumé in a general sense, particularly when such omissions are easily supplied by the subsequent detailed arrangements of the local symptoms. This will, in every instance, be found so complete, that the reader will be enabled either to accept or reject my own general conclusions, provided he will remember that, if a remedy should be enumerated among the general remedies without being mentioned again among the local symptoms, it had not yet been used in their treatment.

One word about the pathological definitions. When Rückert published his repertory of the cutaneous diseases, the work was considered defective, because the diseases had not been classified agreeably to the systems of ***Willan*** or ***Bateman***. But this is by no means so easy. If the cutaneous symptoms had been recorded by the provers with reference to established systems of dermatology, it would not be a difficult task to arrange them agreeably to any other definitive plan; but considering the unsatisfactory and confused state of this portion of our Materia Medica, the most accomplished dermatologist would not be able to produce a satisfactory arrangement of the skin-symptoms according to some definite pathological system. I have, therefore, like my predecessors, retained the expression of the symptoms as we find them in our Materia Medica, and have endeavoured to remedy the defect by appending to this preface a list of the most important pathological names of the cutaneous diseases, mentioning at the same time the remedies which, according to the pure provings and my own observations, correspond to their respective forms. In arranging this list I have endeavoured to simplify it by mentioning the synonyma which have been used for the same disease by the different authors of dermatological systems. This list is arranged alphabetically, and, in defining the particular forms of the different cutaneous diseases, I have, without reference to any particular system, chosen all the truly characteristic symptoms, leaving out, for the sake of brevity, all symptomatic secondary symptoms which were not absolutely necessary. This list is indeed not as complete as I desired it should be, because I have not yet been able to discover, in every case, the exact correspondence between the different names used by different pathologists. It is to be hoped, however, that even this incomplete list will contribute, in a measure, to simplify and render more precise our terminology of the cutaneous diseases, and to lead to more satisfactory results in practice. ***Willan*** and ***Bateman*** being almost entirely contained in ***Biett***, there are, strictly speaking, only three systems to which I have had occasion to refer; these are the systems of ***Biett***, *Alibert* and ***Hebra***. All the other systems only serve to create confusion.

To every pathological form the reader will find appended the remedies which have been used for it with more or less success in practice, or, if the pathological name was evidently identical with the symptoms of the Materia Medica, reference has been made to these symptoms. At the conclusion of the list will be found a résumé of Hebra's system, which, after all, shows more clearly than others, the internal, pathological relationship of the different cutaneous diseases, thereby enabling the practitioner to infer with a tolerable degree of certainty, that a certain remedy which cured one disease, will cure another analogous one. Unfortunately, the system not yet being printed and having been communicated to me in manuscript, I have not been able to mention all the varieties belonging to a class; the omissions, however, are trifling, and would not have justified a suppression of those parts of the system which are really important.

The author of this work offers it to his professional brethren with all due humility, and hopes that, even if it should not prove satisfactory in all respects, it will advance the cause of Homœopathy at least one step farther.

G. H. G. Jahr.

Paris, January, 1850.

ALPHABETICAL LIST

Of the different Pathological Names of the

MOST IMPORTANT CUTANEOUS DISEASES,

Together with their synonyma and the corresponding remedies.

Achor, s. *Tinea.*

Acne. Pustulous eruption, with more or less inflamed pimples, generally suppurating very slowly, and frequently retaining during their whole course, the appearance of hard tubercles. Varieties:

Acne disseminata, *scattered acne.* Numerous pustules, especially on the forehead, cheeks and shoulders, either small and scaling off (acne simplex) or large, hard and secreting a follicular substance (acne indurata).—Corresponding remedies: Ars. ***Bell.*** Calc. ***Carb. veg. Hep.*** Lach. ***Led.*** Natr. m. ***N. vom.*** Nitr. ac. ***N. jugl.*** Phosp. ac. Puls. Sab. Selen. ***Sulph.***

Acne punctata. Black clots occasioned by the dust which gets mixed up with the follicular secretion. Remedies: ***Bell. Hep. Natr.*** Natr. m. ***Nitr. ac.*** Sabin. Selen. ***Sulph.***

Acne sebacea ***Biett,*** *comedones.* Same as the former, except that the follicular secretion looks yellow, not black. Remedies: See the former and those mentioned under "*Comedones,*" in the Repertory.

Acne ROSACEA. Copper colour of the skin, face, with scaly desquamation, with pustules that are more or less large and sometimes entirely wanting. Remedies: ***Ars.*** Aur. m. ***Calc.*** Cann. Canth. ***Carb. an. Carb. veg.*** Caust. Cic. ***Kreas.*** Lach. Led. ***Mez. Rhus t. Ruta.*** Sep. ***Veratr.***

ACNE MENTI, S. MENTAGRA.

ALBINISMUS, ALBINO, the milky-white colour of the skin of the so-called 'Albinos, which Biett numbers among the maculæ.

ALOPECIA, s. *hair, falling off of the,* in the Repertory.

ANTHRAX, s. *furunculus malignus.*

BOILS, s. *Repertory.*

BULLÆ, the same anatomical character as that of furunculi, except that they are more elevated. See PEMPHIGUS and RHYPIA.

CANCER, s. CARCINOMA.

CARCINOMA, s. *the Repertory.*

CRUSTA LACTEA, s. IMPETIGO LARVALIS.

CRUSTA SERPIGINOSA. This crust secretes a greenish-yellow, acrid fluid. It consists of violently-itching, isolated vesicles, with red areolæ, commencing about the ear and thence spreading over the face, neck and trunk, sometimes covering even the extremities and attacking the eyes. It is doubtful whether they are a variety of the itch or not, but it is certain that they are not of a syphilitic nature, for no syphilitic eruption is characterized by such *violent itching.* Remedies: ***Ars.*** Baryt. Calc. ***Cic. Graph.*** Lyc. ***Merc.*** Rhus t. ***Sassap. Sulph.***

DERMATOPHYTA et DERMATOZOA HEBRA, s. TINEA, PITYRIASIS, SCABIES, PHTHIRIASIS.

ECZEMA, HERPES SQUAMOSUS ALIBERT. Very small, agglomerated *vesicles*, upon a more or less inflamed base; the skin is sore and there is at first a considerable secretion of ichor; afterwards scales form, repeating frequently.—Remedies: ***Acon.*** Ars. Aur. ***Bell.*** Carb. veg. Clem. Con. ***Dulc.*** ***Merc.*** N. jugl. Petr. ***Phosph.*** Rhus. t. Sulph. Zinc.

Eczema CAPITIS, s. TINEA AMIANTACEA.

Eczema CHRONICUM. Chronic form of the eczema without fever. Remedies: Clem. Dulc. Merc. Petr. Phosph. Sulph.

Eczema FEBRILE. Acute form of simple diseases.

Eczema IMPETIGENOÏDES. Very much inflamed *vesicles*, almost like the pustules of impetigo, with similar yellow, soft scurfs.—Remedies: *Carb. veg. Con.* ***Rhus t. Zinc.***

Eczema MERCURIALE. Red eczema produced by abuse of Mercury.—Remedies: Acon. Bell. ***Chin.*** Dig. Hep. ***Sulph.***

Eczema RUBRUM. Vesicles upon a very red, very much inflamed base, with almost erysipelatous swelling of the affected parts; afterwards scaly crusts form, yellow and more or less humid. — Remedies: Ars. Aur. Dulc. Merc. Phosph. Sulph.

Eczema SOLARE. This appears upon uncovered parts which are exposed to the summer-heat for a sufficient length of time.—Remedies: *Acon.* ***Bell.*** *Camph.* Clem. Hyos.

ECHTHYMA, ***herpes pustulosus.*** This pustulous eruption is not to be confounded with the pustulous rupia, with dark-green, brownish scurfs, which arise from red, not very numerous pustules, and, on falling off, leave dark spots or even cicatrices.—Remedies: ***Ars.*** Borax. Cham. ***Merc. Rhus t.*** Staph. ***Sulph.***

Ecthyma BATEMAN, s. ECTHYMA.

Ecthyma PLUMBE, s. RUPIA.

Ecthyma SCHŒNLEIN, s. RUPIA.

ELEPHANTIASIS. A variety of LEPRA, s. LEPRA.

Elephantiasis ALBA. LEUKE GRÆCORUM, s. LEPRA ALBA.

Elephantiasis ARABUM. Variety of LEPRA, the joints growing large, deformed and insensible. S. LEPRA ELEPHANTINA.

Elephantiasis GRÆCORUM, LEPRA NODOSA. Variety of lepra; the epidermis and the adipose tissue form tubercles, and become unfit to perform their natural functions. S. LEPRA TUBERCULOSA.

Ephelides, freckles.—S. ***Freckles*** in the Repertory.

Ephelides HEPATICÆ.—Remedies: s. ***Spots, hepatic***, in the Repertory.

Erysipelas, s. ***the Repertory.***

Erythema. ***Redness of the skin without heat.*** Of no importance except when accompanied with soreness. S. INTERTRIGO.

Exanthemata. S. ERYSIPELAS, INTERTRIGO, MORBILLI, SCARLATINA, RUBEOLÆ, URTICARIA.—Some number variola and varicella among the exanthemata, others all acute eruptions, and many all eruptions whatsoever.—***Bateman*** and ***Biett*** number among the exanthemata such eruptions only as are characterized by red spots. *Hebra* limits the exanthemata still more; he numbers *erythema, roseola* and *urticaria* among his HYPERÆMIÆ; and *morbilli, scarlatina, variola, varicella* and *vaccina* among his EXSUDATIONS.

EXSUDATIONES HEBRA.—S. EXANTHEMATA, MORBILLI, SCARLATINA, VARIOLA, VARIOLOIS, VARICELLA, ERYTHEMA, RUBEOLA, URTICAREA, LICHEN URTICATUS, PERNIONES, ERYSIPELAS, FURUNCULUS, HERPES HEBRA, PEMPHIGUS, ZONA, PITYRIASIS, PSORIASIS, LICHEN, ACNE, MENTAGRA, LUPUS, PRURIGO, SCABIES, ECZEMA, PEMPHIGUS, IMPETIGO.

FRAMBOESIA, LEPRA FUNGIFERA, LUES INDICA, RUBULA.—*Fungous eruption* first consisting of pustules which appear in the face, groins, axillæ and around the anus, and become afterwards covered with more or less thick scurfs; these, on falling off, leave fungous, more or less red ulcers, which, on account of their cauliflower or raspberry-shaped appearance, on account of the diseases of the bones with which these ulcers are frequently accompanied, and the fork-shaped cicatrices which they frequently leave behind, have been considered a variety of syphilis by many authors. *Framboesia* is, beyond doubt, contagious; but it is not easily communicated by an embrace, and the sexual organs are never affected by it first.—Remedies?

Framboesia SYCOTICA, SYCOSIS INDICA, YAWS. Generally in the face, on the neck, chest and extremities less on the sexual parts, with large, more or less red pustules, secreting a thick, tenacious, white pus; the hair which is near these pustules is disposed to grow gray.—Remedies?

Framboesia THYMOTICA, THYMOSIS INDICA, PIANS. Generally first appearing on the sexual parts in the shape of small pimples which, on breaking, secrete a yellowish water but no pus; nor does the hair turn gray.—Remedies?

Framboesia SCOTICA, LUES SCOTICA, SIWNENS.—Whitish, bleeding, fungous excrescences in the mouth and corners of the mouth, originating in small raised, white spots, and either drying up, in which case they change to dark-brown scurfs, or else changing to painful ulcers which frequently spread widely and destroy the parts rapidly.—Remedies?

FURUNCULI, s. the repertory.]

Furunculus MALIGNUS, CARBUNCULUS, ANTHRAX.—Remedies: s. ANTHRAX in the Repertory.

GUTTA ROSACEA, s. ACNE ROSACEA.

HÆMORRHAGIA HEBRA, s. PURPURA.

HERPES ALIBERT, s. PITYRIASIS, PSORIASIS, IMPETIGO, LICHEN, ECTHYMA, RUPIA, ECZEMA, LUPUS, ACNE ROSACEA.

Herpes BATEMAN and BIETT.—*Vesicular* eruptions, with *groups* of vesicles, in a few days changing to more or less thin scurfs, or drying without forming scales.—See: HERPES ZOSTER, HERPES PHLYCTÆNOÏDES, HERPES CIRCINATUS, HERPES LABIALIS, HERPES PRÆPUTIALIS, HERPES IRIS.

Herpes CINCINNATUS. Circular rings of red spots, the skin within the rings having a natural appearance; the rings are surrounded by transparent vesicles. — Remedies: Calc.? Caust.? *Clem.* Magn. c. *Natr.* Natr. m. *Sep.* Sulph.?

Herpes CRUSTACEUS, s. IMPETIGO.

Herpes ERYTHEMOÏDES *Alibert*, s. ACNE ROSACEA.

Herpes EXEDENS seu RODENS, s. LUPUS and IMPETIGO RODENS.

Herpes FACIALIS, s. *Herpes* LABIALIS.

Herpes FARINOSOSUS, s. PITYRIASIS.

Herpes FURFURACEUS, s. PITYRIASIS.

Herpes HEBRA. This author only admits the following varieties of herpes: HERPES LABIALIS, HERPES PRÆPUTIALIS and HERPES IRIS.

Herpes IRIS. A species of herpes circinnatus, first consisting of red, circular spots each of which contains four concentric rings, the innermost of which alone becomes, in a few days, covered with vesicles until desquamation sets in, in about 10 or 12 days. They are generally seen on the dorsum of the hands and feet, on the ankles, &c.—Remedies?

Herpes LABIALIS et FACIALIS. Small circular groups of vesicles which, after a few days, become confluent, moist, and finally are covered with brownish scurfs that fall off in the shape of scales.—Appears on the lips, cheeks, eyelids and ears.—Disappears frequently without any treatment, though we may sometimes require to use: *Acon.* Ars. *Bell.* Cic. *Dulc.* *Hep.* Sulph.

Herpes LICHENOÏDES *Alibert*, s. Lichen.

Herpes MILIARIS, s. *Herpes* PHLYCTÆNOÏDES.

Herpes PHAGEDÆNICUS, s. *Lupus*.

Herpes PHLYCTÆNOÏDES seu MILIARIS. Groups of small, millet-sized, hard vesicles, full of a brown or lemon-coloured fluid, upon a red base, arising from small, red, burning, tingling and smarting dots; the vesicles break afterwards and become covered with yellow or blackish crusts.—Remedies: ***Acon.*** Ars. ***Bell.*** Bov. Calc. Lyc. Merc. ***Rhus t.*** Sep. ***Sil. Sulph.***

Herpes PRÆPUTIALIS et VULVARIS. The same as *herpes* LABIALIS, except that it appears upon different parts, and that it is, on this account, accompanied with different consensual symptoms, such as: burning in the surrounding parts, sometimes even swelling of the inguinal glands, &c. Remedies: *Aur.* Dulc. ***Hep.*** *Nitr. ac.* Petr. ***Phos. ac.*** *Sep.* ***Sulph.***

Herpes PUSTULOSUS, s. ECTHYMA.

Herpes PUSTULOSUS *Alibert*, s. ACNE ROSACEA, ECTHYMA, MENTAGRA.

Herpes RODENS, s. IMPETIGO RODENS and LUPUS.

Herpes SQUAMOSUS *Alibert*, s. IMPETIGO, LICHEN, ECZEMA, PSORIASIS.

Herpes VULVARIS, s. *Herpes* PRÆPUTIALIS.

Herpes ZOSTER, ZONA.—Groups of *vesicles* upon a red base, surrounding the trunk like a belt, increasing in a few days to pea-sized pustules which finally become covered with scurfs.—*Bateman, Biett,* and *Hebra*, number the zona among the varieties of herpes, and very properly so, for it is just as little related to vesicular erysipelas as to itch.—Remedies: Ars. *Graph.* Merc. ***Rhus t.*** Puls.— ***Bry. ? Cham. ?*** *Natr. ? Selen. ? Sil. ? Sulph. ?*

HYPERÆMIÆ. *Hebra* numbers among this class: *Erythema, Roseola, Urticaria ephemera.* See these names.

HYPERTROPHIES OF THE SKIN, *Hebra*.—See: VERRUCÆ, ICTHYOSIS, PITYRIASIS, TINEA AMIANTACEA, LENTIGINES, EPHELIDES, PELLAGRA, ELEPHANTIASIS, LEPRA, TYLOMA.

ICHTHYOSIS.—*Hebra* numbers it among the HYPERTROPHIES OF THE SKIN, *Bateman*, *Willan* and *Biett* among the SQUAMÆ. Thick, hard, rough tissue of the skin which prevents all secretion, with scales like those of the fishes, falling off with great difficulty, frequently covering the larger portion of the body, and generally the extremities, without any other derangement of the general health being perceptible or actually existing. It is in most cases congenital or hereditary.—Remedies: *Coloc. Hep. Plumb.*

IMPETIGO, *P. Frank*.—All chronic cutaneous eruptions which are not accompanied with fever.

IMPETIGO, *Bateman* and *Biett*. Pustules with humid yellow or green scurfs, arising from small pustules the largest of which is of the size of a millet-seed; they are crowded together, yellow, upon red, circular or oval spots; on falling off they either leave red, scaly spots, or else a red, porous surface which secretes an ichor.—Remedies: Alum. Amm. Ant. *Ars.* Baryt. *Bell.* CALC. Carb. veg. Caust. *Cic. Clem. Dulc.* GRAPH. Hep. Kreas. Lach. *Lyc. Merc.* Natr. *Natr. m. Nitr. ac.* Oleand. Phosph. Phosph. ac. RHUS T. Sassap. Sep. *Sil. Staph.* SULPH.

IMPETIGO FACIALIS. This is no particular variety, and is so named on account of the locality.—Remedies: Ars. *Calc.* Cic. *Graph.* Lyc. Rhus t.

Sep. *Sulph.* (Compare: IMPETIGO LABIALIS, LARVALIS and RODENS.

IMPETIGO FIGURATA. — Appears mostly on the hands and forearms of bakers and millers; among old people we often see it on the lower extremities. — Remedies: Ars. Calc. Clem. Dulc. Graph. Lyc. Rhus t. Sulph.

IMPETIGO GRANULATA, S. TINEA GRANULATA.

IMPETIGO LABIALIS. Ulcerated eruption on the lips and in the corners of the mouth.—Remedies: Amm. Ant. Arn. *Ars.* Bell. *Calc.* Caust. *Graph.* Hep. Ign. *Kreas.* Merc. Natr. Natr. m. Nitr. ac. Phosph. *Rhus t. Sep. Sil. Staph.* Sulph. Veratr.

Impetigo LARVALIS, PORRIGO LARVALIS *Willan*, CRUSTA LACTEA. — Remedies: Ars. Baryt. Bell.? *Calc.* Carb. veg.? Cic. Dulc.? Graph. Lyc. Merc. Natr. m.? Phosph. r. Phosph. ac.? *Rhus t.* Sassap. Sep.? *Sulph. Viol. tr.*

Impetigo RODENS, HERPES EXEDENS SCROPHULOSUS. Not to be confounded with LUPUS or HERPES EXEDENS IDIOPATHICUS; it is the common herpes phagedænicus. — Remedies: *Ars.* Bell. *Calc. Cic. Graph. Hep. Merc.* Natr. m. Nitr. ac. *Rhus t. Sep. Sil. Staphys. Sulph.*

Impetigo SCABIDA.—The whole length of the limb is covered with a crust.—Remedies: *Dulc.* Lyc. Sulph.

Impetigo SPARSA.—Irregular, scattered, humid scurfs on the whole body, limbs, trunk, and even on the hairy scalp.—Remedies: Cic. Lach. Sulph.

INTERTRIGO. See "SORENESS" in the Repertory.

ITCH, see the Repertory.

LAZARI MORBUS, s. LEPRA TUBERCULOSA.

LEONTIASIS, s. LEPRA TUBERCULOSA.

LEPRA, s. LEPRA VERA.

LEPRA ÆGYPTICA, true lepra, with scaly, cold, wrinkled, bronze-coloured skin of the face, pustules which change to fetid ulcers, with ulceration of the articular ligaments, bones and whole limbs.—Remedies: See "LEPRA VERA."

Lepra ALBA, VITILIGO ALBA, BARAS ALBA, ELEPHANTIASIS ALBA, LEUKE GRÆCORUM.—Remedies: Alum. *Ars.* Phosph. Sep. *Sil.* Sulph.

Lepra ALEPPICA, red, hard blotch, generally in the face, afterwards forming a crust, secreting but a small quantity of ichor, and finally leaving an ugly cicatrix. Remedies?

Lepra ARABUM VERA, s. LEPRA TUBERCULOSA.

Lepra ARETICA, s. LEPRA NORVEGICA.

Lepra ASTURIENSIS. Red, painful spot on the hand or foot, with thickening and roughness of the skin, leaving a smooth spot which develops a new scurf every year; accompanied with a good deal of nightly burning, great debility, frequently even mania, and sometimes with an eruption extending from the neck downwards along both sides of the chest. Remedies?

Lepra CAYENNENSIS, LEPRA RUBRA, MAL ROUGE DE CAYENNE. Spots without sensation, of a dirty red and yellow, or large tubercles with frightful disfiguration of the face, horrid ulcers on the whole body, caries and softening of the bones, thickening of the skin and lead-coloured ulcers.—Remedies?

Lepra CRIMENSIS. Resembling the former, except that the spots on their first appearance are *blue-red*, becoming afterwards brownish, even blackish, accompanied with much itching, creeping, smarting, burning and stinging.—Five or six years sometimes elapses before ulcers form.—Remedies ?

Lepra GRÆCORUM, s. LEPRA SQUAMOSA.

Lepra HOLSATICA. Probably of a syphlitic nature. All sorts of spots, white and brown scurfs and scales, crusts, pustules, tubercles, swelling of bones, rhagades, sycosic excrescences around the anus, ulcers in the buccal cavity, &c.—Remedies ?

Lepra ITALICA, s. LEPRA LOMBARDICA.

Lepra LAZARI, s. LEPRA TUBERCULOSA.

Lepra LOMBARDICA, PELLAGRA, *Lepra* MEDIOLANENSIS seu ITALICA. Some authors consider it a variety of ichthyosis, others of lepra ; according to *Biett* it is an independent disease, and *Hebra* numbers it among his *hypertrophies.*—First we perceive a redness on uncovered parts which are exposed to the heat of the sun, especially on the face and back of the hand, with scaly desquamation, and afterwards, often repeated returns of the disease, with claw-shaped nails, bristle-shaped hairs, aphthous ulcers in the mouth. First a creeping and numb feeling in the limbs, vertigo and melancholy which frequently leads to suicide, afterwards herpes, miliaria, petechiæ, hepatic spots, scaly desquamation, spasms, paralysis, diarrhœa, dropsy.—Remedies ?

Lepra MEDIOLANENSIS, s. LEPRA LOMBARDICA.

Lepra NIGRICANS, BARAS NIGRUM, VITILIGO NIGRI-

CANS. Incipient form of scaly lepra.—Remedies: S. LEPRA VERA.

Lepra NODOSA, S. LEPRA TUBERCULOSA.

Lepra NORVEGICA, LEPRA ARCTICA, SPEDALSKED. First dark-red spots on the nose, with a bluish redness of the face of a peculiar lustre, with violent itching; after which remain lead or copper-coloured tubercles which change to ulcers; accompanied with tubercles and phagedenic ulcers in the mouth and throat, also on the nose and at the anus, sycosic excrescences at the anus or on the whole body, lentil-shaped, copper-coloured or blackish spots and pustules, crusty eruptions.—Remedies?

Lepra PSORICA, S. LEPRA SQUAMOSA.

Lepra RUBRA, S. LEPRA CAYENNENSIS.

Lepra SCORBUTICA, Nakka.—See: LEPRA VERA.

Lepra SQUAMOSA, *Lepra* PSORICA, *Lepra* GRÆCORUM. First we perceive small, round, reddish elevations which become covered with white scales, afterwards forming crusts which, on being detached, soon form again.—Remedies: See "LEPRA VERA."

Lepra TAURICA. See LEPRA CRIMENSIS.

Lepra TUBERCULOSA, LEPRA ARABUM VERA, MORBUS LAZARI, LEPRA NODOSA, ELEPHANTIASIS, GRÆCORUM, LEONTIASIS seu LEPRA LEONINA, TYRIASIS.—This is the most malignant form of lepra, the whole skin with the subjacent adipose tissue degenerates into tubercles, and its functional power is entirely destroyed.—Remedies: LEPRA VERA.

LEPRA VERA. This has many forms, appearing at times as LEPRA ALBA, at others as NIGRICANS,

SQUAMOSA OR TUBERCULOSA.—Remedies: *Alum.* Amm. *Ars.* Baryt. Calc. *Carb. an. Carb. veg. Caust.* Coloc. Con. *Graph.* Iod. Kal. Lach. Lyc. Magn. m. *Merc. Natr.* Natr. m. Nitr. ac. *Petr. Phosph.* Sep. *Sil. Sulph.* Zinc.

LEUKE GRÆCORUM, s. LEPRA ALBA.

LICHEN, HERPES LICHENOÏDES ALIBERT. Small papulæ either colourless or red and inflamed, in more or less numerous, circumscribed or scattered groups; when acute, they are frequently spread over vast portions of the skin; when chronic, they are only seen on the dorsum of the hands, on the arms, face, neck or dorsa of the feet. Scurfs do not form except after violent scratching.—Remedies: *Acon.* Agar. Amm. Ars. *Bry.* Calc. Carb. veg. Caust. Cham. *Cic. Cocc.* Con. *Dulc.* Graph. *Lyc.* Merc. *Mur. ac. Natr. m.* Phos. ac. Puls. Rhus t. Staph. Stront. *Sulph.*

LICHEN AGRIUS. Numerous groups of inflamed tubercles, excoriated at their tips, with more or less thickened skin, especially in chronic cases, appearing principally on the backs of the hands, on the face and wrist-joints; the eruption on these joints frequently resembles the itch.—Remedies: Calc. *Cic.* Dulc. Graph. *Lyc.* Mur. ac. Rhus t. *Sulph.*

Lichen SIMPLEX. Small pimples which start up on the healthy-looking skin and scarcely present any symptoms of inflammation.—Remedies: Acon. Bry. *Cocc. Dulc.* Puls.

Lichen STROFULUS. Generally in the face, in groups, more or less inflamed.—Remedies: *Caust. Cic. Cham. Graph. Merc.* Rhus t. *Sulph.*

LIPOMA, See LUPIA in the Repertory.

LUPIA, See the Repertory.

LUPUS, HERPES EXEDENS IDIOPATHICUS. *Alibert* numbers it among the varieties of HERPES EXEDENS, *Bateman* and *Biett* consider it as an independent class, *Hebra* numbers it among his EXSUDATIONS, though in other respects it is to be considered as a form of tuberculosis. Phagedenic ulcers on the ala nasi, arising from broad, flat tubercles; they become covered with a thick scurf; after one part heals, the adjoining part is affected; it is in this way that even the nasal cartilages are sometimes destroyed. — Remedies: Ars.? Aur.? Calc.? Sep.? Sil.? *Staph.?* Sulph.?

Lupus IDIOPATHICUS, see LUPUS.

Lupus FACIALIS, s. IMPETIGO RODENS.

Lupus NASALIS, s. LUPUS.

Lupus SCROPHULOSUS, s. IMPETIGO RODENS.

MACULÆ, s. ROSEOLA, RUBEOLÆ, SCARLATINA, EPHELIDES, PURPURA, SYPHILIS, NÆVI, VITELLIGO, ALBINISMUS.

Maculæ BATEMAN and BIETT. Eighth order of their dermatoses, among which they number: EPHELIDES, NÆVI, ALBINISMUS, VITELLIGO.

MEASLES, MORBILLI, s. MEASLES in the Repertory.

MENTAGRA, HERPES MENTI, SYCOSIS seu SYCOMA MENTI. *Alibert* ranges it among his HERPES PUSTULOSUS, *Bateman* and *Biett* among their PUSTULOUS ERUPTIONS, *Hebra* among his CHRONIC EXSUDATIONS. It is a species of ACNE, the pustules invading principally the chin, inflaming the skin and sometimes imparting to it the appearance as though it were covered with humid excrescences. — Remedies: *Ant.* Carb. veg.? *Cic.* Clem.? Dulc.? *Graph.* Kreas.? Merc.? Sass.? Sep.? *Sulph.?*

MILIARIA. See RASH in the Repertory.

MILIARIA PURPUREA, s. PURPLE-RASH in the Repertory.

MOLLUSCUM. Sporadic eruption consisting of tuberculous pocks of the size of a pea to that of a pigeon's egg, increasing slowly, not very painful, containing a pappy matter, sometimes redunculated, at others conical or flat.—Remedies?

MORBILLI, see MEASLES in the Repertory.

MORBUS MACULOSUS, see PURPURA HÆMORRHAGICA.

NÆVI. See Repertory.

NEOPLASMATA HEBRA. Eighth class of Hebra's cutaneous diseases, containing: CONDYLOMATA, CANCER OF THE SKIN, BALENS OF THE SKIN, LIPOMA, TELANGICKTASIS, ACNE ROSACEA, NÆVUS VASCULOSUS.

PAPULÆ. Fifth order of the dermatoses according to *Bateman* and *Biett*, containing: LICHEN and PRURIGO.

PELIOSIS, see PURPURA HÆMORRHAGICA.

PELLAGRA, see LEPRA LOMBARDICA.

PEMPHIGUS. Numerous red, erythematous spots with free intervals, almost resembling the blisters which are occasioned by scalding. After the fluid which they contain is discharged, thin, reddish scales form. This is the PEMPHIGUS ACUTUS, or the POMPHOLIX BENIGNUS WILLAN. Remedies: Ars. *Bell.* Canth. Caust. *Dulc.* Hep.

Ran. *Rhus t. Sep.* (Also, and principally, *Acon.*, Hempel.)

Pemphigus CHRONICUS, POMPHOLIX DIUTINUS Willan. Distinguished from the former by the absence of all fever, and by its running a long course.—Remedies: See those of PEMPHIGUS ACUTUS.

Pemphigus SOLITARIUS, POMPHOLIX SOLITARIUS WILLAN. Single blister of the size of an egg, on the back, hand, &c., sometimes succeeded by two or three smaller vesicles near by.—Remedies?

PERNIONES, see CHILBLAINS in the Repertory.

PETECHIÆ. PURPURA PETECHIALIS.

PHTHIRASIS, see Lice-disease in the Repertory.

PIANS, see FRAMBOESIA THYMOTICA.

PITYRIASIS, HERPES FURFURACEUS seu FARINOSUS *Alibert. Bateman* and *Biett* number it among the squamæ, *Hebra* among his anomalies of the secretory organs, especially those of the follicular glands.—Rough, dry spots on the skin, not raised, of various colours, characterized by nothing but their scaly desquamations. —Remedies: Agar. Alum. Anac. ARS. Aur. BRY. Bruc. CALC. Cic. *Dulc. Graph.* KREAS. Lach. Led. *Lyc.* Merc. Natr. m. Petr. *Phosph. Sep.* LIT. SULPH. THUJ.

PLICA POLONICA. See this name under HAIR, DISEASES OF THE.

POMPHOLIX, see PEMPHIGUS.

PORRIGO CAPILLITII, see TINEA CAPITIS.

Porrigo LARVALIS, see IMPETIGO LARVALIS.

PRURIGO. Hard, flat papulæ, exceedingly small and sometimes even scarcely perceptible to the finger, of a healthy skin-colour, accompanied by violent itching, and, although vastly different from the itch, yet it is easily mistaken for it, especially when appearing upon the hands and causing a violent itching.—Remedies: Alum. Amb. Amm. Baryt. *Bry.* CALC. *Carb. veg.* Caust. Cocc. *Con.* Graph. Lyc. MERC. Natr. m. NITR. AC. N. vom. Oleand. *Op.* *Phosph. Puls. Rhus t.* SEP. SIL. SULPH. Thuj.

Prurigo FORMICANS. Attacking principally full-grown persons, with broader, more prominent papulæ and violent itching.—Remedies: Alum. Amb. Amm. Baryt. CALC. *Carb. veg.* Caust. Cocc. *Con.* Graph. Lyc. MERC. Natr. m. NITR. AC. Phosph. Rhus t. *Sep. Sil.* SULPH. Thuj.

Prurigo MITIS. Affecting principally young people in spring and summer.—Remedies: *Bry.* Cocc. *N. vom.* Oleand. *Op. Puls. Rhus. t. Sil.* *Sulph.*

Prurigo MERCURIALIS. See SCABIES MERCURIALIS.

Prurigo PODICUS. See ITCHING OF THE ANUS in the Repertory.

Prurigo SCROTI. See ITCHING OF THE SCROTUM in the Repertory.

Prurigo SENILIS. Itching of old people, frequently accompanied with phthiriasis.—Remedies: Arg.? *Ars.* Bov.? Canth.? Caps.? Laur.? Magn. arct.? Magn. m.? *Mers. Mez.* *Oleann.* Plat.? Rhod.? Ruta.? Sabad.? Staph.? *Sulph.*

Prurigo VENERA. This does not exist, and is always caused by mercury. We may safely assert that, when it is doubtful whether an eruption is syphilitic or not, it is not syphilitic when characterized by violent itching.*

Prurigo VULVARIS. See ITCHING OF THE PUDENDUM in the Repertory.

PSORIASIS, HERPES SQUAMOSUS *Alibert.* Scaly spots of various sizes, sometimes scattered and small, lentil-sized or else confluent and large, sometimes covering a whole extremity, with white, thick, more or less firmly adhering scales, and, in chronic cases, with hard, cracked skin.—Remedies: *Ars.* Aur.? Bry. *Calc.* Caust. *Cic.* *Clem.* Cupr.? *Dulc.* Graph. *Led.* *Lyc.* Magn. c.? *Merc.* Mur. ac. Nitr. ac. Oleand. Petr. Phosph. Rhus t. Sassap.? *Sep.* *Sulph.* Zinc.?

Psoriasis DIFFUSA. Especially on the face and extremities, with large, reddish, rough spots, nightly itching and single scales, after the removal of which the furrows of the uneven, shining cutaneous surface become covered with thin scales.—Remedies: Ars. Calc. *Cic.* Clem. *Dulc.* Graph. *Lyc.* Mur. ac. Rhus. t. *Sulph.*

Psoriasis FACIALIS. — Remedies: CALC. Cic. *Graph.* Led. *Lyc.* Merc. Oleand. Sep. *Sulph.*

Psoriasis GUTTATA. Single, rather large, not inflamed spots, mostly on the chest, nape of the neck, arms, loins, thighs, with scales which are easily detached, leaving a red, shining base. Remedies?

* This is too sweeping. Syphilitic gonorrhœa may be accompanied with intolerable itching of the glans, which is increased by pressure and scratching. It is this itching which is frequently the principal and most characteristic indication for the administration of Mercury. (Hempel.)

3

Psoriasis GYRATA. — Narrow, scaly spots or streaks on different parts of the body, sometimes spiral-shaped.—Remedies ?

Psoriasis INFANTILIS.—Generally like the spots in psoriasis diffusa, sometimes rough, raised, sore, traversed by rhagades.—Remedies : Calc. Cic. Lyc. Merc. Sulph.

Psoriasis INVETERATA.—Large, scaly spots, with rough, cracked skin, also with thickening and distortion of the nails and skin of the fingers. Remedies: Calc. *Clem.* Merc. Petr. Rhus t. Sep. *Sulph.*

Psoriasis LABIALIS.—Scaly spots on the lips and in the corners of the mouth, which are easily detached and then reappear again, generally traversed by rhagades. — Remedies: Calc. Graph. *Merc.* Mez. *Natr. m.* Nitr. ac. Phosph. Sep. Sil.

Psoriasis PALMARIS.—Peeling off of the skin in large scales; the disease commences with rough, scaly, dirty brown or blackish spots, and generally with deep, bleeding rhagades.—Remedies: Aur. Calc. *Clem.* Graph. Hep. Merc. *Mur. ac.* Petr. Sassap. Sil. *Sulph.* Sulph. ac.

Psoriasis SCROTALIS.—Scaly, red, hard and thickened skin of the scrotum, frequently with soreness and painful rhagades.—Remedies : Petr. Nitr. ac. Thuj.

Psoriasis SYPHILITICA.—A kind of PSORIASIS PALMARIS OR PLANTARIS; the scales originally do not consist of spots, but papulæ; there is no trace of psoriasis on any other part of the body.—Remedies: *Merc.* Clem.? *Nitr. ac.?* Thuj.?

PSYDRACIA, see SCABIES SPURIA.

Psydracia VACCINA.—This is frequently a sequel of vaccination.—Remedy: *Sulph.*

PURPLE-RASH, s. Repertory.

PURPURA. Red spots of different sizes.—Remedies: See RED SPOTS in the Repertory, and compare.

Purpura HÆMORRHAGICA, HÆMORRHŒA PETECHIALIS, MORBUS MACULOSUS *Werlhaf, Peliosis.*—Large, round, somewhat raised petechial spots which are filled with a thick blood, sometimes appearing on the whole body and sometimes accompanied with other kinds of hæmorrhage. —*Remedies:* Arn. Bell. Berb. *Bry.* Hyosc. Lach. Ledum, N. vom. Phosph. Ruta. *Rhus t.* Sec. Sil. Stram. Sulph. ac.

Purpura MALIGNA, Puncticulæ. Very small, red stigmata, frequently imparting to the skin a marbled appearance, of a benign character when small, a malignant character when larger. Remedies?

Purpura PETECHIALIS IDIOPATHICA DICTA, see PURPURA TYPHODES.

Purpura ROSEA. Large, flat spots from 2 to 3 inches broad, dark, rose-coloured, without sensation; while running their course the general health is not disturbed.—Remedies?

Purpura SCORBUTICA. The spots are like those of PURPURA HÆMORRHAGICA, except more greenish and accompanied with stomacace, bad ulcers, &c.—Remedies: See Scurvy in the Repertory.

Purpura SENILIS. Like the spots of purpura scorbutica, but there are no other symptoms of scurvy.—Remedies: *Ars.* Baryt.? *Bry.* CON. Lach.? Op.? *Rhus t. Sec.* Sulph. ac.

Purpura SYPHILITICA, s. ROSEOLA SYPHILITICA.

Purpura TYPHODES, PETECHIÆ IDIOPATHICÆ, FEBRIS PETECHIALIS. This is no more nor less than typhus, the petechiæ being a mere symptom. The accidental absence or presence of a particular symptom in typhus is no sufficient reason why we should consider it a particular variety of this disease. Such a symptom frequently depends upon the constitution of the patient, the intensity of the disease, the particular portion of the nervous system which is principally involved, &c. If, however, petechiæ should be present, we may give: Ars. *Bry.* Rhus t.

Purpura URTICANS *Willan.* Seems to be identical with purpura scorbutica, but occurs very rarely in this form.

Purpura URTICATA, s. URTICARIA.

Purpura VENEREA, s. *Purpura* SYPHILITICA.

PUSTULÆ. Sixth order of *Biett,* containing: VARIOLA, VACCINI, ECTHYMA, IMPETIGO, ACNE, MENTAGRA, PORRIGO.

RHYPIA, s. RUPIA.

ROSEOLÆ. Intermediate eruption between measles and scarlatina, so that, if the eruption should resemble the measles, the secondary symptoms frequently resemble the symptoms of scarlatina, and, if the eruption should be like scarlatina, the accompanying symptoms are like the catarrhal symptoms of the measles.—Remedies: Acon. Bell. Nux v. Puls.

Roseolæ SYPHILITICÆ. Dark, violet-red spots, mostly on the abdomen, arms, forehead, &c.; in constitutional syphilis these spots generally are the first symptom, even when the primary chancre is still existing.—Remedies: *Merc.*

RUBEOLÆ. See MEASLES in the Repertory.

RUPIA, RHYPIA. Small, isolated vesicles, upon a red, inflamed base, first containing a serous, afterwards a purulent fluid, generally on the extremities or loins, afterwards covered with brown crusts; the subjacent skin is sore. Is not to be confounded with ECTHYMA, the primary form of which is not vesicular, but pustulous; the scurfs of ecthyma are less broad and more firmly adhering than those of RHUPIA.—Remedies: Alum. *Ars.* Borax. Calc. *Cham.* Clem. *Graph.* Hep. *Merc.* Natr. Nitr. ac. *Petr.* Rhus t. Sep. *Sil.* Staph. *Sulph.*

Rupia HEBRA; this is the syphilitic rupia with pyramidal scurfs, and probably identical with the RUPIA PROEMINENS BATEMAN.

Rupia PROEMINENS, with conical scurfs consisting of several layers, and probably of a syphilitic nature.—Remedies: Alum.? Clem. *Merc.* Nitr. ac.? Sassap.? *Sulph.* Thuj.?

Rupia SIMPLEX, BULLA PHAGEDÆNICA HAHNEMANNI, PHAGEDENIC ULCER of some authors.—Remedies: See BULLA PHAGEDÆNICA in the Repertory.

SCABIES, ITCH. According to modern authors the *acarus* is supposed to be the characteristic diagnostic of the true itch. It is doubtful, however, whether the ancients meant by scabies the acarus-scabies exclusively. Lice, and other kinds of vermin, may likewise cause a species of scabies which is very much like the acarus-scabies, and is likewise characterized by the peculiar voluptuous itching. Though this kind of scabies has been termed SPURIOUS SCABIES, yet it is by no means certain what is the true diagnostic of the real itch.

SCABIES SPURIA. Eruptions which resemble the itch, without being the disease. The different forms of PRURIGO, IMPETIGO, and VESICLES, also HYDRARGYRA and syphiloïd forms of eruption, have been termed SPURIOUS SCABIES.

SCARLATINA, see Repertory.

SPEDELSKHED, see LEPRA NORVEGICA.

SPILOSIS, see MACULÆ.

SQUAMÆ. Sixth order of the dermatoses according to *Bateman* and *Biett*, containing: ICHTHYOSIS, PITYRIASIS, LEPRA, PSORIASIS.

STEATOMA, s. LUPIA in the Repertory.

STROFULUS, s. LICHEN STROFULUS.

SYCOMA, s. MENTAGRA.

SYCOSIS, see the following:

Sycosis BARBÆ seu MENTI, s. MENTAGRA.

Sycosis HAHNEMANNI, s. SYCOSIS VENEREA.

Sycosis INDICA, s. FRAMBOESIA SYCOTICA.

Sycosis LABIALIS, principally affecting persons who take snuff; small, painful blisters changing to ulcers with yellowish lymph; they become covered with scurfs which keep forming, and they are surrounded by hardness and redness.—Remedies: Acon. *Ars. Bell. Cic.* Dulc. Hep. *Sulph.*

Sycosis MENTI, s. MENTAGRA.

Sycosis PALPEBRARUM. Thick, granular, pustulus elevations on the margin and the inner surface of the eyelids.—Remedies?

Sycosis VENEREA, SYCOSIS HAHNEMANNI, CONDYLOMATA.—Remedies: See FIGWARTS in the repertory.

Sycosis VERRUCOSA, see FIGWART.

SYPHILIS, SYPHILOIDES, see the following:

Syphilis BULLOSA, RUPIA HEBRA, see RUPIA PROEMINENS.

Syphilis MACULOSA, ROSEOLA SYPHILITICA, see SYPH. BULLOSA.

Syphilis PUSTULOSA, at times resembling the pustules of smallpox, at others those of acne; in the former case they generally appear on the face and trunk, with brown, thick crusts, beneath which the ulcerative process continues and which leave a round, white, deep cicatrix; whereas, if the pustules resemble acne, they scarcely ever occur on the forehead or in the face, but rather on the rest of the body, and almost without scurfs, and leave only superficial cicatrices and always livid spots.—Remedies: *Merc.* Nitr. ac. Thuj.

Syphilis SQUAMOSA, only in the palms of the hands and on the soles of the feet. See PSORIASIS SYPHILITICA.

Syphilis TUBERCULOSA. The form varies. Sometimes semi-globular, flattened, with ulcerative surface, in which case the disease frequently breaks out primarily at the anus and on the sexual organs; frequently, however, the tubercles are larger, rounder, especially on the neck, forehead and face; sometimes the eruptions are granular and cracked, in which case they appear principally in the corners of the mouth. Principal remedy: *Merc.*

Syphilis ULCEROSA, CUTANEA. Secondary *syphilitic cutaneous ulcers.* Very rare unless the previously mentioned forms are numbered among this class. There is a variety of these ulcers arising from deep-seated cutaneous tubercles, resembling a number of small cutaneous buboes, with semi-globular, sunken, lardaceous base. Always secondary, and existing only in constitutional syphilis. *Carbo veg.* acted as a specific in one case. *Merc.* is a specific for the ulcerated syphilitic rhagades between the toes.

Syphilis VEGETANS, VEGETATIONES SYPHILITICÆ, s. SYCOSIS VENEREA.

SYPHILONYCHIA EXULCERANS. Ulceration of the root of the nail.—Principal remedy: *Merc.*

Syphiloïdes. The syphilitic *cutaneous diseases,* see above. The other syphilitic forms, such as: ANGINA, CORYZA, GUMMA, TOPHUS, DOLORES OSTEOCOPI, BUBONES, OPHTHALMIA, &c., are sufficiently known.

TELANGIEKTASIS, s. ANEURYSMS BY ANASTOMOSIS in the Repertory.

TINEA CAPITIS, s. SCALDHEAD in the Repertory.

Tinea capitis AMIANTACEA seu ASBESTINA, ECZEMA CAPILLITII.—Dry, inodorous scald, with scales which shine like silver, or changing silk, with the hairs united in clusters, with little itching, but red, furrowed skin.—Remedies: Ars. Carb. an. Merc. Rhus t. Staph.

Tinea c. ANNULATA. Circular groups of yellowish pustules, through whose centre a hair passes, very dry.—Remedies?

Tinea c. ASBESTINA, see TINEA AMIANTICEA.

Tinea CRUSTACEA, s. *Tinea* FAVOSA.

Tinea FAVOSA, seu LUPINA seu CRUSTACEA seu MALIGNA, FAVUS.—Dry scurf of a dirty-yellow colour, with deep, scattered holes, like a honey-comb, with pustules depressed at their tips like a funnel.—Remedies: Baryt. Brom. Calc. *Merc. Phosph.* Sulph. (Compare TINEA C. SICCA.)

Tinea c. FURFURACEA seu SQUAMOSA, PITYRIASIS CAPITIS.—Itching scabs on the hairy scalp, well known.—Remedies: *Alum.* Bry. Calc. Graph. Kal. Lach. *Mez. Oleand.* Rhus t. Staph.

Tinea c. GRANULATA, IMPETIGO CAPITIS seu GRANULATA HERPES MILIARIS CAPILLATA. Gray or brown, irregularly scattered crusts, not depressed at their tips as in favus, but arched, arising from small, yellow pustules which secrete a thick, speedily drying humour.—Remedies: Ars. *Calc.* Hep. Merc. Phosph. Rhus t. *Sulph.*

Tinea c. HUMIDA, see *Tinea c.* MUCIFLUA.

Tinea c. IMPETIGINOSA, see *Tinea c.* GRANULATA.

Tinea c. LUPINOSA, s. *Tinea c.* FAVOSA.

Tinea c. MILIARIS, s. *Tinea c.* GRANULATA.

Tinea c. MUCIFLUA, PORRIGO C. WILLAN, *humid scaldhead.* Groups of pustules with copious secretion of humour, which, on drying, covers the hairs like layers and glues them together. Remedies: Baryt. Calc. Cic. Graph. *Hep.* LYC. Oleand. *Rhus t. Sep.* Staph. *Sulph.* Vinc.

Tinea c. PORRIGINOSA, s. *Tinea c.* MUCIFLUA.
Tinea c. SICCA, s. *Tinea c.* GRANULATA.
Tinea c. SQUAMOSA, s. *Tinea c.* FURFURACEA.
Tinea FACIES, s. IMPETIGO LARVALIS and CRUSTA SERPIGINOSA.
Tinea facies LACTEA, s. IMPETIGO LARVALIS.
Tinea f. MUCIFLUA, s. the former.
Tinea f. PORRIGINOSA, PORRIGO LARVALIS WILLAN, s. IMPETIGO LARVALIS.
Tinea f. SERPIGINOSA, s. CRUSTA SERPIGINOSA.
TUBERCULÆ. Seventh order of the cutaneous diseases according to *Bateman* and *Biett*, containing: ELEPHANTIASIS GRÆCORUM and MOLLUSCUM.
TYLOMA, s. CALLOSITIES in the Repertory.
TYRIASIS, s. LEPRA TUBERCULOSA.
ULCERA, s. ULCERS in the Repertory.
URTICARIA, s. NETTLERASH in the Repertory.
VARICELLÆ.—Remedies: ACON. ANT. *Ars.* Asa. BELL. *Canth. Carb. veg.* Caust. *Con.* Cycl. *Ipec.* Led. *Merc.* Natr. Natr. m. PULS. RHUS T. Sec. *Sep.* Sil. Sol. m. Sulph. TART. Thuj.
Varicellæ AGNOSÆ seu EMPHYSEMATICÆ, according as the fluid in the vesicles is more or less thick or evaporates.—Remedies: *Acon. Ant. Bell.* Canth. Con. Merc. *Puls.* Sec. Sil. Sol. m. *Tart.* Thuj.
Varicellæ CONOÏDES. — Remedies: *Acon. Ant.* Ars. *Bell.* Carb. veg. Ipec. *Puls. Rhus t.* Sep. *Tart.* Thuj.
Varicellæ MILLÆ seu OVALES. Oblong, large pustules, changing to dark crusts.—Remedies:— Acon. Bell. Led. Puls. Rhus t.
VARICES, see Repertory.

VARIOLÆ. See Smallpox in the Repertory.
VARIOLOÏDES.—Remedies: Ant. *Ars. Bell.* Bry. *Merc.* Puls. *Rhus t.* Sulph. Tart. *Thuj.*
VESICULÆ. Second order of the cutaneous diseases according to *Bateman* and *Biett*, containing: HERPES, ZONA, ECZEMA, SCABIES, MILIARIA, VARICELLÆ.
VITELLIGO ALBA, s. LEPRA ALBA.
Vitelligo NIGRICANS, s. LEPRA NIGRICANS.
YAWS, s. FRAMBOESIA SYCOTICA.
ZONA, s. HERPES ZOSTER.

CONCISE VIEW
OF
HEBRA'S SYSTEM OF CUTANEOUS DISEASES.

(From the manuscript copy of one of his disciples.)

I. *Class:* HYPERÆMIÆ.—1) ACTIVE: *Erythema, Roseola variolosa, Urticaria ephemera.*—2) PASSIVE: *Cyanosis, Morbus cœruleus.*
II. *Class:* ANÆMIÆ: *Chlorosis,* &c.
III. *Class:* ANOMALIES OF THE SECRETORY ORGANS.—1) ANOMALIES OF THE SECRETION OF SWEAT: *Deficient exhalation, Sudor anglicus, Coloured sweat, Bloody sweat,* &c.—2) ANOMALIES OF THE SECRETION OF THE FOLLICULAR GLANDS: *Seborrhœa, Lichen simplex, Grutum milecum, Comedo* seu *Acne punctata, Strofulus albidus, Molluscum, Pityriasis.*
IV. Class: EXSUDATIONS, *either* ACUTE or CHRONIC:
1) ACUTE; *a*) *contagious: Exanthemata, Morbilli, Scarlatina, Varioli, Varioloïdes, Varicellæ, Varicella fimbriata, Vaccina.*—*b*) *Non-contagious: Erythema exsudativum, Erythema nodosum, Intertrigo, Decubitus Roseolæ, Dermatitis* (*Cutitis*) *Burns, Congelations, Ery-*

sipelas, Pseudo erysipelas, Furunculus, Anthrax, Herpes labialis, Zona (*Herpes zoster*), *Herpes præputialis, Herpes iris, Pemphigus acutus.*

2) *Chronic exsudations; a) solid: Pityriasis rubra, Psoriasis, Lichen ruber, Acne simplex, Mentagra, Lycosis, Lupus.—b) fluid: Prurigo, Scabies, Eczema, Tinea muciflua, Porrigo* seu *Impetigo larvalis, Crusta, serpiginosa, Elephantiasis Arabum.—c) vesicular: Pemphigus chronicus, Pompholix, Rupia.—d) pustulous: Impetigo achor, Porrigo, Erysipelas pustulosum, Maliasmus, Psydracium, Phlycacium.*

V. *Class:* HÆMORRHAGES.—1) *Idiopathic: Purpura traumatica, Purpura senilis, Purpura simplex afebrilis.*—2) *Symptomatic: Purpura, Roseola, Paliosis rheumatica, Purpura simplex febrilis.*

VI. *Class:* HYPERTROPHIES.—1) *Syloma* (*Tylosis*) *Verruca, Nævus verrucosus, Ichthyosis, Pityriasis capitis* seu *Tinea asbestina.*—2) *Of the pigmentum: Lentigines, Ephelis, Chloasma, Pellagra, Lepra lombardica, Nævus spilosus.*—3) *Of the chorion: Elephantiasis Græcorum, Lepra norvegica, Lepra tuberculosa, Leuke Græcorum,* (*Lepra alba*), *Morphea* (*Lepra alba et nigricans*), *Spilop laksia* (*Alibert*) *Ophiasis.*— 4) *Elephantiasis Arabium dermatokeras* (*Callus*), *Polytrichia, Orychia, Polynychia.*

VII. *Class:* ATROPHIES.—*Leukopathica, Achromasia, Argyria. Stopecia* (*Calvities*).

VII. *Class:* NEOPLASMATA.—*Condylymata, Cancer of the skin, Keloïdes, Baleus of the skin, Lipoma, Telangiektasia, Acne rosacea, Nævus vasculosus.*

IX. *Class: Pseudoplasmata.*

X. *Class:* ULCERA.—*Ulcera syphilitica, scrophulosa, cancerosa, scorbutica, varicosa, herpetica,* &c.

XI. *Class: Dermatophyta, Dermatozoa, Favus, Tinea tondens, Porrigo decalvans,* (*Alopecia circumscripta*), *Pityriasis versicolor, Epizoa* (*Pediculi*) *Acarus scabiei, Filaria medinensis.*

XII. *Class:* NEUROSES: *Hyperæsthesis, Pruritus, Dermathalgia, Anæsthesis, Anomalies of motion, Cutis anserina.*

Appendix: Syphilitic forms. Well known.

Blackness, Acon. Vip. torv.
Boils, *Phosph. Zinc. ox.*
Brownish spots, °Sep.
Buboes, s: glands, affections of.
Burning of skin, Berb. Carb. veg. Caust. Kreos. Led. N. vom. *Ol. an.* Sabad. Sassap.
Eruption, Bell. Bry. Merc.
Erysipelas, °*Graph.*
Glands, inguinal, affections of, °*Aur.* °Ars. *Calc.* °*Carb. veg.* Clem. **Dulc. Graph.* Lyc. **Merc.* Natr. **Nitr. ac.* Phosph. Stann. Stram. **Staph.* **Sulph.* °Thuj. Tereb.
Glands, inguinal, suppuration of, °Aur. °*Merc.* **Nitr. ac.* °*Sulph.*
Glands, ulcerated, *Hep.*
Glands, inflamed, Graph. **Sil.*
Hernia, inflamed, Baryt. Jod.
Abdominal integuments, °Graph.
Spots, inflamed, Ars. Bell. Canth. *Kal. *Lach.* Led. Lyc. °Natr. m. **Phosph. Sabad.* °*Sep.*
—, pit of stomach, Natr. m.
Rash, Bruc. Selen.
—, hepatic region, Selen.
Spots, yellow, Canth. **Phosph.*
Swelling, Acon. Bell. Canth. Caust. Oph. Puls. Sep.

Swelling, glands, inguinal, °*Aur.* °Ars. *Calc.* ° *Carb. veg.* Clem. **Dulc. Graph.* Lyc. **Merc.* Natr. **Nitr. ac.* Phosph. **Staph.* Stann. Stram. **Sulph.* Tereb. °Thuj.

—, umbilical region, Caust. Lyc. Lach.

Hernia, °*Acon.* Alum. Amm. Asar. °*Aur. Cocc.* °*Coloc.* Con. Lach. °Laur. ? °Lyc. ? °*Magn. art.* °Magn. c. Natr. m. Nitr. ac. **N. vom.* °Op. °Petr. °Phosph. °Spig. °Staph. °*Sulph.* Zinc.

—, incarcerated, °*Acon.* Alum. °Cocc. ? °*N. vom.* °Op. Phosph. °*Sulph.*

Itching, Agar. Alum. Arn. Aur. Baryt. **Bell.* Berb. Bov. Can. Coloc. Con. Ign. Kal. Kal. hdr. Laur. Led. Magn. arct. Magn. c. Magn. s. *Merc. Natr.* N. vom. *Ol. an. Petr.* Phosph. *Puls.* Sassap. Sep. Spig. Stront. Sulph. Tereb. Zinc.

—, hernia, Baryt.

—, inguinal region, Berb. Laur. Magn. c. Magn. m. Magn. s. Sep. Spig.

—, umbilical region, Ign. Kal. Kal hdr. Magn. arct. Ol. an. Phosph. *Puls.*

Osseous tumour, pelvis, °Aur.

Pain as if ulcerated, Amm. m. *Bov.* Dig. Hell. *Kreos.* Magn. c. Mang. °Nitr. ac. *Ran. Rhus.*

—, umbilical region, Magn. c.

Pimples, Ars. Bar. m. Bry. Cham. Dulc. Natr. Natr. m. Petr.

Pock-shaped pustules, *Puls.*

Pustules, inguinal region, *Puls.*

Red skin, Amm. °Graph. **Rhus.*

Red spots, Bell. Lach. *Sabad.*

" rash, Bruc.

Red swelling of glands, Lyc. **Merc.*
Soreness, abdomen, Rhus t.
—, inguen, Phosph. ac.
Sore pain, Cann. Carb. veg. Croton. Euphorb. °Hyos. Lyc. Phosph.
Sore, inguinal region, Bry. Calc. Chin. Spig.
Scarlet-redness, **Bell.* **Rhus.*
Stinging, Berb. Mur. ac. Phos. ac.
Streaks, umbilical region, Phos. ac.
Swelling, black and blue, Aeth. Vip. red.
Swelling, painful, °Lach. Tereb. Thuj. Vip. torv.
—, inguinal region, Agar. Ant. Croton. **Graph.* Hep. **Therid.*
Swelling, sensation of, glandular region, Con. Sil.
Tumours, Natr.
Ulcers, °*Ars.* Bar. m. Chin. Cupr. *Hep.* Plumb.
—, inguinal region, Bar. m. *Hep.*
—, inguinal glands, *Hep.*
—, umbilical region, °*Ars.*
Vesicles, Caust. Merc.

Abscesses.

Head, °*Calc.* Lyc.
Canthi, lachrymal, sac., Bry. Nat. *Puls.* Stann.
Mouth, Amm. Canth. °Caust. Natr. *Sulph.*
—, tonsils, Bar. c. **Bell.* Berb. °Gran. ? °Ign. °*Lach.* **Merc.* Nicc. Sep. °Hep. °*Sulph.*
—, gums, Amm. Canth. °Caust. °Sulph.
—, tongue, Natr.
Dorsal region, axilla, Petr.
—, nape of neck, Sil.
—, neck, Hyos.
—, back, Lach.
—, loins, °Sil. °Staph.

Aching-pressing.

Blood-vessels, swelling of, Ign. Phosph.
Pimples, Stann.
Swelling, Magn. aust. °*Merc.* Mosch. N. vom. Phosph. Seneg. Sep. Stann.
Ulcers, Camph. Carb. veg. Chin. **Graph.* Par. **Sil.*
Corns, Anac. **Ant.* Bry. Calc. Caust. Graph. Ign. °*Lyc.* Magn. arct. Magn. aust. Phosph. Phos. ac. **Sep.* °*Sil.* Staph. °*Sulph.*
Nails, Calc. Caust. Magn. art. Magn. aust. Sassap. Sulph.

Dorsal region, eruptions, Merc.
—, swelling, °Merc.
Lower limbs, eruptions, Kal.

Acne punctata.

In general, Dig. Dros. Graph. °*Natr.* **Nitr. ac.* Sabad. Sabin, **Sulph.*

Nose, °Dros. Graph. Selen. **Sulph.*
Face, Dig. °Dros. °Nitr. ac. Sabin. °Selen. **Sulph.*

Acne-shaped.

Pimples, **Bell.* **Carb. veg.* Hep. *Lach. Sulph.*

Head, eruptions, Bov.
Face, blisters, **Bell.* **Carb. veg. Hep.* °Lach.
Comp: ACNE OF DRUNKARDS, ACNE ROSACEA, PUNCTATA, &C.

Acuminated.

Pimples, *Ant.* Ars. Tart.
Pustules, Dulc. Thuj.

Adhesion of the skin.

In general, Arn. Par.
—, sensation of,
In caries, °Arn.? °*Asa.* °Aur.? °Chin.? °Hell.? °Merc.? °*Phos. ac.* °Puls.? Ruta. °Sabin.? °*Sil.* °Staph.?

Head, Arn. Berb. Magn. arct. Par.
Face, Sabin.

Air, containing.

Blisters, vesicles, Kal. Vip. torv.

Canthi, Natr. m.

Air, passing through, sensation as of.

Glands, Spong.

Anal region.

Black, eruption, Carb. veg. Sassap.
Black, swelling, black and blue, **Carb. veg.* *Mur. ac.*
Bleeding, Alum. **Amm.* **Amm. m.* °*Anac.* Ant. Ars. Asar. Baryt. Borax. Calc. Caps. *Carb. an.* **Carb. veg.* Cast. **Caust.* Chinin. Coloc. **Con.* Croc. Crotal. *Cupr. Ferr.* Graph. Hep. Ign. *Kal.* °*Lach.* Lam. Led. Lyc. Magn. art.

Magn. m. **Merc.* Mercurial. **Merc. corr.* Mur. ac. Natr. m. Nitr. Nitr. ac. **N. vom.* Oph. **Petr.* **Phosph.* Plat. Prun. *Puls.* Raph. Ratanh. Sabad. Sabin. °*Sassap.* Selen. **Sep.* Sil Stram. **Sulph.* Tart. Thuj. Val. Vip. torv. Zinc.

Bleeding varices, Acon. Amm. Bell. **Calc.* Cham. Chin. Cupr. Electr. *Ferr.* Galv. Hyos. *Kal.* Magn. a. Men. Nitr. ac. **Puls.* **Sep.* Stram. **Sulph.*

Bloody pus, discharge of, Natr. m.

Blotches, Carb. veg. Hep. Ign. Stann. Staph. Thuj.

Boil, Carb. an.

Burning, Aloë. ***Alum.*** Amm. Amm. m. Ant. **Ars.* Aspar. Baryt. Berb. Bov. Bry. *Calc.* Canth. **Caps.* *Carb. an.* **Carb. veg.* Cast. Caust. Chen. Chin. °*Cocc.* *Colch.* Con. Crot. Elect. Euphorb. Ferr. Gins. Gran. Graph. Grat. Hell. Hep. Ign. Ipec. Jod. *Kal.* Lach. Lact. Laur. Lyc. Magn. art. Magn. c. Magn. m. Magn. s. **Merc.* Mur. ac. Natr. c. **Natr. m.* Natr. s. Nitr. *Nitr. ac.* *N. vom.* Oleand. Ol. an. Onisc. Paeon, Petr. Phell. *Phosph.* Plumb. Prun. *Puls.* Ran. Ratanh. Sabad. Sassap. Senn. **Sep.* Sil. Staph. Stront. **Sulph.* *Sulph. ac.* Tab. Tart. Tereb. Thuj. Veratr. Vinc. Zinc.

—, perineum, Gran. Nitr. ac. Plumb. Sil.

Burning varices, Alum. Ant. Ars. Berb. **Calc.* Carb. an. Caust. Graph. Kal. Nitr. ac. N. vom. Phosph. Plat. Sulph. ac.

Creeping, Agar. Alum. Baryt. Berb. Calc. Carb. veg. Caust. Chin. Cocc. *Colch.* *Croc.* Ferr.

magn. Hep. Ign. Ipec. Kal. Laur. Magn. aust. Mosch. Mur. ac. Natr. *N. vom.* Ol. an. Phosph. Plat. Plumb. Rhus. *Sabad.* Sabin. Sep. Spong. Sulph. Tereb. Teucr. Zinc.

Eruption, Calc. Carb. veg. Ipec. Lyc.

Figwarts, * *Thuj.*

Fistulous ulcer, ° *Caust.* Petr. °Thuj.

—, perineum, Agn. Ars. Tarax.

Gnawing, Agn. Ars. Ferr. Phosph. Phos. ac. Stann. Tarax.

Grape-shaped, eruption, Calc.

Herpes, Ipec. Natr. m. Petr.

—, perineum, Petr.

Humour, Amm. Calc. Carb. an. *Carb. veg. Caust.* Led. Natr. m. *Nitr. ac.* Rhod. Sil. Sulph. Zinc.

Humid varices, Alum. Amm. Baryt.

Ichor, Hep. Natr. m.

Inflamed varices, ° *Cham.* Kal.

—, eruption, Calc.

Itching, Agar. **Alum.* Amb. **Amm.* Amm. m. **Anac.* Ant. Ars. Bell. Berb. Borax. Bruc. Bry. * *Calc.* Canth. Caps. * *Carb. veg.* * *Caust.* Cham. Chin. Cin. Cocc. Coloc. Con. Croc. Ferr. magn. Gran. Graph. Grat. Ign. Jod. **Kal.* Lach. Led. **Lyc.* Magn. art. Magn. aust. Magn. m. Men. Merc. Mur. ac. Natr. Natr. m. Natr. s. Nicc. **Nitr. ac. N. vom.* Ol. an. Petr. Phell. **Phosph.* Phos. ac. Plat. Prun. Rhus. *Sabad.* Sassap. **Sep.* ° *Sil. Spig.* Squill. Stann. Staph. **Sulph.* Tereb. Teucr. Zinc.

—, between butt ends, Alum. Con. Gran. Seneg.

—, perineum, Agn. Alum. Ars. Carb. veg. Gran. Ign. Mur. ac. N. vom. Plumb. Tarax.

Itching, eruptions, Ipec. Ign. Lyc. Staph.

Pain as if contused, Alum. Lact. Staph.
—, perineum, Alum.
Pain as if inflamed, Sulph.
—, perineum, Alum.
Pain as if ulcerated, Magn. c.
Painful eruptions, Lyc.
—, swelling, Aur.
—, ulcers, Sassap.
—, varices, Amm. °*Anac.* Ars. Calc. Caps. **Carb. veg.* *Caust.* Coloc. Ferr. °*Graph.* Grat. Kal. Lach. Lyc. Magn. art. Magn. c. Magn. m. Mur. ac. °*Natr. m.* *Nitr.* Nitr. ac. N. vom. Phosph. Puls. Sabin. Sep. Sil. Stront. Sulph ac. Thuj. Zinc.
Pimples, Carb. veg. Kal. Nitr. ac.
—, perineum, Nitr. ac. Caust. Natr. m. Sep. Sulph. Sulph. ac.
Pocks, black pocks, Sassap.
Prolapsus, Ant. °Asar. Canth. Dulc. Gran. Graph. **Ign.* Lach. Lyc. Magn. art. Magn. m. °*Merc.* Mur. ac. Natr. m. Nitr. ac. °*N. vom.* *Ruta. **Sulph.*
Pustules, Calc.
Rhagades, °*Agn.* °*Cham.* Graph.
Smarting, Agar. Alum. Amb. Baryt. Canth. Caps. Carb. veg. Caust. Chin. Dulc. Hell. Kal. Lach. Led. Lyc. Mercurial. Mez. Natr. c. N. vom. Phosph. Phos. ac. Rhod. Sabin. Sep. Sulph.
Soreness, Berb. Calc. *Carb. an.* *Carb. veg.* Ferr. Grat. Kal.. Lach. Merc. Natr. m. Nitr. ac. N. vom. Phosph. Sep. Zinc.
—. between buttocks, *Carb. veg.* Natr. m. Nitr. ac. Sep.

Soreness, perineum, Carb. veg.
Sore as if excoriated, Alum. Amm. Amm. m. Ang. Ant. *Ars.* Aspar. Baryt. Berb. Calc. Cann. Carb. veg. *Caust.* Croton. Euphorb. *Graph.* Grat. Hep. °*Ign.* Jod. Kal. Lach. Led. Lyc. Magn. art Magn. c. Magn. m. Mez. Mill. *Merc.* *Mur. ac.* Natr. °*Natr. m.* Natr. s. Nitr. ac. *N. vom.* Petr. Phell. Phosph. Prun. °*Puls.* Rhod. Rhus. Sabin. Sassap. Sep. *Spong.* Stann. Staph. *Sulph.* Tab. Veratr. Zinc.
—, eruptions, Stann.
Stinging eruption, Nitr. ac.
—, varices, Alum. *Ars.* Baryt. Caust. Grat. Kal. Merc. Natr. m. Nitr. N. vom. Phosph. Puls. Sil. Sulph. Sulph. ac.
Stricture, Ign. Lyc. Magn. aust. **N. vom.*
Suppuration, °Lach. Sulph.
—, ulcer, Sassap.
Swelling, Aur. Borax. Croton. Graph. *Hep.* Ign. Lach. Sep. Sulph.
Swollen, sensation as if, Camph. Graph. Hep. N. mosch. Teucr.
Tickling, Grat. Hep. °*Ign.* Jod. Kal. Lach. Led. Lyc. Magn. art. Magn. c. Magn. m. Mez. Mill. *Merc.* Mur. ac. Natr.
Tumours, tubercles, Carb. veg. Ipec.
Ulcers, Paeon. Sassap.
—, perineum, Paeon.
Varices, Acon. °Aloë.? *Alum.* Amb. **Amm.* °Anac. Ang. *Ant.* Arn. *Ars.* Baryt. Bell. *Berb.* Bruc. **Calc.* *Caps.* *Carb. an.* Carb. veg. *Caust.* Cham. Chin. Chinin. Coloc. Cupr. Electr. Ferr. **Graph.* Grat. Hell. **Ign.* **Kal.* °*Lach.* Lact. Lyc. Magn. art. Magn. aust. Magn. c. Magn.

m. *Mur. ac.* *Natr. m.* Nitr. **Nitr. ac.* **N. vom.* *Phosph.* Plat. °Plumb. **Puls.* Ran. Rhus. **Sabin.* **Sep.* Sil. Stram. Stront.**Sulph.* Sulph. ac. *Tart.* Therid. Thuj. Veratr. Zinc.

Varices, swollen and blue, *Carb.

Aphthæ.

Lips, Ipec.

Sexual organs, labia, Agar. **Borax.* °Cham. °Hell. Jod. °*Merc.* °N. mosch.? °N. vom. °*Sulph.* **Sulph. ac.* Sassap. Thuj. Vinc.

Arms and parts of arms.

Anthrax. °*Lach.* *Sec.*

Arthritic, arms, *Caust.*

—, elbow, °*Lyc.*

—, upper arm, Veratr.

Black, pocks, *Ars.*

Blisters, bloody, Sec.

Boils, Amm. °*Calc.* Carb. veg. Lyc. Magn. m. *Mez.* *Nitr.* Petr. Phos. ac. *Sil.* *Zinc.*

—, shoulder, Amm. *Nitr.* Phos. ac.

—, arm, *Mez.* *Sil.*

—, upper arm, Carb. veg. *Zinc.*

—, forearm, °*Calc.* Lyc. Magn. m. Petr.

Bones, affection of, Acon. Anac. °*Ang.* °*Calc.* *Indig.* Jod. Lact. °*Lyc.* Meph. Merc. *Natr.* *Natr. m.* Natr. s. Nicc. *Nitr. ac.* Plumb. Raph. °*Rhus.* Ruta. **Sil.* Staph. °*Sulph.* Tereb. *Thuj.*

—, elbow, °Amb. °Lyc. Phosph.

—, upper arm, Baryt. *Bell.*

—, forearm, Natr. m. Plumb. Spig. Spong.

Blueness, arms, Bism. Plat. Sep.
Blue spots, Berb. Sulph. ac.
—, swelling, Oph. Vip. torv.
Brown, eruptions, Ant.
Brown, spotted, swelling, *Sep.*
Bubbling, arm, Amb. Magn. aust.
—, shoulder, Berb. Mang. Puls.
—, elbow-joint, Kreos. Mang. Rhab. Spong.
—, upper arm, Berb. Colch. Zinc.
—, forearm, Zinc.
Burning, Alum. Amm. Amm. m. Arg. Arn. Asa. *Berb.* Borax. Bov. °*Bry.* Calc. Carb. an. *Carb. veg.* Caust. Coccul. Colch. Coloc. Dig. Dulc. Euphorb. *Graph.* Indig. Kal. Kreos. *Lach.* Laur. Led. *Magn. art.* *Magn. arct.* Magn. m. Mang. Men. Merc. Mez. Mill. Mosch. Mur. ac. Natr. m. *Natr. s.* N. vom. Oleand. *Ol. an.* Par. Petr. Phosph. Phos. ac. *Plat.* *Puls.* Ran. sc. Ratanh. **Rhus.* Sep. Spong. Staph. Stront. **Sulph.* Tarax. Teucr. Tong. Vip. torv. *Zinc.*
—, shoulder, Amm. m. Berb. *Carb. veg.* Coccul. Graph. Kal. Magn. m. Men. mill.
—, shoulder-joint, Graph. Stront.
—, arm, Alum. Bov. °*Bry.* Calc. Cocc. Dig. Kreos. Lach. Led. *Magn. art.* Magn. m. Merc. *N. vom.* Ol. an. Petr. Phell. Phos. ac. Plat. *Puls.* Rhus. Staph. *Sulph.* Vip. torv.
—, elbow, Amm. m. Arg. Berb. Carb. an. Carb. veg. Dulc. Indig. Laur. Merc. Mill. Natr. s. Nitr. Phos. ac. Plat. Rhus. Staph. Sulph. Teucr. Tong.
—, elbow-joint, Asa. Magn. art. Merc.
—, upper arm, Arg. Asa. Berb. Borax. Carb. veg. Caust. Colch. Coloc. Dig. Dulc. Graph.

Kal. Magn. arct. Mang. Mur. ac. Natr. m. Phosph. Sep. Zinc.
—, forearm, Amm. Amm. m. Arn. Asa. *Berb.* Carb. an. Carb. veg. Caust. Dig. Euphorb. *Graph.* Laur. Magn. m. Mosch. Mur. ac. Natr. s. Oleand. *Ol. an.* Ran. sc. Ratanh. *Rhus.* Staph. **Sulph.* Tarax. *Zinc.*
Burns, that which, (eruptions, pimples, vesicles, &c.,) Alum. Berb. Canth. Dulc. *Laur.* Magn. arct. Merc. *Mur. ac.* Natr. s. Phosph. Sabad. Sep. Staph. *Sulph.*
—, herpes, °*Con.*
—, swelling, Rhus. *Sulph.*
—, scaldhead, Amm. m.
—, erysipelas, Petr.
Carbuncle, s. Anthrax.
Chapped, arm, Sil.
Cold swelling, PULS.
Contracted tendons, see: Muscles.
Crawling, arm, Amm. Arn. *Bell.* Caps. Cham. Cocc. Croc. Gran. Natr. m. °*Nitr.* Paeon. *Sec.* °*Sulph.*
—, shoulder, Ammoniac. Berb. Coccul.
—, elbow, Berb. Canth. Merc.
—, upper arm, Lach. Sep. Thuj.
—, forearm, Arn. Bry. Con. Plumb.
Creeping, arm, Bell. Magn. aust.
—, forearm, Caust.
—, arm, °*Bell.* °Ign. Lach.
Cuts, see: Chapped.
Eczema, Mez. Phosph. *Sil.*
Eruption, (in general,) Alum. Berb. Bry. *Carb. an.* **Caust.* Lach. Led. Lyc. *Merc.* Phosph. Rhus. Sabin. Tart. Tax. Val. Zinc.

Eruption, shoulder, Alum. Berb.
—, arm, °Caust. Rhus. Val. Tart.
—, upper arm, Led. Vip. torv.
—, elbow, *Merc.* Phosph. *Sabin.* Zinc.
—, forearm, Bry. *Carb. an. Caust.* Lach. Lyc. TAX. Zinc.

Erysipelas, arm, Petr. **Rhus.*
Erysipelatous swelling, **Rhus.*
Fetid pocks, °*Ars.*
Flesh, as if beaten loose, arm, *Dros.* Ign. *Staph. Thuj.*
—, shoulder-joint, Staph.
—, upper arm, Thuj.
Furfuraceous, eruptions, Agar.
—, tetters, °Phosph.
Gangrene, arm, *Ran.* Sec.
Gnawing, arm, Ars. Hell. Led. Lam. °*Lyc.* Phell. Phosph. Plat. Ruta. **Sulph.*
—, shoulder, Berb.
—, axilla, Agn.
—, elbow, Berb. Dulc. Phosph. Puls.
—, upper arm, Led.
—, forearm, Rhus.

Hardness, upper arm, Magn. c.
—, forearm, Carb. an.
Hard eruptions, Mez. Sep. Sil.
—, swelling, Led.

Hepatic spots, arm, Ant.
Herpes, *Con. Cupr.* °*Dulc.* Grat. *Hell.* Kreos. Lach. Magn. s. *Mang.* **Merc.* °*Phosph. Sep.*
—, arm, °*Dulc. Hell.* Lach. Merc. Natr. m. °*Phosph.*
—, elbow, *Cupr.* Kreos. *Sep.*

Herpes, upper arm, Grat. Magn. s.
—, forearm, *Con.* Magn. s. *Mang.* **Merc.*
Herpetic eruptions, Natrum m. SEP.
Humid herpes, °*Con.* Hell.
—, scald, °*Alum.*
Induration of muscles, upper arm, Petr.
—, forearm, cellular tissue, °*Sil.*
Inflammation, °*Arg.* *Petr.* *Ran.*
Inflamed (swelling,) *Bry.* **Lyc.* Sep.
—, erysipelas, *Petr.*
Itching, arm, Agar. Ang. Ant. Ars. Aur. *Bov.* Calc. Carb. veg. **Caust.* Chin. Con. Cupr. Graph. Hell. Kal. *Lach.* Lam. Led. °*Lyc.* Natr. N. vom. Ol. an. Op. Phell. *Phosph.* Phos. ac. Plat. *Puls.* Rhus. Rut. Sep. Sulph. Tab. Tart. Teucr. Thuj. Veratr. Zinc.
—, elbow, Agar. Amm. m. Berb. Canth. Coloc. Dulc. Hep. Lach. *Laur.* Merc. Natr. Nitr. ac. *Oleand.* Petr. Phosph. Puls. Rhus. Sep. *Spig.*
—, upper arm, Ant. *Berb.* Bov. Carb. veg. Dig. Dulc. Euphorb. Kal. hdr. Lach. *Laur.* Led. Lyc. Magn. arct. Magn. aust. Mang. N. vom. Oleand. Phell. Phos. ac. Ran. sc. Rut. Stront. Thuj.
—, forearm, Amm. Amm. m. Berb. Bov. Carb. an. Carb. veg. *Caust.* Con. Dulc. Euphorb. Hyos. *Laur.* Magn. c. Magn. m. Magn. s. Merc. Mill. Nitr. Puls. *Ran.* *Ratanh.* Sassap. Spig. Stront. *Sulph.* Tax. Verbasc.
Itching eruptions, *Agar.* Berb. Bov. Canth. Carb. an. Carb. veg. *Caust.* Cupr. Dulc. Euphorb. Kal. Kal. hdr. *Laur.* Lyc. Magn. c. Mang. *Merc. Mez. Mur. ac. Natr. Natr. m. Natr.

s. Phosph. *Puls.* Ratanh. Sabad. Sabin. Staph. *Sulph.* Tart. Zinc.

Itching, herpes, Mang. **Merc.*

Itch-shaped, pimples, Tart.

—, herpes, Grat.

Lymphatic swelling, *Berb.*

Marbled appearance, arm, *Berb.*

Mosquito-bite, like, Ant.

Muscles, contraction of, arm, Bell.

—, elbow, *Caust.* Sass. Sulph.

Nettlerash, like, itching and eruption, *Berb.*

Numbness, arm, Acon. *Amb.* Calc. ph. *Cham.* °*Ign.* *Kal.* *Meph.* Natr. m. °*Natr.* Phosph. Puls. °*Rhus.* Sec.

—, elbow, Sulph.

—, forearm, Berb. Caps. Nitr. *Stront.* Sulph.

Pain as if bruised, shoulder, Sassap.

—, elbow, Baryt. Caust. Hep. Magn. art. Ruta.

—, upper arm, Cycl. Hell. Kreos. Mez.

—, forearm, Mur. ac. Sulph. ac.

Pain, as if contused, *Dros.* Dulc.

—, shoulder, Acon. Berb. Dros.

—, elbow, Dros. Plat.

—, upper arm, Cycl. Merc.

—, forearm, Dros. Hep.

Pain as if dislocated, arm, Coloc. Merc.

—, elbow, Lach.

—, upper arm, Caust.

Pain as if sprained, arm, Bov. Ign. Nitr. ac. Phosph. Stann.

—, shoulder and joints, Alum. Amb. Anac. Asar. Bry. Caps. Caust. Croc. Hep. Ign. Magn. arct. Magn. c. Mang. Mur. ac. Oleand. Petr. Phosph. Puls. Ruta. Sabin. Sep. Spig. Stann. Staph. Tart.

Pain, elbow, Alum. Mang. Tab.
—, upper arm, Alum. Euphorb. Lact. *Rhod.* Tereb.
—, forearm, Cocc. Led. Natr.
Pain as if ulcerated, Sep. Staph. Tab. Thuj.
—, elbow, Natr. s.
—, upper arm, Baryt.
—, forearm, Stront.
Painful eruptions, Ars. Kal. °Lyc. Petr.
—, swelling, N. vom. Rhus.
Pale swelling, Sec. Vip. torv.
Peeling off of skin, forearm, Merc. Stront. Tax.
Peels off, that which, vesicles, Puls.
Petechiæ, Berb.
Pimples, Amm. Amm. m. Ant. Baryt. Bell. Berb. Bov. Bry. Canth. Carb. veg. *Caust.* Chin. Cocc. *Dulc. Hyos. Kal.* Lac. Laur. *Magn. c.* Magn. s. Mosch. Natr. Natr. s. *Nitr.* °*Phos. ac.* Ratanh. Rhod. Sabad. *Sabin.* Sassap. Sep. *Staph.* Sulph. Tart. *Tax. Zinc.*
—, shoulder, Berb. Cocc. *Kal.* Magn. c. Nitr. *Zinc.*
—, arm, Baryt. Canth. Chin. Kal. Lach. Magn. c. °*Phos. ac.* Tart.
—, elbow, Amm. m. Ant. Bell. Berb. Bry. *Dulc. Hyos.* Lach. Natr. Nitr. *Sabin.* Sep. *Staph.*
—, upper arm, Carb. veg. *Dulc. Kal.* Lach. *Laur.* Mosch. Tax.
—, forearm, Amm. Amm. m. Bov. *Caust.* Lach. Laur. Lyc. Magn. c. *Magn. s. Natr. s.* Nitr. Ratanh. Rhod. Sabad. Sassap. Sulph. *Tax. Zinc.*

Pocks, arm, *Ars.* Hydroc.
—, upper arm, Sep.
Prickling, Alum. Coloc. Magn. arct. Plat.
—, arm, Magn. arct. Plat.
—, forearm, Alum. Coloc.
Pustules, Anac. Merc. Mez. *Rhod.* Rhus. *Staph.* *Sulph.*
—, upper arm, Anac. Merc.
—, forearm, *Rhod.* Rhus. *Staph.*
—, elbow, Sulph.
Raised, eruption, *Merc.* *Mez.* *Natr. m.* Sabin. Staph.
Rash, arm, Alum. Bry. Galv. Mez. N. vom. **Sulph.* Tart.
—, elbow, Zinc.
—, upper arm, Ant.
—, forearm, Amm. Bry. Calad. *Merc.* Selen.
Redness, arm, Arg. **Bell.* Lach. Ruta. Sabad.
—, upper arm, Dulc.
—, forearm, Tax.
Red, eruptions, Amm. Arg. Bry. Dulc. Magn. c. *Merc.* Natr. m. Phosph. *Sabad.* *Staph.*
—, spots, Berb. Dulc. Kal. hdr. Plat. *Rhus.* Sep. *Sulph.*
—, swelling, **Bell.* °*Bry.* Sep.
—, streaks, Sabad.
Red areola, with, eruptions, Anac.
Rheumatic, arm, *Agar.* Ammoniac. **Bell.* **Bry.* **Calc. ph.* *Grat.* Jod. Meph. Rhus. v. Sil. **Thuj.*
—, shoulder and shoulder-joint, Amm. m. **Calc. ph.* Graph. Grat. Ign. Jod. Lach. Lyc. N. vom. Ol. an. *Phosph.* Phos. ac. Puls. Ran. Rhod. Rhus v. Sabin. *Sulph.* Tart. Teucr.

Rheumatic, elbow, Grat. Mez. Ran. Rhus. v. Tart. Teucr. Zinc.
—, upper arm, Coff. N. vom. Phosph. Ran. Stram. *Zinc.*
—, forearm, Gran. Lach.
Ridges, Euphorb. *Sabad.*
Roughness, forearm, Mill.
Sarcoma, elbow, °*Hep.*
Scaly, herpes, Cupr. Merc.
Scrofulous ulcer, °*Lach.*
Scarlet redness, **Bell.*
—, ridges, Euphorb. *Sabad.*
Scurfs, elbow, *Sep.*
—, forearm, °*Alum.*
Scurfy ulcer, Electr. Sabin.
Shining swelling, **Bry.*
Smarting, Amm. m. Berb. Bov. Canth. Carb. veg. Hell. Lach. Magn. arct. Mur. ac. Natr. Nitr. Ol. an. Phos. ac. Zinc.
—, shoulder, Berb. Mur. ac. Phos. ac.
—, arms, Bov. Hell.
—, elbow, Berb, Natr. Nitr.
—, upper arm, Canth. Carb. veg. Lach. Magn. arct. Ol. an. Zinc.
—, forearm, Amm. m. Berb.
Smarting eruptions, pimples, &c., Lyc. Zinc.
Smarting as if excoriated, eruption, Berb.
Sore, as if, eruption, Hyos.
—, swelling, Bov.
Sore pain, arm, Bov. Dig. Phosph.
—, shoulder, Arn. Aur. Cic. Con. Magn. arct. Sep.
—, elbow, Carb. an. °*Crotal. Plat.* Stann.
—, upper arm, Graph.

Sore, forearm, Cupr.
Spots, arm, Ant. Bry. Crotal. *Cupr.* Lach. Led. *Natr. m.* Petr. *Sabad.* **Sulph.*
—, shoulder, Berb. Sulph. ac.
—, elbow, Calc. *Sep.* Vip. torv.
—, upper arm, Berb. Kal. hdr. *Plat. Rhus.* Tax.
—, forearm, Amm. Berb. Magn. m. *Merc. Sulph. ac. Thuj.*
Stinging swelling, **Bry.*
Suppurating eruption, Lyc.
—, tumour, Crotal.
—, swelling, Galv.
Swelling, arm, Alum. °*Ars.* Baryt. **Bell.* Bov. °*Calc. ph.* **Chin.* Crotal. Elect. Oph. °*Puls.* **Rhus.* Sep. °*Sulph.* Vip. torv.
—, shoulder, Acon. **Bry.* °*Calc. ph.*
—, upper arm, Berb. **Bry.* °*Sep. Sulph.* Vip. torv.
—, elbow-joint, Bry. Puls.
—, elbow, °*Hep.* °*Lach.* Merc. Puls. °*Veratr.*
—, forearm, *Berb.* Calc. *Caust.* Dig. Lach. *Lyc. N. vom. Sep.* °*Sulph.* Vip. torv.
Swollen, sensation as if, shoulder, Kal. hdr. Laur.
Tearing and swelling, **Bry.*
Thickening of skin, arm, Lach.
Throbbing, swelling, Magn. aust.
Tickling, arm, Plat.
—, upper arm, Canth.
Tickling, eruption, Agar.
Tight, swelling, **Bry.* Calc. Sulph.
—, scurf, Amm. m.
Tubercles, blotches, Ars. Caust. Cocc. Dulc. Mang.
—, shoulder-joint, *Crotal.* Kal. chl. Phosph.

Tubercles, elbow, Caust. Magn. c. Mur. ac.
—, forearm, *Agar.* Amm. *Mur. ac. Nitr.* Phos. ac.
Tumour, forearm, Crotal.
—, arm, *Natr. m.*
—, upper arm, Berb.
Ulcers, arm, *Electr.* Rhus.
—, upper arm, °*Lach.*
Vesicles, Amm. m. Ant. Caust. Daph. Kal. chl. Magn. c. Mang. Merc. Natr. *Natr. m. Puls.* Sassap. *Sil. Spong. Staph. Sulph. Vip. torv.*
—, shoulder, Amm. m. Magn. c. Mang. Vip. torv.
—, arm, Ant. Caust. Daph. Mang. Merc. *Natr. m. Puls.* Vip. torv.
—, elbow, Natr. *Sulph.*
—, forearm, Caust. Sassap. *Sil. Spong. Staph. Sulph.*
Vesicles, watery, arm, Natr. s. Nitr. Sulph.
Warts, arm, °*Caust.* Nitr. ac. °*Sep.* °*Sulph.*
—, upper arm, Nitr. ac.
—, forearm, °*Calc.*
White, eruptions, Agar. Kal. Merc. Natr. m.
Yellow, eruptions, Hell. Sulph.
—, herpes, Cupr. Hell.
—, spots, Petr.

Arthritic.

In general, **Acon.* °Agn. °Alum. °*Ant.* °Arn. °*Aur.* °Bell. °*Bry.* **Calc.* °*Carb. an.* °*Caust.* °*Cic.* °Cocc. **Colch.* **Daph.* °*Dig.* °Ferr. °*Graph.* °Hep. °Jod. °Kal. °Kreos. °Lach. **Led.* **Lyc.* °Men. °*Merc.* °Nitr. ac. °Ol. jec. °Phosph. °Phos. ac. °*Puls.* °Ran. °Ran. sc.

°*Rhod.* °*Rhus.* °Sabin. °*Staph.* °*Sulph.* °Tarax. °*Thuj.*

Arms, swelling, *Caust.*
—, elbow, °*Lyc.*
—, upper arm, Veratr.
Hands, (swelling,) °*Calc.* °*Carb. an.* Carb. veg. Caust. *Cocc.* Gent. Grat. Graph. Hep. **Lyc.* Magn. art. Mur. ac. Petr. Sep. Teucr. Veratr.
Lower limbs, Ars. Asa. ? °*Bry.* °*Calc.* Canth. Cham. Chinin. ? Crotal. Croton. *Graph.* Hep. ? Lach. **N. vom.* Phosph. °*Rhus.* °*Sep.* °*Spong.* Staph. ?
Feet, *Amb.* Arn. °*Bry.* °*Chin.* *Graph.*
—, toe (gout,) Amm. ? °*Arn.* °*Bry.* Con. Led. ? *Sabin.* °*Sulph.* Veratr.
Bones, °Asa. °Aur. Bell. Bry. °*Calc.* °*Chin.* Dig. ? °*Hep.* °*Lyc.* °*Merc.* °*Mez.* °Puls. °Sabin. °*Staph.* °*Sulph.*

Inflammations, °Acon. °*Arn.* °Bell. °*Bry.* °*Carb. an.* °*Chin.* °*Cocc.* °*Colch.* °Cycl.? °Graph. °Hep. °*Kreos.* °Led. ? °Lyc. °Nitr. °*N. vom.* °*Puls.* °*Rhus.* °*Sulph.*
Swelling, °*Acon.* °*Ant.* °*Arn.* °*Bry.* °*Chin.* °Chinin. °*Cocc.* °*Colch.* °Hep. °Kreos. °*Merc.* °N. vom. °Rhus. °*Sulph.*
Nodosities, (s: arthritic.)

Beating, throbbing.

Bones, Asa. Berb. °*Calc.* Carb. veg. Lyc. °*Merc.* Mez. Nitr. Nitr. ac. Phosph. Rhod. Ruta. *Sabad.* Sep. Sil. °*Sulph.* *Thuj.*

Nails, *Amm. m.* Con. Magn. aust. Sep.
Glands, Amm. m. Arn. Asa. Bell. Bov. Bry. Calc. Caust. Cham. Clem. Kal. Lach. Lyc. Magn. art. Merc. Natr. Nitr. ac. Phosph. Rhod. Sabad. Sep. Sil. Sulph. Thuj.

BITING ON THE SKIN.

In general, Agn. Alum. Amm. *Amm. m.* Ant. Arn. Bar. m. Bell. *Berb.* Bov. *Bry.* *Calc.* Camph. Canth. Caps. Carb. an. *Carb. veg.* *Caust.* Cham. Chel. Chin. Cocc. *Colch.* Coloc. Con. Dros. *Euphorb.* Grat. Hell. Ipec. Lach. Lact. Lam. *Led.* *Lyc.* Magn. art. Magn. aust. Magn. c. Mang. Merc. Mez. Mur. ac. Natr. c. Natr. m. Nicc. Nitr. Nitr. ac. *N. vom.* Oleand. Ol. an. Op. Phosph. Phos. ac. Plat. **Puls.* Ran. *Ran. sc.* Rhod. Rhus. Ruta. Selen. Sep. Sil. Spig. *Spong.* Stront. *Sulph.* Tart. Thuj. Veratr. Viol. tr. Zinc.

Head, Agn. Bry. Coloc. Dros. Grat. Jod. Magn. arct. Merc. Mez. Ran. Rhod. Thuj. Zinc.
Eyes, **Agar.* Agn. *Alum.* *Amb.* Amm. Ars. Aur. **Bell.* Bry. Calc. Camph. Canth. Carb. an. Carb. veg. Cast. Caust. *Chin.* *Clem.* Colch. **Con.* Croc. *Dros.* Eugen. Euphorb. Euphr. *Graph.* Hell. Kal. Kal. hdr. Kreos. Lact. Laur. Lyc. Magn. arct. Magn. c. Mang. **Merc.* Mez. Mosch. Mur. ac. Natr. Nicc. Nitr. ac. **N. vom.* Oleand. Ol. an. Par. Petr. Phosph. Phos. ac. Ratanh. **Ran.* Ran. sc. Rhab. Rhod. **Rhus.* Sabad. Sep. **Sil.* Stann. Staph. Stront. **Sulph.* *Sulph. ac.* Tart. Teucr. Thuj. **Val.* Viol. tr. Zinc.

Eyelids, Aur. Camph. Carb. veg. Caust. Clem. Ign. Nitr. Rhus. Spig.

Canthi. *Ant.* Bry. Camph. Carb. an. *Carb. veg.* Colch. *Con.* Graph. Hell. Ign. Kal. Lact. Magn. aust. Magn. c. Mang. Mez. Mosch. Mur. ac. Nicc. Nitr. *N. vom.* Ol. an. *Ran. Ran. sc.* Rhus. Ruta. *Sep.* Sil. °*Staph.* Sulph. Tart. Teucr. Zinc.

Ears, Grat. Lach. Lyc. Ol. an.

Nose, Arn. Berb. Chen. Chin. Euphorb. Grat. Hell. Lyc. Nitr. Plat. Sabad. °Spig. Teucr. Thuj.

Chin, Stront.

Buccal cavity, *Acon. Amb. Arn.* Ars. Asar. Bell. Calc. Carb. an. *Cham.* Chen. *Chin.* Cocc. *Dros. Ipec. Kal.* Mez. Natr. Ol. an. Phell. Ran. sc. Rhod. Seneg. *Sep.* Sulph. Teucr. Zinc.

—, palate, Cham. Chen. *Chin. Kal.* Ran. sc. Seneg. Sep. Zinc.

—, fauces, Amb. Dros. Ran. sc. Sep. Teucr.

—, gums, Asar. Calc. Carb. veg. Cocc. Phell. Rhod.

—, tongue, *Acon. Arn.* Ars. Asar. Bell. Cham. Chin. Ipec. Mez. Natr. Ol. an. Sulph.

Anus, Agar. Alum. Amb. Baryt. Canth. Caps. Carb. veg. Caust. Chin. Dulc. Hell. Kal. Lach. Led. Lyc. Mercurial. Mez. Natr. c. N. vom. Phosph. Phos. ac. Rhod. Sabin. Sep. Sulph.

Sexual parts, Graph. Hep. Heracl. *Magn. art. Puls.* Ran. sc. Staph. Thuj.

—, inguen, Hep.

—, scrotum, Heracl. Ran. sc.

—, labia, Staph.

—, vagina, Graph. Thuj.

Sexual parts, prepuce, *Magn. art. Puls.*
Thoracic region, Amm. Amm. m. Kal. Natr.
Dorsal region, axilla, Ruta.
—, neck, Magn. c. Nitr.
—, small of back, Canth. Phell.
—, nape of neck, Grat. Kal. hdr. Magn. c. Nitr. ac. Ol. an.
—, back, Magn. aust. Mur. ac. Natr.
—, scapular region, Stront.
Arms, Amm. m. Berb. Bov. Canth. Carb. veg. Hell. Lach. Magn. arct. Mur. ac. Natr. Nitr. Ol. an. Phos. ac. Zinc.
—, shoulder, Berb. Mur. ac. Phos. ac.
—, arms, Bov. Hell.
—, elbow, Berb. Natr. Nitr.
—, upper arm, Canth. Carb. veg. Lach. Magn. arct. Ol. an. Zinc.
—, forearm, Amm. m. Berb.
Hands, Berb, Natr. m. Zinc.
—, finger, Berb. Mez.
Lower limbs, Lyc.
—, hips, Amm. m.
—, thigh, Alum. Amm. m. Berb. Chel. Grat. N. vom. Phell.
—, knee, Berb. Bry. °*Lyc.* Nitr. Ol. an. Phell. Ran. sc. *Thuj.*
—, legs, calves, Amm. m. Berb. Grat. Tart. Veratr.
Feet, Merc.
—, heel, Lam. Sep.
—, toe, Berb.

Black, blackish.

Eruption, Ant. **Ars.* Asa. **Bell.* **Bry.* Chinin.

(Con.) *Crotal.* Electr. *Lach.* °Mur. ac. °Nitr. ac. *Oph.* °*Rhus.* *Sec.* Sep. °*Sil.* Spig. Vip. red.
Blisters, vesicles, °*Ars.* °Lach. *Natr.* Petr. Vip. torv.
Pimples, Carb. veg. Spig.
Blood, Amm. Arn. Asar. Canth. Carb. veg. **Chin.* **Croc.* Electr. Ferr. Kreos. *Magn. c.* Magn. m. Magn. s. Natr. *Natr. m.* Natr. s. Nitr. Nitr. ac. Ol. an. **Puls.* Sec. Stram. Sulph.
Pustules, Bry. Rhus.
Spots, Ars. *Crotal.* °*Lach.* °*Rhus.* Sec. *Vip. red.*
Swelling, *Acon.* Aeth. Amm. °*Arn.* **Ars.* Aur. °*Bell.* *Carb. veg.* Con. °*Dig.* Hep. **Lach.* Mang. °*Merc.* N. vom. °Op. Oph. *Phosph.* Phos. ac. *Plumb.* **Puls.* *Samb.* Sec. Seneg. *Sil.* *Sulph. ac.* °*Veratr.*
—, black-spotted, N. vom.
Scurfs, crusts, °*Bell.* Chinin. Vip. torv.
Pocks, Ant. **Ars.* **Bell.* Bry. Hyos. **Lach.* Mur. ac. °*Rhus.* *Sec.* Sep. Sil. Spig.

Nose, skin, °Merc.
—, pores, °Dros. Graph. Selen. **Sulph.*
Face, Spig. Vip. torv.
—, pores, Dig. Dros. °Nitr. ac. Sabin. °Selen. **Sulph.*
Lips, Spig.
Buccal cavity, blisters, Petr.
—, swelling, Vip. torv.
—, ulcers, Mur. ac.
Arms, eruption, Carb. veg. Sassap.
—, swelling, black, **Carb. veg.* *Mur. ac.*
Sexual parts, eruption, Bry.
Arms, pocks, °*Ars.*

Hands, swelling, Lach. Vip. torv.
Lower limbs, swelling, N. vom.
—, ulcer, °*Lach.*
Feet, blisters, °*Ars.* Natr. m.
—, pocks, *Sec.*
—, ulcer, °Ipec.

Blackish colour of the skin.

In general, Acon. Ant. Asa. Nitr. ac. Oph. Sec. Spig. Vip. red. Vip. torv.

Nose, °Merc.
Face, Spig. Vip. torv.
Lips, **Acon.* **Ars.* Bry. Chin. Merc. Phos. ac. °Rhus. °Squill. Tart. ac. °Veratr.
Abdomen, Acon. Vip. torv.
Lower limbs, Vip. torv.
Feet, Ant.

Bleeds, that which.

Blisters, vesicles, Graph.
Bloodvessels, swelling of, Acon. Amm. Bell. **Calc.* Cham. Chin. Cupr. Electr. Ferr. Galv. Hyos. *Kal.* Magn. arct. °Men. Nitr. ac. **Phosph.* **Puls.* °*Sep.* Stram. **Sulph.*
Bloat, rhagades, **Merc.* Nicc. **Petr.* Puls. Sassap. **Sulph.*
Eruption, Merc. Par.
Exudations, Arn. *Calc.* Cham. Clem. Cocc. *Crotal. Lach.* N. mosch. °*N. vom. Oph.*
Figwarts, Magn. aust. *Thuj.*
Herpes, °Dulc. °Lyc.

Nails, Crotal.
Pimples, Stront. Thuj.
Pustules, Tart.
Rash, Alum.
Scabies, itch, *Calc.* ? Dulc. ? °*Merc.* °*Sulph.*
Scars (cicatrices) of old ulcers and wounds, Lach. Oph. Phosph.
Scurfs, crusts, *Merc.* Mez
Swelling, Canth. °*N. vom.* Ran. sc. Sep. **Sulph.*
Ulcers, Alum. Arn. **Ars.* Asa. Bell. Bov. **Carb. veg.* Caust. °*Con.* Croc. Dros. **Hep.* Hyos. Jod. **Kal.* Kreos. **Lach.* **Lyc.* Magn. art. *Merc.* Mercurial. Mez. Natr. m. **Nitr. ac.* **Phosph.* **Phos. ac.* **Puls.* Rhus. Ruta. Sabin. Sec. Sep. °*Sil.* °Sulph. ac. Thuj. Zinc.
Warts, Magn. aust. °*Natr.* Nitr. ac. Thuj.

Nose, Amm. m. Ferr. Stront.
Lips and mouth, region of, °Bry. **Merc.* Nicc. Thuj.
Buccal cavity, eruptions and ulcers, Alum. Bov. Canth. Graph. *Merc.* Phosph. Zinc.
—, swelling, °N. vom. Ran. sc. Sep.
Arms, varices, Acon. Amm.Bell. **Calc.* Cham. Chin. Cupr. Electr. *Ferr.* Galv. Hyos. *Kal.* Magn. art. Men. Nitr. ac. **Puls.* **Sep.* Stram. **Sulph.*
Hands, rhagades, **Alum.* *Merc.* **Petr.*
Lower limbs, ulcers, °Carb. veg. Phos. ac.
—, scurf, Mez.
Feet, ulcers, **Ars.*

Blisters, phagedænic.

In general, Amm. °*Ars.* Borax. Caust. °*Cham.* °*Clem.* °*Graph.* *Hep.* *Kal.* *Magn. c.* Merc.

°*Natr. Nitr. ac.* Oph. **Petr.* °*Sep.* **Sil.* **Sulph.* (Comp: ULCERS, PHAGEDÆNIC.)
Burning, Graph. Sil.
Suppurating, Graph.
Ulcerated, Natr.
Itching, Graph. Sil.
Beating, Sil.
Humid, Kal.
Stinging, Graph. Magn. c.

Hands, °Clem. Magn. c.
—, fingers, °*Clem. Graph.* Hep. *Kal. Magn. c.* Nitr. ac. *Sil.* Sulph.
—, finger-joints, Hep.
—, thumb, *Hep.* Nitr. ac.
Lower limbs, nates, Borax.
Feet, *Con. Selen.* °*Sulph. Zinc.*
—, heels, Caust. *Natr.* °*Sep. Sil.*
—, toes, °*Ars.* °*Graph. Nitr. ac.* °*Petr.*

BLOATED.

In general, **Acon.* Amm. *Amm. m.* **Ant.* **Arn.* **Ars. Asa.* Aur. Baryt. **Bell.* **Bry.* **Calc.* **Caps.* **Cham.* *Chin. Cin. Cocc. Colch. Coloc. Con. °*Crotal.* **Cupr.* Dig. Dros. Dulc. **Ferr.* Graph. Guaj. Hell. **Hyos.* °Ipec. °Kal. Lach. Laur. Led. Lyc. Magn. c. Merc. Mez. Mosch. Natr. Nitr. ac. N. mosch. **N. vom.* Oleand. **Op.* **Phosph.* Plumb. **Puls.* Rhab. **Rhus.* **Samb.* Sassap. *Seneg.* **Sep.* **Sil.* **Spig.* **Spong.* Staph. Stram. **Sulph.* °Tart. *Teucr.*
Head, Acon. Berb. Rhus. Ruta. Staph. Sulph.

Eyes, *Ars.* Bry. Cham. Ferr. **Kal.* N. vom. Oleand. **Phosph.* Puls. Rhab. Ruta. **Sep.*

Face, **Acon.* Ammon. °Arn. *Ars. Aur. Baryt. Bell. **Bry.* **Cham.* **Chin.* Cin. Cocc. °Crotal. Dig. Dros. Dulc. °Ferr. **Hyos.* °Ipec. °Kal. Laur. Led. Lyc. Merc. Natr. **N. vom.* **Op.* **Phosph.* Plumb. °*Puls.* Rhus. **Samb.* Sep. °*Sil.* °Spig. °*Spong.* Staph. °Sulph. °Tart. Teucr.

—, around the eyes, **Ars.* **Bry.* *Cham. °*Ferr.* **N. vom.* Oleand. **Phosph.* °*Puls.* Rhab. Ruta. Sep.

—, glabella, Kal.

Blood, according to character.

Acrid, corrosive, Amm. Ars. Baryt. Bov. Canth. Carb. veg. Graph. Hep. *Kal. Nitr.* Rhus. Sassap. *Sil.* Sulph. Sulph. ac. Zinc.

Badly-coloured, Oph.

Black, Amm. Arn. Asar. Canth. Carb. veg. **Chin.* **Croc.* Electr. Ferr. Kreos. *Magn. c.* Magn. m. Magn. s. Natr. *Natr. m.* Natr. s. Nitr. Nitr. ac. Ol. an. **Puls.* Sec. Stram. Sulph.

Brown, brownish, *Bry. Calc. *Carb. veg.* Con. Puls. Rhus.

Dark, black-red, Acon. *Amm. Ant.* Arn. *Asar.* Bell. *Bism.* Bry. Canth. Carb. veg. **Cham.* **Chin.* Cocc. Con. Croc. Cupr. Dig. Dros. Ferr. Graph. Ign. *Kreos. Lach.* Led. Lyc. Magn. c. Magn. m. Nitr. Nitr. ac. N. mosch. *N. vom.* Phosph. Phos. ac. Plat. **Puls.* Sec. Selen. Sep. Stram. Sulph.

Decomposed, Cic. *Crotal. Lach. Oph. Vip. red. Vip. torv.*

Fetid, Ars. *Bell. Bry. Carb. an.* Carb. veg. Caust. *Cham.* Chin. *Croc.* Ign. Kal. Merc. Phosph. Plat. Rhab. Sabin. Sec. Sil. Sulph.

Flesh, like pieces of, Rhus. v.

Frothy, Oph.

Glue, like, Puls.

Gray-shining, Berb.

Light-coloured, Amm. *Arn. Ars.* Baryt. *Bell.* Borax. Bov. Bry. Calc. Canth. Carb. an. Carb. veg. Chin. °*Crotal.* Dig. Dros. Dulc. **Ferr.* **Graph.* **Hyos.* °*Ipec.* Kreos. Laur. Led. *Magn. aust.* Magn. m. Natr. Nitr. Nitr. ac. N. mosch. **Phosph.* **Puls.* **Rhus.* Sabad. *Sabin. Sec.* Sep. Sil. Stram. Stront.

Lumpy, coagulated, Amm. Arn. **Bell.* Bry. Canth. Carb. an. Caust. **Cham.* **Chin.* Con. Croc. Ferr. *Hyos. Ign.* **Ipec.* Magn. m. Merc. Natr. s. Nitr. Nitr. ac. N. vom. Phos. ac. **Plat.* **Puls. Rhus.* Rhus. v. *Sabin.* Sec. Sep. *Stram.* Stront. Zinc.

Oil, like, Laur. Oph.

Pale, watery, Alum. Amm. Berb. Borax. Bov. Carb. veg. °*Crotal.* Dulc. **Ferr.* **Graph.* °*Kal.* Kreos. Magn. art. Magn. m. Nitr. ac. Phosph. Prun. °*Puls.* Stram. °*Sulph.* Tart.

Pitch-like, Magn. c.

Tenacious, **Croc.* Cupr. Magn. c. Sec.

Thick, Carb. veg. Electr. Kreos. Lach. Laur. Magn. c. Magn. s. Nitr. N. mosch. Plat. **Puls.* Sulph.

Thin, watery, Berb. Bov. Crotal. Dulc. Ferr. Graph. Kreos. Laur. Magn. aust. Magn. m.

Natr. s. Phosph. Prun. Puls. °*Rhus.* Sabin. Sec. Stram. Tart.

Viscous, Kal. chl. Sec.

Watery, Alum. Amm. *Berb.* Borax. Bov. Carb. veg. Crotal. Dulc. **Ferr.* **Graph.* Kal. Kreos. Laur. Natr. s. Nitr. ac. Phosph. Prun. *Puls.* Rhus. Sabin. Sec. Stram. Sulph. Tart.

Bloody crust, that which has a.

Ulcers, Bell.

Bloodvessels, swelling of.

In general, **Acon.* Alum. **Amm.* Ang. **Arn.* **Ars. Baryt.* **Bell. Bry.* **Calc.* Camph. *Carb. an.* **Carb. veg.* **Caust.* Chel. *Chin.* Cic. Coloc. Con. *Croc.* Cycl. *Ferr.* **Graph.* Hyos. Lach. Lyc. Magn. art. Magn. aust. Men. Mosch. **Mur. ac.* Natr. m. Nitr. **N. vom.* Oleand. Op. **Phosph.* Phos. ac. **Puls.* Rhod. *Rhus.* Sassap. **Sep.* Sil. Spig. Spong. Staph. Stront. **Sulph.* Thuj. Zinc.

Aneurysms, °*Carb. veg.* °Lyc. ? °*Lach.* °Puls. ? Spig. ?

Aneurysms by anastomosis, *Berb.* °*Carb. veg.* °*Caust.* Lyc. Plat. °*Thuj.*

Congested capillaries, **Acon.* Aeth. **Amb.* Amm. °*Ars.* **Bell.* Bruc. Electr. Eugen. *Kal.* °*Lach.* Laur. Meph. **Merc.* Phosph. °Phos. ac. Spig. **Sulph.*

Cutaneous veins, swelling of, Acon. Alum. **Amm.* **Arn.* Ars. *Baryt. Bell.* Bry. Calc. Camph. Chel. **Chin.* Cic. Coloc. Con. *Croc.* Cycl. *Ferr.* Graph. Hyos. Lach. Lyc. Magn. arct. Magn. aust. Men. Mosch. Natr. m. N. vom. Oleand. Op. *Phosph.*

Phos. ac. *Puls.* Rhod. Rhus. Sassap. Sep. Sil. Spig. Spong. Staph. Stront. *Sulph. Thuj.* Zinc.
Swelling with smarting, Grat. Tart.
Swollen and blue, **Carb. veg.* **Mur. ac.*
Swollen and bleeding, Acon. Amm. Bell. **Calc.* Cham. Chin. Cupr. Electr. Ferr. Galv. Hyos. *Kal.* Magn. arct. °Men. Nitr. ac.**Phosph.***Puls.* *Sep.* Stram. **Sulph.*
Swollen, with pressure, Ign. Phosph.
Swollen and inflamed, **Arn.* **Ars.* Calc. °*Cham.* Kal. Kreos. Lyc. N. vom. °*Puls.* °*Sil.* °*Spig.* **Sulph.* Thuj. Zinc.
Swollen and ulcerated, °*Ars.* °*Cham.* Kreos. °*Lach.* °*Lyc.* °*Puls.* °*Sil.* Sulph. Tart.
Swollen and indurated, °*Sep.*
Swollen and itching, Berb. Bruc. *Caps.* Carb. veg. Caust. Graph. Lach. Magn. art. Magn. aust. N. vom. Plumb. Puls. *Sep.* Sil. **Sulph.* Sulph. ac. Tart.
Swollen and itching, Carb. veg.
Swollen and creeping, Ant. Kal.
Swollen and crampy-painful, Graph.
Swollen and humid, Alum. Amm. Baryt. Caust. Natr. m. Sep. Sulph. Sulph. ac.
Swollen, with tearing, Sulph. ac.
Swollen and red, **Acon.* Aeth. **Amb.* Amm. °*Ars.* **Bell.* Bruc. Electr. Eugen. *Kal.* °*Lach.* Laur. Meph. **Merc.* Phosph. °Phos. ac. Spig. **Sulph.*
Swollen and painful, **Caust.* Coloc.
Swollen and cutting, Carb. an. Plat.
Swollen and tight, Graph.
Swollen and stitching, Alum. *Ars.* Baryt. *Caust.* Graph. Grat. Kal. Merc. Natr. m. *Nitr.* N.

vom. Phosph. Puls. *Sil.* Sulph. Sulph. ac. Tart.

Swollen and sore, Amm. Ang. Baryt. *Caust. Graph.* Grat. (Hep.) Ign. *Kal.* Magn. arct. Merc. Mur. ac. Natr. m. Nitr. N. vom. *Phosph. Puls.* Rhus. Sil. *Sulph.* Sulph. ac.

Varices, hæmorrhoidal, *Alum.* Amb. *Amm.* Amm. m. Anac. Ang. **Ant.* Arn. **Ars.* Baryt. Bell. **Calc.* Canth. **Caps. Carb. an.* **Carb. veg.* Caust. Cham. Chin. Coloc. Cupr. Euphr. *Ferr.* **Graph.* Grat. Hell. Hep. Hyos. *Ign. Kal.* Lach. Led. Lyc. Magn. art. Magn. aust. Magn. c. Merc. **Mur. ac. Natr. m. Nitr. ac.* **N. vom.* Petr. **Phosph.* Phos. ac. Plat. Plumb. **Puls.* Ran. Rhod. Rhus. Sabin. **Sep.* Sil. Spig. Stann. Staph. Stram. Stront. **Sulph. Sulph. ac.* Tart. Veratr. Zinc.

Varices, *Amb. Arn.* **Ars.* Berb. Calc. °*Carb. veg.* **Caust.* Coloc. °*Ferr.* °*Graph.* °*Kreos.* °*Lach.* °*Lyc.* °*Magn. aust.* Magn. c. °*Natr. m.* N. vom. °*Puls. Spig.* Sil. *Sulph.* Sulph. ac. °Tart. Thuj. °*Zinc.*

Eyes, **Acon.* Aeth. *Amb. Amm. °*Ars.* **Bell.* Bruc. Electr. Eugen. *Kal.* °Lach. Laur. Meph. **Merc.* Phosph. °Phos. ac. Spig. **Sulph.*

Back, neck, Bell. Thuj.

Anus, Acon. °Aloë. ? *Alum.* Amb. **Amm.* °Anac. Ang. *Ant.* Arn. *Ars.* Baryt. Bell. *Berb.* Bruc. **Calc. Caps. Carb. an.* Carb. veg. *Caust.* Cham. Chin. Chinin. Coloc. Cupr. Electr. Ferr. **Graph.* Grat. Hell. **Ign.* **Kal.* °*Lach.* Lact. Lyc. Magn. art. Magn. aust. Magn. c. Magn. m. **Mur. ac.* **Natr. m.* Nitr. **Nitr. ac.* **N. vom. Phosph.* Plat. °Plumb. **Puls.* Ran. Rhus. **Sabin.* **Sep.*

Sil. Stram. Stront. **Sulph.* Sulph. ac. *Tart.* Therid. Thuj. Veratr. Zinc.
Sexual parts, °Calc. °Lyc. °N. vom. ? Zinc.
Lower limbs, thighs, *Calc. Zinc.*
—, leg, **Caust. Coloc.* Ferr. Graph. Puls. Sulph. °*Zinc.*
—, knees, aneurysm, °*Carb. veg.*
Feet, Sulph.

Blotches, tubercles.

In general, Anac. *Ant.* Arn. **Ars.* °*Asa.* Baryt. **Bell.* Berb. *Bry.** *Calc.* Caps. Chel. Cic. Cocc. Con. Croc. *Crotal.* Dulc. Electr. Hell. **Hep. Hyos.* Ign. Kal. Kreas. *Lach. Led.* Lyc. *Magn. c.* °*Mang.* **Merc.* Natr. Natr. m. Nitr. ac. *N. vom. Oph.* Op. *Petr.* °*Phosph.* Phos. ac. °*Puls.* Rhus. *Rhus. v.* Ruta. Sabin. *Sassap. Sec.* Selen. Sep. **Sil.* Spig. Squill. Staph. Stram. Sulph. Sulph. ac. Tart. Val. Veratr. Vip. torv.
Bloody, Arn. Bry. Sec.
Blotches, Berb. Kreos. Lach. Lyc. Natr. Natr. m. Nitr. ac. Op. Sassap. Sep. Spig. Stram. Sulph. Veratr.
Burning, Lach. Sassap.
Chilblains, like, s.: Chilblains.
Feet, on the, Sep. Sulph.
Gangrenous, anthrax, **Ars.* °Bell. Caps. Electr. *Hyos.* Lach. Rhus. *Sec.* °*Sil.* Tart. Vip. torv.
Gray, Nitr. ac.
Inflamed, °Hep. °Mang. **Merc.* °*Phosph.* °*Sil.*
Itching, Electr. *Magn. c.* Natr. Natr. m. Nitr. ac. Op. *Rhus. v.* Sassap. Sep. Stann. Stram. Sulph.
Large, Crotal. Natr. m. Nitr. ac.

Like nettlerash, Berb. Kreos. Lach. Sassap. Veratr.
Painful, °Ars. Caust. Lyc. *N. vom.* Oph.
Like plague, °N. mosch. ?
Red, Electr. Ipec. Natr. m. Op.
With red areola, Ant.
Smarting, gnawing, Lach. °Sulph.
Soft, Ant. Carb. veg. Daph. Petr. Rhus. Sil.
Sore, as if, Hep.
From stings of insects, as if, *Ant.*
Stinging, *Petr.* Sassap. Stram. Zinc.
Suppurating, abscesses, Ant. °*Ars.* °*Asa.* Bry. **Calc.* Caust. Cic. Cocc. Con. Croc. *Crotal.* Dulc. °*Hep.* Kal. *Lach.* Magn. c. °*Mang.* **Merc.* Natr. Natr. m. Petr. °*Phosph.* °*Puls.* *Sassap.* Sec. Sep. °*Sil.* Staph. Sulph. Tart.
Tuberculous, Lach.
White, Lach. Natr. m.

Head, Anac. Baryt. **Calc.* Carb. an. °*Daph.* Hell. Kal. *Lyc.* Natr. m. N. vom. Puls. Phosph. Phos. ac. Ruta. Sil.
Eyes, Sassap.
Ears, in front of, Bry.
—, behind, Bry. **Calc.* Carb. an. Caust. Staph.
—, on the, Spong.
Nose, **Bell.* Jod.
Face, Alum. Ant. Ars. Baryt. Calc. Canth. Carb. veg. Chel. Cic. Con. Dig. Dulc. Graph. Hell. Hep. Jod. Kal. Lach. Led. Lyc. Magn. arct. Magn. Magn. m. Merc. Natr. N. vom. Op. Puls. Sep. Viol. tr. Zinc.
Lips and mouth, region of, Hep. Magn. m.
Lower jaw, Stann. Staph.

Mouth, Alum. Berb. **Calc.* Canth. Caust. Jod. Lyc. N. mosch. °Phos. ac. **Staph.* °*Sulph.*
—, buccal cavity, Jod. Lyc. N. mosch. Phosph. **Staph.*
—, gums, Alum. Berb. **Calc.* Canth. ***Caust.*** °Phos. ac. Plumb. **Staph.* °*Sulph.*
—, tongue, Graph. Lyc.
—, under the tongue, Amb.
Abdomen, Natr.
Anus, Carb. veg. Ipec.
Sexual parts, Natr.
Thorax, Natr. Sassap.
Dorsal region, blotches, axilla, Petr.
—, neck, Graph. Natr. m. Sassap. Sep.
—, nape of neck, °Sil.
—, back, Lach. Mez.
Arms, forearm, Crotal.
—, arm, *Natr. m.*
—, upper arm, Berb.
Hands, Ars.
—, finger, Ant.
Lower limbs, Ant. Spig.
—, nates, Ant. Sassap.
—, thighs, Crotal. Merc. Zinc.
—, knee, Ant.
—, legs, Carb. veg. Lach.
Feet, Lyc.
—, toes, *Sulph. Zinc.*

Blue, that which is.

Blisters, vesicles, **Ars.* Bell. Con. **Lach. Ran. Rhus.* Vip. torv.
Spots, Amm. *Ant.* °*Arn.* Ars. Baryt. Berb. Con. Crotal. **Ferr.* Lach. Led. Merc. Nitr. ac. N.

mosch. °*N. vom.* Op. Phell. Phosph. *Plat.* Ruta. *Sulph.* **Sulph. ac.*
Swelling, Acon. Aeth. Aur. Lach. Oph. Vip. torv.
—, black-blue, *Acon.* Amm. °*Ant.* *Ars. Aur. °*Bell. Carb. veg.* Con. °*Dig.* Hep. **Lach.* Mang. °*Merc.* N. vom. °*Op.* Oph. **Puls. Samb.* Sec. Seneg. *Sil. Sulph. ac.* °*Veratr.*
Ulcers, *Ars.* °*Asa.* °*Aur.* Bell. °*Con.* °*Hep.* **Lach. Mang. Merc.* Sec. Seneg. *Sil. Veratr.*
Face, spots, Ars. *Ferr.
Buccal cavity, herpes, °Zinc.
Abdomen, swelling, Aeth. Vip. red.
Anus, swelling of varices, **Carb. veg. Mur. ac.*
Dorsal region, spots, neck, Phell.
Arms, spots, Berb. *Sulph. ac.*
—, swelling, Oph. Vip. torv.
Hands, eruption, *Ran.*
—, swelling, Lach.
Lower limbs, spots, Amm. Ant. Con. °*Lach.* Phosph. *Sulph.*
—, swelling, °*Lach.* °*Sil.*
Feet, spots, *Sulph.*
—, chilblains, Kal.
—swelling, Ars.

Blue colour

Of the skin in general, Acon. Amm. Ang. *Arn. *Ars. Aur. Bell. Bism. Bry. Calc. **Camph.* °*Carb. veg.* Cocc. Con. *Crotal. Cupr.* °*Dig.* **Lach.* Led. Merc. Natr. m. **N. vom.* Oph. **Op.* Phosph. Phos. ac. Plumb. Puls. Rhus. Samb. Sec. Sil. Spong. Sulph. ac. Thuj. °*Veratr. Vip. red. Vip. torv.*

Cyanosis, °Ars.? °Bell.? °*Camph.* °*Carb. veg.* °Con. °Cupr.? °*Dig.* °*Lach.* °Op.? °Samb. °Sec.? ° *Veratr.*

Eyes, sclerotica. Veratr.
Eyelids, °Dig.
Canthi, Aur. Sassap.
Nose, alæ, Hydroc.
Lips, Agar. Alum. Ang. **Ars.* Berb. Calc. Caust. Cin. Con. Cupr. °*Dig.* **Lyc.* Merc. Op. Phosph. Stram, Veratr. Vip.
Buccal cavity, °*Dig.* Oleand. Plumb. Sabin.
—, gums, Oleand. Plumb. Sabin.
—, tongue, °*Dig.*
Thorax, clavicles, Thuj.
Arms, Bism. Plat. Sep.
Hands, Acon. Amm. Cocc. Lach.**N. vom.* Spong. Zinc.
Lower limbs, Bism. Con.
—, thighs, Bism.
—, legs, con.
Feet, Vip. torv.
Nails, Amm. °*Aur.* Carb. veg. Chel. **Chin.* Cocc. *Dig.* Dros. Lyc. °*Natr. m.* **N. vom.* Petr. Phos. ac. Sassap. °*Sil.*
Glands, Arn. Ars. Aur. Carb. an. Carb. veg. Con. Hep. Lach. Mang. Merc. Puls. Sil. Sulph. ac.

Blue-red, that which is.

Spots, Ferr. magn. Lach. Phosph.
Chilblains, Arn. Bell. Kal. °*Puls.*
Swelling, **Arn.* *Ars.* **Bell.* **Cham.* Canth. Con. *Kal.* **Lach.* °*Sil.*

Face, swelling, Bell. °Bry. **Cham.* °Lach.
Chin, Plat.
Buccal cavity, swelling, Canth. Con. Lach.
—, gums, Con. Lach.
Sexual parts, swelling, °Arn. Ars.

Boils.

In general, *Acon. Alum. Amm. Amm. m. Anac. *Ant.* **Arn.* Ars. Aur. Baryt. **Bell.* Bry. **Calc.* Carb. an. Carb. veg. Chin. Cocc. *Euphorb.* Graph.
Grat. **Hep.* *Hyos.* Ign. Kreos. *Lach.* Laur. **Led.* **Lyc.* Magn. art. Magn. m. **Merc.* Mez. **Mur. ac.* Natr. *Natr. m.* Nitr. **Nitr. ac.* °*N. mosch.* **N. vom.* *Petr.* **Phosph.* **Phos. ac.* Puls. Rhus. *Sec.* **Sep.* **Sil.* Spong. **Staph.* Stram. **Sulph.* Sulph. ac. Tart. Thuj. Vip. red. Zinc.
Large, *Hep. Hyos. **Lyc.* Natr. **Nitr. ac.* Phosph.
Small, **Arn.* Baryt. Grat. Lyc. Magn. c. Magn. m. Natr. m. *N. vom.* Sulph. Zinc.
Periodically recurring, Hyos. **Lyc.* **Nitr. ac.* **Staph.*

Head, Baryt. Bell. Calc. Kal. *Led. Magn. m. Mur. ac. Nitr. ac. Rhus.
Ears, Sil. Sulph.
Nose, Amm. Carb. an. Magn. m.
Face, Alum. Amm. Arn. Baryt. Bell. °Bry. Calc. Carb. veg. Chin. Cin. Laur. Led. Mez. Mur. ac. Natr. Natr. m. Nitr. ac. Sil.
Lips and mouth, region of, Natr. Petr.
Chin. Hep. Nitr. ac. Sil.

Abdomen, *Phosph. Zinc. ox.*

Arms. Carb. an.

Chest, Amm. Chin. Magn. Phosph.

—, small, Amm.

Dorsal region, axilla, Borax. Lyc. °Phos. ac.

—, neck, Magn. c. Natr. m. Sep.

—, nates, Agar.

—, small of back, Aeth. Thuj.

—, nape of neck, Electr. Nitr. ac. Phosph.

—, back, Caust. Electr. Mur. ac. Sulph. ac. Zinc.

—, scapulæ, Amm. Bell. Led. Lyc. Nitr. ac. Zinc.

Arms, Amm. °*Calc.* Carb. veg. Lyc. magn. m. *Mez. Nitr.* Petr. Phos. ac. *Sil. Zinc.*

—, shoulder, Amm. *Nitr.* Phos. ac.

—, arm, *Mez. Sil.*

—, upper arm, Carb. veg. *Zinc.*

—, forearm, °*Calc.* Lyc. Magn. m. Petr.

Hands, °*Calc.* Lyc.

—, finger-joints, Calc.

—, thumb, *Nitr.*

Lower limbs, Nitr. ac.

—, nates, hips, Alum. Amm. Baryt. Graph. *Hep.* Lyc. Nitr. ac. **Phos. ac.* °*Ratanh.* Sabin.

—, thigh, Clem. *Cocc. Hyos. Ign. Lyc.* Magn. c. *Nitr. ac.* N. vom. Petr. Phosph. Sep. **Sil.*

—, knee, Natr. m. N. vom.

—, legs and calves, °*Magn. c.* Nitr. ac. **Sil.*

Feet, *Stram.*

—, heel, Calc.

—, soles, *Ratanh.*

BONES AND PERIOSTEUM, AFFECTIONS OF.

In general, *Acon.* Aeth. Agar. Alum. **Amb.* **Amm.* Amm. m. Anac. **Ang.* Anis. **Arg.* *Ars.* **Asa.* Atham. **Aur.* **Baryt.* Bell. Berb. Bism. Borax. Bov. **Bry.* **Calc.* Canth. Caps. Carb. an. **Carb. veg.* **Caust.* Chel. **Chin.* Cic. Clem. Cocc. Coff. Con. Croc. Crotal. **Cupr.* °*Daph.* Diad. Dros. Euphorb. Euphr. Graph. Grat. **Guaj.* Ign. *Indig.* **Jod.* Kal. Kreos. °*Lach.* Lact. Laur. Led. **Lyc.* Magn. arct. Magn. c. Magn. m. Magn. s. **Mang.* Men. Meph. **Merc.* *Merc. corr.* **Mez.* Mur. ac. *Natr.* *Natr. m.* Natr. s. Nicc. Nitr. **Nitr. ac.* Oleand. Ol. an. Par. **Phosph.* °*Phos. ac.* Plat. Plumb. Poth. Prun. **Puls.* Ran. sc. Raph. Rhod. **Rhus.* **Ruta.* Sabad. **Sabin.* Samb. Sassap. Sec. Sep. °*Sil.* *Spig.* Spong. Stann. **Staph.* Stront. **Sulph.* Sulph. ac. Tax. Tereb. Teucr. Thuj. Vinc. *Zinc.* Zinc. ox.

Arthritic pains, °Asa. °Aur. Bell. Bry. °*Calc.* °*Chin.* Dig.? °*Hep.* °*Lyc.* °*Merc.* °*Mez.* °Puls. °Sabin. °*Staph.* °*Sulph.*

Boring, Anac. Ang. Asa. Aur. **Bell.* **Calc.* Carb. an. Dulc. Hell. Hep. Lach. Lyc. Mang. **Merc.* Mez. *Natr.* *Natr. m.* Phosph. Phos. ac. °*Puls.* Ran. sc. Rhod. Rhus. Sabad. Sabin. °*Sep.* °*Sil.* °*Spig.* Staph.

Burning, Arn. Ars. Asa. Bry. Carb. veg. Caust. Con. Euphorb. Lyc. Mang. Merc. Nitr. ac. Phosph. Phos. ac. **Rhus.* **Ruta.* **Sabin.* Sil. Sulph. Tart. Zinc.

Caries, Ars. Asa. Euphorb.? Phosph.? Plumb. *Sabin.* *Sec.* °*Sil.* (Comp: GANGRENE.)

Coldness, feeling of, Ars. °*Calc.* °*Lyc.* Sep. Sulph. °*Zinc.*

Contusive pain, Ign. Ruta.

Crampy feeling, Ang. Asa. *Aur.* Bell. Calc. *Euphr.* Ign. Lact. Mez. Petr. *Phos. ac.* Plat. Spig.

Creeping, Acon. Arn. Cham. Colch. Merc. Plat. Plumb. Puls. Rhus. Sec. Sep. Sulph.

Curvature, Amm.? °*Asa.* Bell.? °*Calc.* Cic.? Ferr.? °*Hep.* Jod.? Ipec.? °*Lyc.* °*Merc. Mez.* °*Nitr. ac.* °*Phosph.* °*Phos. ac.* Plumb.? °*Puls.* Rhod. °*Rhus.* Ruta. °*Sep.* °*Sil.* °*Staph.* °*Sulph.*

Cutting, Anac. Dig. Sabad.

Digging, Asa. Calc. *Carb. an. Cocc.* Diad. Dulc. Mang. Natr. Rhod. *Ruta.* Sep. Spig. Thuj.

Distention, interstitial, °*Asa.* °*Calc.* °Lyc. °*Merc.* °*Mez.* Nitr. ac.? °*Phosph.* °*Phos. ac.* Puls.? Rhus.? Ruta.? *Staph.* Sep.? *Sil. Sulph.*

Drawing, Acon. Agar. Anac. Ang. Asa. Atham. Aur. *Baryt.* Bry. **Carb. veg.* **Caust. Chin.* Crotal. Cupr. Ign. Indig. Kal. Kreos. **Lyc.* Magn. arct. Mang. Men. Merc. Par. Phos. ac. Plumb. Rhod. *Sabin.* Samb. Seneg. Stann. Staph. Tereb. Thuj. Zinc. ox.

Flesh, as if loose, **Bry.* Canth. *Dros.* Electr. **Ign.* Kreos. Led. Mosch. Natr. *Nitr. ac. N. vom.* Ol. an. **Rhus. Stann. Staph. Sulph. Thuj.* Zinc.

Fractures, °*Calc.* °*Lyc.* °*Ruta.* °*Sil.* °*Sulph.*

Gnawing, *Amm. m.* Arg. Bell. Canth. *Con. Dros.* Graph. *Lyc. Mang. Phosph. Phos. ac.* Puls. °*Ruta.* Samb. Staph. Stront.

Griping, Natr.

Inflammation, Acon.? Ang.? Ars.? °*Asa.* °*Aur.* °*Bell.* Bry.? °*Calc.* °*Chin.* Clem.? Con.? Cupr.? Euphorb.? °*Hep.* °*Jod.* °*Lach.* °*Lyc.* Magn. m.? °*Mang.* °*Merc.* °*Mez.* °*Nitr. ac.* °*Phosph.* °*Phos. ac.* °*Puls.* Rhus.? Sep.? *Sil.* °*Staph.* °*Sulph.* Thuj.? Veratr.?

Itching, *Cycl.* Nitr. *Phosph. Veratr.*

Jerking, Anac. **Asa.* Aur. Bell. °*Calc.* Caust. **Chin.* Clem. Colch. Lyc. Merc. *Natr. m.* N. vom. Petr. Phosph. °*Puls.* Rhod. Rhus. Sep. Sil. Sulph. ac. Val.

Jerks, Amm. Phosph. Rhod. Sulph. ac.

Laming pain, *Aur.* Bell. *Chin. Cocc. Crotal.* Cycl. *Lach.* Led. Mez. Natr. m. N. vom. Petr. Puls. Rhus. Sabin. Sil. Staph. Veratr. Zinc.

Marrow, as if coagulated. Ang.

Marrow, as if without, Lyc.

Mercurial pains, °Asa. °Aur. Calc.? Carb. veg.? Caust.? °*Chin.* °*Guaj.* °*Hep.* °*Lach.* °*Lyc.* °*Mez.* °Nitr. ac. °Phosph. °*Phos. ac.* °Staph. °*Sulph.*

Pain as if broken, Cocc. *Cupr.* Hep. Magn. m. Natr. m. Puls. °*Ruta.* Samb. Sep. Veratr.

Pain as if bruised, Agar. Amm. M. Ang. Asa. Aur. Baryt. Bov. Calc. Cann. Chin. **Cocc.* Graph. °*Hep.* °*Ign.* °*Ipec.* *Led.* Magn. aust. Magn. c. Meph. Mez. Natr. m. N. vom. Par. Petr. *Phosph.* °*Puls.* **Ruta.* Sabad. Sabin. Sep. Val. °*Veratr.* Zinc.

Painfulness and simple pain, Acon. Agn. °*Amb.* Agar. Alum. Amm. Amm. m. Anac. Ang. Ant. **Arg.* Arn. **Ars.* **Asa.* **Aur.* Baryt. Bell. Bism. Bry. °*Calc.* Camph. Cann. Canth. Caps.

Carb. an. Carb. veg. Caust. *Cham.* Chel. **Chin.* Chinin. Cic. Clem. °*Cocc.* Colch. Coloc. °*Con.* **Crotal.* **Cupr.* **Cycl.* °*Daph.* Dig. *Dros.* Dulc. *Euphorb.* **Ferr.* Graph. Guaj. Hell. °*Hep.* Ign. Jod. Ipec. *Kal.* **Kreos.* **Lach.* Led. °*Lyc.* Magn. art. Magn. arct. Magn. c. Magn. m. **Mang.* **Merc.* **Mez.* **Mur. ac.* Natr. *Natr. m.* **Nitr. ac.* N. mosch. N. vom. Oleand. Op. Petr. **Phosph.* **Phos. ac.* Plumb. Poth. **Puls.* Ran. sc. **Rhod.* **Rhus.* **Ruta.* Sabad. **Sabin.* Samb. Sassap. Sec. Sep. **Sil.* *Spig.* Spong. **Staph.* Stront. **Sulph.* Thuj. Val. *Veratr.* Viol. tr. °*Zinc.*

Pressure, Alum. Amm. *Anac.* Ang. Anis. **Arg.* Arn. Ars. Asa. *Aur.* **Bell.* *Bism.* Bry. Cann. Canth. Carb. veg. Cham. Chel. Cocc. *Colch.* Coloc. Con. °*Cupr.* **Cycl.* °*Daph.* Dros. *Graph.* Guaj. Hell. Hep. Ign. **Kal.* Led. Magn. arct. Magn. aust. *Merc.* *Mez.* Nitr. N. mosch. N. vom. **Oleand.* Phosph. *Plat.* *Puls.* Rhod. **Rhus.* **Sabin.* Sil. Spong. Stann. **Staph.* Teucr. *Thuj.* Val. *Veratr.* Viol. tr. Zinc.

Rolling, Phos. ac.

Scraping, **Asa.* Berb. °*Chin.* Coloc. *Phos. ac.* Puls. **Rhus.* **Sabad.* Spig.

Softening, °*Asa.* Bell.? °*Calc.* Cic.? °*Hep.* **Lyc.* °*Merc.* Mez.? °*Nitr. ac.* Petr. °*Phosph.* Phos. ac.? Puls.? Ruta.? °*Sep.* **Sil.* Staph.? °*Sulph.*

Sore, as if raw, °*Con.* Graph. Hep. Ign. Merc. °*Phos. ac.* Sep.

Stinging, Aeth. Acon. Agn. Agar. Amm. Anac. Ant. Arg. Ars. Asa. Aur. **Bell.* Berb. Bry. **Calc.* Canth. Carb. veg. **Caust.* Chel. **Chin.* Cocc. Colch. **Con.* Daph. **Dros.* Dulc. Euphorb. Euphr. Graph. **Hell.* Jod. Kal. **Lach.* Laur. Lyc. Magn. art. Magn. m. Mang. **Merc.* Mez. Mur. ac. Natr. Natr. s. Nitr. Nitr. ac. N. vom. Ol. an. Par. Phell. Petr. Phosph. Phos. ac. Prun. **Puls.* Raph. *Ran. sc.* **Ruta.* Sabin. Samb. **Sassap.* °*Sep.* Sil. Spig. Staph. Stront. Sulph. Thuj. Tarax. Tax. *Val.* Verb. Viol. tr. Zinc.

Suppuration, Caries, °*Ang.* Ars. °*Asa.* °*Aur.* Calc. Caps.? Chin. Con. Cupr. Euphorb.? Graph.? °*Hep.* Jod. °*Lach.* °*Lyc.* **Merc.* °*Mez.* °*Natr. m.* °*Nitr. ac.* Op.? Phosph. Phos. ac. Puls.? Rhus.? °*Ruta.* °*Sabin.* Sec.? Sep.? °*Sil.* Spong.? °*Staph.* °*Sulph.* Thuj.?

Swelling, Amb. Amm. Ant. °*Asa.* °*Aur.* Bell. Bry. °*Calc.* Carb. an. °*Clem.* Coloc. Con. °*Daph.* Dig. Dulc. °*Guaj.* Hep. Jod. °*Lach.* Led. °*Lyc.* **Merc.* °*Mez.* Natr. Natr. m. **Nitr. ac.* Petr. °*Phosph.* °*Phos. ac.* °*Puls.* Rhod. °*Rhus.* °*Ruta.* *Sabin.* Sep. °*Sil.* Spig. **Staph.* °*Sulph.* Thuj. Veratr.

Syphilitic affections, °*Aur.* °Carb. veg.? °*Merc.*

Tearing, **Agar.* Alum. °*Amm. m.* Ang. **Arg.* Arn. Ars. Asa. °*Aur.* **Baryt.* °*Bell.* Berb. Bism. Bov. Bry. Cann. **Carb. veg.* °*Caust.* Cham. Chel. **Chin.* **Cocc.* Coloc. **Cycl.* °*Cupr.* Dig. Dulc. Graph. Hell. Ign. Jod. Kal. Lach. Lact. Laur. °*Lyc.* °*Magn. c.* Magn. m. Mang. Meph. *Merc.* Mur. ac. Natr. Natr. m. Nicc. °*Nitr.* Nitr. ac. N. vom. °*Phosph.* °*Phos. ac.* Puls. °*Rhod.* °*Ruta.* Sabad. **Sabin.* Sassap. Sep. **Spig.* Spong. Stann. **Staph.* Stront. *Teucr. Thuj. Veratr.* Verb. Zinc. (Comp: Drawing.)

Throbbing, Asa. Berb. °*Calc.* Carb. veg. Lyc. °*Merc.* Mez. Nitr. Nitr. ac. Phosph. Rhod. Ruta. *Sabad.* Sep. Sil. °*Sulph.* Thuj.

Wandering pains, Lact. Sil.

Head, bone-pain, *Ant. Ang.* **Aur.* Baryt. *Bell.* Bry. *Calc.* Canth. Carb. veg. Caust. Cham. **Chin.* Cocc. Cupr. Graph. Guaj. **Hep.* Ign. Ipec. *Lyc.* Mang. **Merc. Mez.* Natr. **Nitr. ac.* N. vom. *Phosph. Phos. ac.* Puls. Rhod. Rhus. **Ruta.* Sabad. Sabin. Samb. **Sep. Sil.* Spig. Staph. Sulph. Veratr. Viol. tr. Zinc.

—, tumours, **Aur.* °*Daph.* °*Merc.*

Ears, pain, Baryt. Indig. Kal. Lach. Raph. Ratanh. Sil. Staph.

—, caries, °Asa. ? °*Aur.* °*Nitr. ac.* °*Sil.* °Staph. ?

—, swelling, °Carb. an. °Puls.

—, —, behind the ear, periosteum, °Carb. an.

Nose, caries, °Aur.

—, pain, Ars. **Aur.* Corall. Hep. Indig. Laur. *Merc.* Natr. m. Nitr. Thuj.

Face, inflammation, °Aur. °Staph.

—, caries, °Cist. °Sil.

—, swelling, °Aur. °Sil. °Spig.

—, pains, °Alum. Asa. °Aur. **Calc.* °Caps. Carb. veg. **Caust.* °Chel. *Chin. *Colch.* °Con. °Dros. **Hep.* **Mez.* **Natr. m.* **Nitr. ac.* N. mosch. **Phosph.* Ruta. Samb. *Spig.* **Staph.*

Lower jaw, caries, °Cist. *Merc.* °Sil.

—, swelling, **Merc.* **Sil.*

Mouth, palate, caries, °*Aur. Merc.*

Abdomen, pelvis, tumour, °Aur.

Chest, caries, Con.

Dorsal region, °*Calc.* Lyc. °*Puls.* °*Rhus.* °*Sil.* °Staph. **Sulph.*

Dorsal region, swelling, °Calc. °Puls. °Rhus. °Sil. Sulph.

—, curvature, °Calc. °Lyc. °Puls. °Rhus. °Sil. °Staph. ? **Sulph.*

Arms, Acon. Anac. °*Ang.* °*Calc.* *Indig.* Jod. Lact. °*Lyc.* Meph. Merc. *Natr.* *Natr. m.* Natr. s. Nicc. *Nitr. ac.* Plumb. Raph. °*Rhus.* Ruta. **Sil.* Staph. °*Sulph.* Tereb. *Thuj.*

—, elbow, °Amb. °Lyc. Phosph.

—, upper arm, Baryt. *Bell.*

—, forearm, Natr. m. Plumb. Spig. Spong.

Hands, Aeth. Agar. Anac. Anis. Arg. Asa. Atham. *Aur.* Bell. *Berb.* *Bism.* Carb. an. °*Carb. veg.* Caust. *Chel.* *Chin.* *Euphr.* Ign. Jod. Kal. Lach. Lact. Laur. Led. Magn. c. Magn. m. *Mang.* *Merc.* Mez. Natr. Natr. s. Nitr. Ol. an. Par. *Phosph.* Phos. ac. Ran. sc. Rhod. *Sabin.* Samb. Sassap. *Spig.* *Stann.* Staph. Sulph. Sulph. ac. Tax. *Teucr.* Zinc.

—, fingers, Crotal. Daph.

Lower limbs, Amm. Ang. Asa. **Baryt.* *Berb.* **Caust.* *Chin.* Crotal. Dros. Kal. Lach. Magn. m. Mez. Nitr. Nitr. ac. Poth. Sulph.

—, hips, *Berb.* Calc. Caust. Cic. Kal. *Kreos.* Magn. c. Natr. s. *Oleand.* *Ruta.*

—, thighs, Aur. Baryt. Berb. Borax. *Canth.* Carb. an. Chin. Cocc. Coff. Euphorb. Graph. Guaj. *Indig.* Lach. Lyc. Magn. c. Magn. s. Men. Mez. Mur. ac. *Puls.* *Ruta.* Sep. Sil. Sulph. Zinc.

—, knee, Bov. Carb. an. Carb. veg. Grat. Indig. Magn. c. Phosph. Prun. Rhod. Stann. Zinc.

—, legs, Ang. Baryt. *Berb.* Bry. *Chin.* Croc. Crotal. Graph. Ign. Indig. *Kal.* Lach. Lyc. Magn. m. Nitr. ac. Puls. °*Sil.* *Thuj.* Zinc.

Lower limbs, tibia, Ang. *Berb.* Lach. Lyc. Magn. m. °*Sil. Thuj.*
—, fibula, Berb. Crotal.
—, caries, °*Lach.* °*Sil.*
Feet, Acon. Agar. *Alum.* Ars. *Asa. Aur.* Bell. Bism. *Carb. veg. Chin.* Cocc. *Cupr.* Lach. °*Merc.* Nitr. ac. Plat. *Rutr. Sabin.* Spig. Stann. *Staph.* Teucr. Veratr. Zinc. Zinc. ox.
—, heel-bone, Berb. Caps. Coloc. Crotal. Diad. Ign.
—, toes, Mez. Sep.

Boring.

Bones, periosteum, Anac. Ang. Asa. Aur. **Bell.* **Calc.* Carb. an. Dulc. Hell. Hep. Kal. Lach. Lyc. Mang. **Merc.* Mez. *Natr. Natr. m.* Phosph. Phos. ac. °*Puls.* Ran. sc. Rhod. Rhus. Sabad. Sabin. °*Sep.* °*Sil.* °*Spig.* Staph. Sulph. Thuj.
Nails, Colch.
Glands, Bell. Lyc. Puls. Sabin.

Boring pain in.

Swelling, Bell.
Ulcers, Ars. Aur. *Bell.* Calc. Caust. Chin. Hep. Kal. Natr. Natr. m. Puls. Ran. sc. Sep. **Sil.* °*Sulph.* Thuj.
Corns, *Borax.* Calc. *Caust.* Hep. Kal. *Natr.* Natr. m. *Phosph.* Puls. °*Ran. sc.* Rhod. °*Sep.* °*Sil.* Spig. Thuj.
Nails, Colch.
Erysipelas, Euphorb.

Breaking again.

Old cicatrices of ulcers and sores, Carb. veg. *Crotal. Lach.* Sil.

Brown, that which is.

Eruption, Cann. *Nitr. ac.* Phosph. Phos. ac.
Blisters, vesicles, Vip. red.
Herpes, °Dulc. Veratr.
Pimples, Veratr.
Pustules, Tart.
Spots, *Ant.* °*Ars.* Aur. Berb. Cann. °*Carb. veg.* °*Con.* Crotal. Hyos. Natr. m. °*Nitr. ac.* °*Petr.* °*Phosph.* Plumb. **Sep.* °*Sulph.* Tax. Thuj.
Swelling, Lach. Vip.
Scurfs, Amm. m. Ant. Berb.
Scars (of ulcers, wounds,) Lach.
Streaks, ridges, *Ars.* °*Carb. veg.*

Head, spots, °Ars.
Nose, red-brown, Aur. Tax.
Face, °Bry. °Dulc. Veratr.
Hips, streaks, *Ars.
—, eruptions, Berb. Phos. ac.
Buccal cavity, swollen and black-brown, Vip. torv.
Abdomen, spots, °Sep.
Sexual parts, spots, Nitr. ac.
Chest, spots, °Carb. veg. °Sep.
Dorsal region, spots, Thuj.
Arms, eruptions, Ant.
—, spots, swelling, *Sep.*

Hands, eruptions, Natr. m.
—, spots, Natr. m. °Petr.
—, scurfs, Amm. m. Ant.
—, swelling, Lach.
Lower limbs, spots, Cann.

Bruised by blows, painful as if.

Ulcers, Ang. Arn. Cham. Chin. Cocc. Con. **Graph.** Hep. Hyos. Natr. m. N. vom. Rhus. **Ruta.** Sulph.

Bones, Agar. Amm. m. Ang. Asa. Aur. **Baryt.** Bov. Calc. Cann. Chin. **Cocc.* Graph. °***Hep.*** °*Ign.* °*Ipec.* °*Led.* Magn. aust. Magn. c. **Meph.** Mez. Natr. m. N. vom. Par. Petr. ***Phosph.*** °*Puls.* **Ruta.* Sabad. Sabin. Sep. Val. °***Veratr.*** Zinc.

Bruised, pain as if.

Arms, shoulder, Sassap.
—, elbow, Baryt. Caust. Hep. Magn. art. **Ruta.**
—, upper arm, Cycl. Hell. Kreos. Mez.
—, forearm, Mur. ac. Sulph. ac.
Hands, Bov. Calc. Graph. Jod.
—, finger, Cin. Cupr. Ruta.
—, thumb, Cin.
Lower limbs, Laur.
—, hips and nates, Cic. Cin. Euphorb. *Kal.* Laur. *Ruta.*
—, thighs, *Arn.* Kreas. Lach. Lyc. *Natr. s. N. mosch. Plat.* Sulph.
—, knees, Arn. Bov. Magn. aust. Mez. Petr. ***Plat.*** Rhod. Sulph. ac.

Lower limbs, legs, calves, Ant. Arn. Caust. Cupr. Euphorb. Natr. m. Prun. Ruta. Sep.
Feet, Hell. Ol. an. Tart.
—, heel, Caps. Magn. m.
—, toe, Ruta.

BUBBLING.

In the skin, in general, with dizziness. ° *Calc.*

Arms, Amb. Magn. aust.
—, shoulder, Berb. Mang. Puls.
—, elbow-joint, Kreos. Mang. Rhab. Spong.
—, upper arm, Berb. Colch. Zinc.
—, forearm, Zinc.
Hands, Berb. Rhus.
—, finger, Berb. Par. Spig. Teucr.
Lower limbs, Squill.
—, nates, Amb. Ant. Zinc.
—, thigh, Berb. Men. Oleand.
—, knee, Arg. Asa. Asar. Bell. Berb. Natr. m. Rhab.
—, legs, Ant. Arn. Berb. Con. Crotal. Rhab. Rhus. Spig.
Feet, Berb. Chel. Lach.

BUBBLES, THROBS, THAT WHICH.

Swelling, N. vom. (Comp: throbbing.)
Ulcers, Mur. ac.

Buccal cavity, swelling, N. vom.

BURNING.

In general, on the skin, **Acon.* **Agar.* Alum. **Amb.* Amm. Amm. m. Anac. Ant. Arg. *Arn.* **Ars.* Aur. Baryt. Bar. m. **Bell.* Berb. Bism. Bov. **Bry.* Calad. **Calc.* Calc. ph. Camph. Cann. Canth.**Caps.* Carb. an. Carb. veg. *Caust. Cham.* Chel. Chin. Chinin. Cic. Cin. Clem. Cocc. Coff. Colch. Coloc. Con. Croton. Cupr. Cycl. Dig. Dros. **Dulc.* **Euphorb.* Even. Ferr. Graph. Grat. Guaj. Hell. *Hep. Hyos. Ign. Kal.* Kreos. **Lach.* Led.**Lyc.* Magn. art. Magn. arct. Magn. aust. Magn. sc. Magn. m. Magn. s. Mang. Men. **Merc. Mercurial.* **Mez.* Mosch. Mur. ac. *Natr. Natr. m. Natr. s.* Nicc. Nitr. Nitr. ac. *N. vom.* Oleand. Ol. an. Oph. *Op. Par.* Phell. Petr. **Phosph.* Phos. ac. Plat. Plumb. *Puls.* Ran. Ran. sc. Raph. Rhod. *Rhus.* Ruta. Sabad. Sabin. Samb. Sassap. Sec. Selen. Seneg. *Sep.* **Sil.* Spig. Spong. *Squill.* Stann. Staph. Stram. Stront. *Sulph.* Sulph. ac. Tab. Tart. Thuj. Veratr. Viol. od. Viol. tr. Zinc.

As if from fire, Tart. Viol. od.

—, from sparks, Phell. Sec. Selen.

—, burning coal, Puls.

—, vesicatory, Kal.

Scalp, Ars. Baryt. ****Bry.*** ****Calc.*** ***Caps.*** Clem. Coloc. Cupr. Dros. Grat. Indig. Lach. Laur. Lyc. ***Merc.*** Mur. ac. Natr. m. Oleand. ***Ol. an.*** Par. Phell. Phosph. Phos. ac. Plat. Ran. Ruta. Sep. Spig. Spong. Staph. Sulph. Thuj. Veratr. Viol. tr. Zinc.

Eyes, ****Acon.*** Aeth. Agar. Agn. Alum. Amm.

Amm. m. Ang. ***Arn.*** **Ars.* ***Asa.*** °*Asar.* Aur. Baryt. **Bell.* Berb. Bism. Bov. Bruc. **Bry.* Calad. **Calc.* Cann. Cant. Caps. Carb. an. **Carb. veg.* Cast. Caust. Cham. Chen. Chin. Cic. Cin. Clem. **Coloc.* Con. Corall. **Croc.* **Crotal.* Dig. ***Dros.*** Eugen. **Euphr.* Ferr. Graph. Grat. Hell. Ign. Indig. ***Kal.*** **Lach.* Lact. *Laur.* Led. **Lyc.* Magn. art. Magn. arct. Magn. c. Magn. m. **Merc.* *Mur. ac.* *Natr.* Natr. m. Nicc. ***Nitr.*** Nitr. ac. N. mosch. **N. vom.* Ol. an. Par. Petr. Phell. *Phosph.* **Phos. ac.* Plat. Plumb. Puls. Ratanh. ***Rhod.*** °*Rhus.* °Ruta. Sabad. Sassap. Seneg. *Sep.* Sil. Spig. **Spong.* Stann. Staph. Stram. Stront. **Sulph.* Sulph. ac. Tab. ***Tarax.*** Tart. Therid. Thuj. Tong. Val. Viol. od. Zinc.

Eyebrows, Asa. Dig. Dros. Merc. Spig.

Eyelids, Alum. Amb. Ars. Asar. Bell. Berb. °*Bry.* **Calc.* Caps. *Caust.* Cin. Clem. Coloc. Con. Graph. Kal. Laur. Magn. arct. Magn. aust. Merc. Nitr. °*N. vom.* Oleand. Phell. Phosph. *Phos. ac.* Rhab. Ran. Ran. sc. Rhus. Sassap. *Seneg.* Sep. *Spig.* Spong. Stann. Sulph.

Canthi, *Agar.* Alum. *Amm. m.* Ang. Asar. °*Aur.* Baryt. Bell. *Calb.* Carb. an. Carb. veg. Chel. Chin. Clem. Coloc. Graph. Hell. Kal. Laur. Magn. c. Natr. m. Nitr. N. vom. *Par.* °*Phosph.* *Phos. ac.* Ran. Rhod. Sep. Squill. Stann. Staph. *Stront.* *Sulph.* Tarax. Tart. Thuj.

Ears, Acon. *Agar.* Amm. m. Ang. Ant. Arn. Ars. Bry. Calc. Canth. Caps. Carb. an. Carb. veg. Caust. Chel. Clem. Dros. Grat.

Ign. ***Kreos.*** ***Laur.*** Magn. c. Magn. m. Merc. Natr. m. Oleand. ***Ol. an.*** Sabad. ***Sabin.*** Spig. Spong. Zinc.

Nose, Agar. Alum. ****Ars.*** ****Bell.*** Bov. Caps. Carb. an. Chen. Cin. Cist. Gran. Graph. Jod. Kal. Led. Magn. art. ****Magn. m.*** Natr. m. Nicc. Nitr. Nitr. ac. Petr. Phosph. Phell. Sulph. ac. Tab.

Face, Alum. Arg. Ars. Berb. Caps. Caust. Graph. Kal. Natr. Nitr. Sep. Stann. Viol. tr.

Lips and mouth, region of, Agar. Amm. Amm. m. Anis. ***Arn.*** Asa. Baryt. Berb. Borax. Bov. °Bry. Caps. Carb. an. Dros. Gran. Graph. Hep. Kal. Kreos. Magn. c. Magn. s. ****Merc.*** ***Mez.*** ***Mur. ac.*** Natr. Natr. m. Natr. s. °N. vom. Oleand. ***Phosph.*** ***Phos. ac.*** Puls. Rhod. ***Sabad.*** Selen. Sep. °Spig. ***Staph.*** Sulph. Tab. Tarax. Tart. ac. Thuj. Veratr. Zinc.

—, corners of mouth, Arn. Coloc. Dros. Mez. Natr. Zinc.

Chin, Anac. Ant. Berb. Bov. Canth. Caust. Magn. c. Mang. Merc. Ol. an. Rhus. Spig. Spong.

Lower jaw, Caust. Par.

Mouth, ****Acon.*** Alum. Amm. Amm. caust. Ang. Arn. ****Ars.*** Asa. Asar. Baryt. ****Bell.*** Berb. ***Bism.*** Borax. Bov. ***Calc.*** Calc. ph. ***Camph.*** Cann. ***Canth.*** Carb. an. ****Carb. veg.*** ***Cast.*** ***Caust.*** °Cham. Chel. Chen. Chinin. ***Cinn.*** Cocc. ***Coff.*** ***Colch.*** Con. Croc. Dig. Euphorb. Galv. ***Grat.*** ***Hydroc.*** ***Indig.*** Iod. ***Kal.*** Kal. chl. Kal. hydr. ****Lach.*** Lact. ***Laur.*** Led. Lob. °Magn. arct. Magn. aust. ***Magn. c.*** Magn. m.

__Merc.__ *__Mez.__* Mosch. Mur. ac. Natr. *__Natr. s.__* Nitr. **Nitr. ac. N. vom.* Oleand. *__Ol. an.__* Par. Petr. Phell. **__Phosph.__* *__Phos. ac.__* Poth. Plumb. Prun. °*__Puls.__* Ran. Ran. sc. Raph. *__Ratanh.__* Rhod. Rhus. **__Sabad.__* Sec. Seneg. Sep. Sil. Spig. Squill. Staph. Stront. **__Sulph.__* **__Tereb.__* Tong. *__Veratr.__* Zinc.

—, palate, Camph. *__Caust.__* Chen. *__Cinn.__* *__Cocc.__* Euphorb. *__Grat.__* *__Hydroc.__* *__Indig.__* Lach. *__Laur.__* Magn. c. Mur. ac. *Natr. s.* Par. Phosph. Rhod. Sabad. Seneg. Spig. Squill. Staph. Tong.

—, velum palati, Phos. ac. Ran.

—, buccal cavity. Asa. Baryt. Bov. Calc. Kal. *__Lach.__* Merc. Mez. Natr. s. *__Op.__* Plumb. **Sabad.* Sulph. *__Tereb.__* *__Veratr.__*

—, fauces, **__Acon.__* Alum. Amm. Amm. caust. Arn. **__Ars.__* Asa. Baryt. **__Bell.__* *__Bism.__* Borax. Bov. Calc. Calc. ph. *__Camph.__* Cann. *__Canth.__* **__Carb. veg.__* Cast. Caust. Chel. Chen. Chinin. Cocc. Dig. Galv. Hydroc. Jod. **__Lach.__* Lact. Laur. Led. Lob. Magn. aust. Magn. c. **__Merc.__* *__Mez.__* Mosch. Mur. ac. Nitr. **__Nitr. ac. N. vom.__* Oleand. *__Ol. an.__* **__Phosph.__* Poth. °*__Puls.__* Ran. Ran. sc. Raph. Rhod. Rhus. Sabad. Sec. Seneg. Sep. *__Sulph.__* Veratr. Zinc.

Mouth, gums, Cast. Con. °Cham. Lach. °Magn. arct. *__Merc.__* Mur. ac. Natr. s. N. vom. Petr. Phell. Phosph. Puls. Rhus. Sep. Sil. Stront. °Tereb.

—, tongue, *__Acon.__* Amm. Ang. Asar. Bell. Berb. Bov. *__Calc.__* Carb. an. *__Cast.__* *__Caust.__* *__Coff.__* *__Colch.__* Croc. Hydroc. Ign. *__Indig.__* *__Kal.__* Kal. chl. Kal. hdr. *Lach. Laur. *__Magn. c.__* Magn. m. Mez. Natr. Natr. s. Ol. an. Phell. Phosph. *__Phos.__*

ac. Plumb. Prun. Ran. sc. Ratanh. Rhod. **Sabad.* Seneg. Sulph. Tereb. Veratr.

Abdomen and stomach, region of, Berb. Carb. veg. Caust. Kreos. Led. N. vom. ***Ol. an.*** Sabad. Sassap.

—, Anus, Aloë. ***Alum.*** Amm. Amm. m. Ant. ****Ars.*** Aspar. Baryt. Berb. Bov. Bry. ***Calc.*** Canth. °***Caps.*** ***Carb. an.*** ****Carb. veg.*** Cast. Caust. Chen. Chin. °***Cocc.*** ***Colch.*** Con. Croton. Electr. Euphorb. Ferr. Gins. Gran. Graph. Grat. Hell. Hep. Ign. Ipec. Jod. ***Kal.*** Lach. Lact. Laur. Lyc. Magn. art. Magn. c. Magn. m. Magn. s. ****Merc.*** Mur. ac. Natr. c. ****Natr. m.*** Natr. s. Nitr. ***Nitr. ac.*** ***N. vom.*** Oleand. Ol. an. Onisc. Pæon. Petr. Phell. ***Phosph.*** Plumb. Prun. ***Puls.*** Ran. Ratanh. Sabad. Sassap. Senn. ****Sep.*** Sil. Staph. Stront. ****Sulph.*** ***Sulph. ac.*** Tab. Tart. Tereb. Thuj. Veratr. Vinc. Zinc.

—, perinæum, Gran. Nitr. ac. Plumb. Sil.

Sexual parts, Amb. ***Amm.*** Anac. Ars. Baryt. ***Berb.*** Bov. ***Calc.*** ***Cann.*** ***Canth.*** ****Carb. veg.*** ***Caust.*** Cham. Euphorb. Hyos. Kal. Kreos. ***Laur.*** °Lyc. ***Magn. arct.*** Magn. aust. Merc. ac. Mez. ***Nitr. ac.*** N. vom. Petr. Puls. Sep. Spong. Stann. ****Sulph.*** Tereb. Thuj.

—, glans, °Anac. Calc. Stann. Viol. tr.

—, testicles, Baryt. Berb. Nitr. ac. °***Puls.*** Tereb.

—, scrotum, Berb. Euphorb. Plat. Spong. Sulph.

—, penis, Caust. Merc. ac. Sep. Spong. Stann.

—, labia, Amm. Calc. Canth. ****Carb. veg.*** Kal. °***Lyc.*** Magn. aust. ****Sulph.***

Sexual parts, vagina, Berb. Cham. Hyos. Lyc. Sulph. Thuj.

Chest, Baryt. Bov. Caps. Cic. Croc. Graph. Laur. Mez. Mur. ac. Natr. c. Nicc. Phell. Phosph. *Phos. ac.* Ratanh. Sulph. Sulph. ac. Zinc.

Mammæ and nipples, *Laur.* Mez. °Sulph.

—, nipples, °Sulph.

Dorsal region, axilla, Carb. veg. Caust. Kal. Natr. m. Sep. Spig. Zinc.

—, neck, Caust. Grat. Nicc. Ol. an. Phell. Stront. Tab.

—, small of back, Aeth. Amm. Asar. Berb. Borax. Kal. Lach. Magn. aust. Natr. Phosph. Phos. ac. Rhus, Stann. Sulph. Sulph. ac.

—, loins, Aeth. Baryt. Berb. Nitr. ac.

—, nape of the neck, Amm. Calc. Ign. Merc. Nat. Nitr. Ol. an.

—, back, Amm. Arn. Bism. Bry. Calc. °*Carb. an.* *Carb. veg.* Lyc. Magn. m. Merc. Mur. ac. Natr. *Nitr. ac.* N. vom. Oph. Raph. Seneg. Sil. ***Sulph.*** Tart. Zinc.

—, vertebræ, Asa. Tart.

—, scapulæ, Alum. Amb. Baryt. Bry. Cann. Carb. veg. Caust. Elect. Galv. Jod. Kal. Laur. Lyc. Magn. m. Merc. Natr. Natr. m. Seneg. Sil. Sulph. Tab. Teucr. Veratr. Zinc.

Arms, Alum. Amm. Amm. m. Arg. Arn. Asa. ***Berb.*** Borax. Bov. °***Bry.*** Calc. Carb. an. ***Carb. veg.*** Caust. Cocc. Colch. Coloc. Dig. Dulc. Euphorb. ***Graph.*** Indig. Kal. Kreos. ***Lach.*** Laur. Led. ***Magn. art.*** ***Magn. arct.*** Magn. m. Mang. Men. Merc. Mez. Mill. Mosch. Mur. ac. Natr. m. ***Natr. s.*** N. vom. Oleand. ***Ol. an.*** Par. Petr. Phosph. Phos. ac. ***Plat.*** ***Puls.*** Ran. sc. Ratanh.

Rhus. Sep. Spong. Staph. Stront. **Sulph.* Tarax. Teucr. Tong. Vip. torv. *Zinc.*

Arms, shoulder, Amm. m. Berb. *Carb. veg.* Cocc. Graph. Kal. Magn. m. Men. Mill. Mur. ac. N. vom. Par. Phos. ac. °*Rhus.* Spong.

—, shoulder-joints, Graph. Stront.

Arm, Alum. Bov. °*Bry.* Calc. Cocc. Dig. Kreos. Lach. Led. *Magn. art.* Magn. m. Merc. N. vom. Ol. an. Petr. Phell. Phos. ac. Plat. *Puls.* Rhus. Staph. *Sulph.* Vip. torv.

—, elbow, Amm. m. Arg. Berb. Carb. an. Carb. veg. Dulc. Indig. Laur. Merc. Mill. Natr. s. Nitr. Phos. ac. Plat. Rhus. Staph. Sulph. Teucr. Tong.

—, elbow-joints, Asa. Magn. art. Merc.

—, upper arm, Arg. Asa. Berb. Borax. Carb. veg. Caust. Colch. Coloc. Dig. Dulc. Graph. Kal. Magn. arct. Magn. Mur. ac. Natr. m. Phosph. Sep. Zinc.

—, forearm, Amm. Amm. m. Arn. Asa. *Berb.* Carb. an. Carb. veg. Caust. Dig. Euphorb. *Graph.* Laur. Magn. m. Mosch. Mur. ac. Natr. s. Oleand. *Ol. an.* Ran. sc. Ratanh. *Rhus.* Staph. **Sulph.* Tarax. *Zinc.*

Hands, Anac. Anis. Arg. Asar. Baryt. Berb. Bry. Calc. *Canth.* Carb. an. Cham. Cop. Dulc. Graph. Galv. *Hep.* Kal. °*Lach. Laur.* Lyc. Magn. c. Merc. Natr. Natr. m. *Natr. s.* Nicc. N. mosch. *N. vom.* Ol. an. *Petr.* **Phosph.* Phos. ac. Plat. Ran. Rhod. Rhus. Sassap. *Sec.* Spig. Spong. Stann. *Stront.* Sulph. Tab. Tax. Zinc.

Hands, wrists, Arg. Asar. Berb. Mez. Phosph. Plat. Plumb. *Stront.* Thuj. Zinc.

—, fingers, **Agar.* Asa. *Berb.* Borax. Calc. Carb. veg. *Caust.* Coloc. Con. Croc. Dig. Euphorb. Gran. Graph. *Kal.* °*Lach.* Laur. Lyc. Magn. art. Magn. arct. Magn. m. Mang. Merc. Mez. Mill. Mosch. *Natr.* Natr. s. Nicc. Nitr. ac. N. vom. *Oleand.* Ol. an. Petr. Ran. Ran. sc. *Rhod.* Sabad. Sabin. Sassap. Sil. Spig. Staph. *Sulph.* Sulph. ac. Tarax. *Teucr.* Therid. Veratr. Vip. torv. *Zinc.*

—, finger-joints, Berb. Carb. veg. Caust. Sabin. Spig.

—, thumb, Gran. Graph. Lach. Laur. Magn. art. Merc. N. vom. Oleand. Ol. an. Sassap. Staph.

Lower limbs, Carb. an. Chin. *Kal.* Kreos. Magn. art. Nitr. ac. Prun. Ratanh. Thuj.

—, nates, hips, Amm. Baryt. Bell. Calc. **Carb. veg.* Caust. Chel. Cic. Croton. Hell. Led. Lyc. Magn. c. *Magn. m. Mang.* Merc. Mez. Natr. Natr. s. Nicc. Nitr. N. vom. Rhus. *Sep.* Staph. Stront. Thuj. Verb.

—, thigh, Alum. Anac. Asa. Baryt. *Berb. Borax. Bov.* Calc. Cann. Carb. an. *Carb. veg. Chin.* Cic. Cocc. *Colch.* Croton. Dulc. *Euphorb.* Graph. Grat. Laur. Lyc. Mang. Men. *Mez.* Mur. ac. N. vom. Oleand. *Phosph.* Phos. ac. Rhod. Rhus. Ruta. Sabin. Samb. Sassap. Spig. Staph. Sulph. Sulph. ac. *Zinc.*

—, knees, Amm. Anac. Asa. Baryt Berb. Bry. Cann. Carb. veg. Grat. Kal. °*Lyc.* Mur. ac. Natr. Oleand. Petr. Phell. Phos. ac. Plat.

Plumb. ***Rhus.*** Sabad. Stann. Staph. ***Sulph.*** Sulph. ac. Tab. ***Tarax.*** Tart. ***Thuj.***

Lower limbs, legs, calves, shins, ***Agar.*** Alum. ***Anac.*** Ang. Arg. ***Ars.* Asa. Bell. Berb. Borax. Calc. Calend. Cann. Caust. ***Chell.*** Chin. ***Crotal.*** Cycl. Dig. Graph. Kal. °***Lyc.*** Magn. arct. Magn. aust. Magn. c. Mang. Men. Mez. ***Natr.*** *Natr. s.* N. vom. Phell. Phosph. ac. Puls. Ran. Rhus. Sabad. Sassap. Sep. Stront. ***Sulph.*** Sulph. ac. ***Tarax.*** Thuj. Veratr. Zinc.

—, tendo Achilles, Berb. Chell. Chin.

Feet, Ammoniac, Ang. Ant. Arn. ***Berb.*** ***Bov.*** ****Calc.*** Carb. an. Caust. Cham. Chin. Con. Croc. Crotal. Dulc. ***Electr.*** ****Graph.*** ***Hep.*** Heracl. *Ign.* Kal. Kreos. Laur. ***Lyc.*** ***Magn. m.*** Merc. *Mez.* ***Natr.*** ****Natr. m.*** Natr. s. ***Nitr. ac.*** ***Ol. an.*** Petr. ***Puls.*** Ratanh. ***Rhab.*** Rhus. Sabin. ***Sec.*** *Sep.* ***Sil.*** ***Spig.*** Squill, ***Stann.*** Staph. ***Stram.*** Stront. Sulph. ***Tarax.*** Thuj. Veratr. Zinc. Zing.

—, heels, Cycl. Graph. ***Ign.*** Magn. art. ***Nitr.*** Puls. Rhus. Sabin. Sep. Sulph. ac. Veratr. Zinc.

—, soles, Alum. ****Amb.*** Amm. ****Anac.*** Asar. Baryt. Bell. Berb. Bov. ****Calc.*** ***Canth.*** ***Carb. veg.*** Caust. Croc. Crotal. °***Cupr.*** ***Graph.*** Hep. Kal. Kreos. Lach. Led. ***Lyc.*** ***Magn. m.*** Merc. Mur. ac. ***Natr.*** Natr. s. Nitr. ***N. vom.*** Petr. ***Phos. ac.*** Puls. ***Sil.*** ***Sulph.*** Tab. Tarax. Zinc.

—, toes, **Agar.* °***Alum.*** Ammoniac. Amm. Ant. Asa. Atham. ***Berb.*** ***Borax.*** Calc. Carb. an. Caust. ***Con.*** Dulc. Hep. °***Kal.*** Lach. Laur. ***Lyc.*** Magn. c. Meph. Merc. Mez. Mosch. Mur.

ac. Natr. Nitr. ac. ***N. vom.*** Oleand. Pæon. Par. Phosph. Phos. ac. Plat. ***Puls.*** Ran. sc. Ratanh. Rhus. Ruta. Sabin. Sep. *Staph.* *Tarax.* Zinc.

Bones, periosteum, Ars. Asa. Bry. Carb. veg. Caust. Con. Euphorb. Lyc. Merc. Nitr. ac. Phosph. Phos. ac. ****Rhus.*** ****Ruta.*** **Sabin.* Sil. Sulph. Tart. Zinc.

Nails, Alum. Calc. ***Caust.*** Con. Kal. Merc. Nicc. Nitr. ac. Vinc.

Glands, Ars. Bell. Cann. Carb. veg. Cocc. Hep. Laur. Merc. Phosph. ****Puls.*** Rhab. Sil. Tereb.

Burn, as after a.

Blisters, vesicles, Amb. Bell. Carb. an. Clem. Lyc. Natr. Phosph. Sep. Sulph.

Spots, Ant. °***Ars.*** Carb. veg. °*Caust.* °*Cycl.* Euphorb. Hyos. Kreos. Lach. Rhus. Sec. Stram.

Ulcers, Alum. Ant. °***Ars.*** Baryt. °*Carb. veg.* Caust. °***Cycl.*** Ign. Kreos. Lach. N. vom. Puls. Sabad. Sec. Sep. Stram.

Face, eruption, Clem. N. vom.

Lips, blisters, Ars. Plat. Rhus. v. Sabad.

Buccal cavity, blisters, Amb. Bell. Carb. an. Lyc. Sep. Sulph.

Burns, that which.

Blisters, vesicles, ***Amm.*** ***Amm. m.*** ***Aur.*** ****Baryt.*** Bell. Bov. ****Bry.*** Calc. Canth. Caps. Carb. an. Caust. Cyc. ***Graph.*** Hep. Lach. Magn. c. Magn.

9

m. Mang. ***Merc. Mur. ac. Natr. Natr. m.*** Natr. s. Nitr. Nitr. ac. Phell. Phosph. Plat. ***Ran.*** Ratanh. Sabad. Seneg. Senn. Sep. ***Spig.*** Spong. Staph. Sulph.

—, phagedænic, Graph. Sil.

Blotches, tubercles, Amm. Amm. m. Calc. Carb. an. Cocc. Dulc. Kal. hdr. Magn. m. Magn. s. Mang. Merc. Mur. ac. Nicc. Nitr. ac. Phosph. Staph.

Chilblains, **N. vom.* °***Puls.*** Spig.

Corns, Alum. Amm. Bruc. ****Bry.*** Calc. Carb. veg. Caust. Chen. Graph. Hep. Ign. Kal. Lyc. Magn. art. Meph. Petr. Phosph. Phos. ac. Puls. Ran. sc. Rhus. **Sep.* Sil. Spig. **Sulph.* Thuj.

—, cracked, chapped, Zinc.

Eruption, Agar. Alum. Amb. Amm. Amm. m. Anac. Ant. Arg. **Ars.* Aur. Baryt. ***Bell.*** Bov. ***Bry.*** Calad. ***Calc.*** Cann. Canth. Caps. ***Carb. an. Carb. veg. Caust.*** Chin. Cic. Cin. Clem. Cocc. Coff. Colch. ***Con.*** Dulc. Euphorb. Guaj. Hell. ***Hep.*** Heracl. Ign. Kal. Kreos. Lach. Laur. Led. Lyc. Magn. art. Magn. arct. Magn. aust. Mang. **Merc.* ***Mercurial.*** Mez. Mosch. Natr. Natr. m. Nitr. Nitr. ac. *N. vom.* Oleand. Par. Petr. Phosph. Phos. ac. Plat. Plumb. ***Puls.*** Ran. Ratanh. ****Rhus.*** Sabad. Sassap. Seneg. Senn. Sep. ***Sil.*** Spig. Spong. Squill. Stann. Staph. Stram. Stront. **Sulph.* Teucr. Thuj. Veratr. Viol. od. ***Viol. tr.*** Zinc.

Erysipelas, Ars. Carb. veg. Petr. Phosph. Rhod. ****Rhus.***

Figwarts, Thuj.

Herpes, °Amb. Amm. Anac. **Ars.* °Bov. °Bry. Calad. Calc. °Carb. veg. °*Con.* Led. Magn. arct. ***Merc.** Mosch. Rhus. °Sep. ***Staph.*** °Sulph.

Lupia, °Baryt.

Nails, Alum. Calc. ***Caust.*** Con. Kal. Merc. Nicc. Nitr. ac. Vinc.

Pimples, Alum. Amm. Arg. ***Ars.*** Bell. Bov. Bry. ***Canth. Caust.*** Cinn. Dig. Dulc. ***Graph.*** Grat. ***Kal.*** Kal. chl. Lyc. Magn. art. Magn. aust. Magn. m. ***Merc. ac.*** Mosch. ***Natr.*** Natr. m. Natr. s. Nicc. Nitr. Nitr. ac. Ol. an. Phell. Petr. Phosph. °***Phos. ac.*** Puls. Ratanh. Rhus. Sabad. ***Squill.*** Stann. ***Staph. Stront. Sulph.*** Thuj.

Pocks, °Ars. Lach. Merc.

Pustules, ***Amm.*** Berb. Cic. Crotal. Graph. Mez. °***Petr.*** Tart.

Ridges, Rhus.

Rash and like rash, Bry. Calad. Euphr. Merc. N. vom. Phos. ac. Teucr.

Scars, old, Ars. Carb. veg. Graph. Lach.

Scurfs, crusts, Amm. m. Calc. Cic. Puls. Sassap.

Spots. Amm. *Amm. m.* **Ars.* Bell. Berb. Canth. Caust. ***Chel.*** Croc. Cupr. Electr. Ferr. Jod. °*Ipec.* °***Kal.*** Lach. Lyc. Magn. c. Magn. m. ***Merc.*** ****Mez.*** Phos. ac. ***Rhus.*** Samb. Squill. Sulph. ***Sulph. ac.*** Tab. Thuj. Zinc.

Stinging, ***Acon.*** Alum. *Anac.* Arg. Arn. Ars. ***Asa.*** Aur. ***Baryt.*** Bell. Berb. ***Bry.*** Cann. Caps. Caust. ***Cin. Cocc.*** Con. ***Dig. Hep. Hyos.*** Ign. ***Lach. Lyc.*** Magn. art. Magn. arct. Magn. aust. Magn. c. Men. ***Merc. Mez.*** Mur.

ac. Natr. s. Nicc. *N. vom.* Phell. Phosph. ***Phos. ac.*** Plat. ***Puls. Ran. Ran. sc. Rhus.*** Sabad. Selen. ***Sep. Sil.*** Spig. ***Spong.*** Squill. *Stann. Staph. Sulph. Sulph. ac. Thuj. Viol. tr.*

Swelling, Acon. Ant. °*Arn.* **Ars.* Asa. °Baryt. ****Bell.*** **Bry. Calc.* ***Carb. an. Carb. veg. Caust.*** °*Cham. Chin. Cocc.* Colch. Coloc. Con. Crotal. ***Dulc.*** *Euphorb.* Hell. ***Hep. Hyos.*** Jod. ***Kal. Lach. Led.*** **Lyc.* Mang. ****Merc. Mez.*** Natr. Natr. m. Nicc. ***Nitr. ac.*** *N. vom.* ***Op.*** **Petr.* **Phosph. Phos. ac.* °*Puls.* ****Rhus.*** Samb. Sec. Seneg. ****Sep.*** °*Sil. Spig.* Spong. Stann. ****Sulph.*** Vip. torv.

Tumors, Lach. Sassap.

Ulcers, Amb. **Ars.* Asa. Aur. Baryt. ***Bell.*** Bov. Bry. Calc. Carb. an. **Carb. veg.* Caust. ***Cham. Chin.*** Clem. Con. Dros. Graph. ***Hep.*** Ign. Kal. Lach. °*Lyc.* Mang. **Merc.* **Mez.* Mur. ac. ***Natr.*** Natr. m. Nitr. ac. N. vom. ***Phosph.*** Phos. ac. Plumb. **Puls.* ***Ran.*** ****Rhus.*** Ruta. Sassap. Sec. Selen. Sep. **Sil.* ***Staph.*** Stront. °*Sulph.* Sulph. ac. Thuj. Zinc.

Warts, Nitr. ac.

—, Ars. Lyc. °*Petr.* ***Phosph.*** °*Rhus.* Sep. Sulph. Thuj.

Head, eruptions, Ars. Baryt. Nitr. ac.

Ears, eruptions, Mosch. Puls. Sassap.

—, herpes, Merc.

—, swelling, Natr. m. Phos. ac.

—, scurfs, Merc.

Face, ***Amm.*** Ant. **Ars.* Asa. Aur. Bell. Bry. Calc. Canth. Caust. Cic. Cin. Crotal. Dig.

Euphr. Kal. Kal. chl. Kal. hdr. Led. Merc. Natr. Nitr. ac. Ratanh. Rhus. Samb. Sassap. Seneg. Senn. Teucr.

Lips, eruptions, &c., Amm. Aur. Bell. Bov. Bry. Caust. Chin. Graph. Magn. m. Mur. ac. Nicc. Phell. Plat. Ratanh. Seneg. Senn. *Staph.* Sulph.

Chin, Bell. Canth. Hep. Rhus.

Buccal cavity, eruptions, Amb. Amm. Amm. m. Arg. ***Baryt.*** Bry. Calc. ***Caps.*** Carb. an. Graph. Kal. hdr. Magn. c. Merc. Mez. Mur. ac. Natr. m. Natr. s. Nitr. ac. Phosph. ***Spig.*** Spong. ***Sulph.***

—, swelling, *Bell. °Cham. Lach. Sil.

—, ulcers, ***Merc.*** Natr. N. vom. Sep.

Anus, varices, Alum. Ant. Ars. Berb. **Calc.* Carb. an. Caust. Graph. Kal. Nitr. ac. N. vom. Phosph. Plat. Sulph ac.

Sexual parts, eruptions, Calc. Kal. Nitr. ac. Phosph.

—, ulcers, Hep.

Chest, eruptions, Heracl. Mez.

—, pimples, Staph.

—, herpes, Staph.

—, spots, Amm. m. °Ipec. °Mez.

Dorsal region, eruptions, Cinn.

—, blotches, Lach.

—, pimples, Cinn. Lyc. Magn. aust. Phosph. Ratanh. Squill.

—, spots, Thuj.

—, swelling, °Baryt. Phosph.

Arms, eruptions, pimples, vesicles, &c., Alum. Berb. Canth. Dulc. ***Laur.*** Magn. arct. Merc.

Mur. ac. Natr. s. Phosph. Sabad. Sep. Staph. *Sulph.*

Arms, herpes, °***Con.***
—, swelling, Rhus. *Sulph.*
—, scurf, Amm. m.
—, erysipelas, Petr.
Hands, eruptions, itching, &c., **Agar.* Amm. m. Berb. Carb. an. Cic. Gran. Graph. Jod. ***Laur.*** Lyc. Magn. arct. Magn. m. Merc. Natr. m. Natr. s. Nitr. ac. N. vom. Oleand. Plumb. Rhus. Sassap. Sil. Spig. *Stront.* Sulph.
—, blisters, phagedænic, Graph. Sil.
—, swelling, Oleand. Vip. torv.
—, ulcers, °*Ars.* Ran.
—, erysipelas, Rhod.
Lower limbs, eruptions, Aur. Mang. N. vom.
—, vesicles, Sabad.
—, pimples, Arg. Phos. ac. Puls. Staph. Thuj.
—, spots, Amm. *Chel.* Magn. c. ***Rhus.*** Sulph. ac.
—, rash, N. vom.
—, swelling, ***Crotal.***
—, ulcers, **Ars. Lyc.*
—, streaks, ***Rhus.***
Feet, spots, **Ars.* Lach.
—, swelling, Caust. Con. Kal. Merc. Nitr. ac. Petr. Phos. ac. **Puls.*
—, ulcers, Caust.

Burnt, Pain as if.

In general, °***Acon.*** Agar.? °*Alum.* Amb.? °***Ant.*** °*Ars.* ***Baryt. Bell. Bry.*** Calc.? Cann. °***Carb. veg.*** **Caust.* Chin. Cycl.? ***Euphorb.?*** Ferr. Hyos. ***Ign.*** Kal. Lach.? ***Magn. m.*** Merc.

Natr. *N. vom.* Op. Par. Phosph. Plat. ***Puls.*** Ruta. Sabad. ****Sec.*** Sep. Stram. ****Sulph. ac.*** Thuj. °*Urtic.* Veratr.
Head, Lach.
Lower limbs, tibia, Lach.
Feet, Amm. Zinc.

Callosities.

In general, Amm. *Ant. Borax. **Graph.* Lach. ***Phosph.*** Ran. Rhus. Rhus v. Sep. Sil. Sulph.
Horny, **Ant.* °Graph.
Red, *Sabad.*

Face, Rhus v.
Chest, Rhus v.
Dorsal region, neck, Rhus v.
Arms, Sabad.
Hands, °*Graph.*
Lower limbs, °*Lach.* ***Phosph.***
Feet, Lyc.
—, soles. °*Sil.*

Cancer.

In general. °Bell. ? Chinin. ? *Clem. ? °Con. °Hep. °Lach. Squill.

Nose, °*Ars.* °Aur. ? °Carb. an. ? °Sep. ? °***Sulph.***
Lips and mouth, region of, **Ars.* °Bell. ? °Clem.? °Con. °Sil. °*Sulph.*

Cancerous.

Ulcers, °***Amb.*** Ant. °*Ars.* °*Aur.* °***Bell.*** °*Calc.*

Carb. an. ***Carb. veg.*** Caust. °Chel. °Chinin. °*Clem.* ***Con.*** °***Hep.*** Kreas. °***Lac.*** °***Merc.*** Nitr. ac. Rhus. °*Sep.* °***Sil.*** °***Squil.*** Staph. °***Sulph.*** Thuj.

Face, ulcers, °***Ars.***
Mammæ and nipples, ulcers, °Bell. °Clem. ? °Con. ? °***Hep.*** °***Lach.*** °Sil. ? °Sulph. ?

Canthi.

Bluish colour, Aur. Sassap.
Burning, ***Agar.*** Alum. ***Amm. m.*** Ang. Asar. °*Aur.* Baryt. Bell. ***Calc.*** Carb. an. Carb. veg. Chel. Cin. Clem. Coloc. Graph. Hell. Kal. Laur. Magn. c. Natr. m. Nitr. N. vom. ***Par.*** °***Phosph.*** ***Phos. ac.*** Ran. Rhod. Sep. Squill. Stann. Staph. *Stront.* ***Sulph.*** Tarax. Tart. Thuj.
Emphysema, Natr. m.
Fistulous ulcer, (lachrymal gland,) °Bry. ? °*Calc.* °Natr. °Petr. ? °Phosph. °*Puls.* ? °Sil. °Stann. ?
Herpes, Tax.
Inflammation, *Acon.* Agar. Alum. Ars. Bell. *Calc.* Cham. Clem. °***Euphr.*** Ign. Merc. ***Petr.*** Phosph. Puls.
Itching, Alum. Ant. Arg. Arn. ***Bell.*** Berb. Borax. Bruc. Bry. *Calc.* Carb. veg. *Caust.* Cin. ***Con.*** Crotal. Euphorb. Ferr. magn. Hell. Hyos. Ign. Jod. Lam. Laur. Led. ***Lyc.*** ***Magn. art.*** ***Magn. c.*** Magn. m. Mur. ac. ***Natr. m.*** Nitr. ac. N. vom. Phell. Prun. ***Puls.*** Rhus. ***Ruta.*** Sep. Squill. *Staph.* *Stront.* Sulph. Tax. Tong.

Livid colour, Plumb.
Pus, Cham. Chin. Graph. N. vom. Puls. Staph.
Pustule at the puncta lachrymalia, Bry. Natr. ***Puls.*** Stann.
Redness, °***Ars.*** °*Aur.* Bell. Bism. Bov. Bruc. Bry. Calc. Eugen. Grat. ***Magn. c.*** Nitr. ac. Ran. Rhus. ****Sulph.*** Teucr. Val. Zinc.
Smarting, ***Ant.*** Bry. Camph. Carb. an. ***Carb. veg.*** Colch. ***Con.*** Graph. Hell. Ign. Kal. Lact. Magn. aust. Magn. c. Mang. Mez. Mosch. Mur. ac. Nicc. Nitr. ***N. vom.*** Ol. an. ***Ran. Ran. sc.*** Rhus. Ruta. ***Sep.*** Sil. °***Staph.*** Sulph. Tart. Teucr. Zinc.
Styes, Natr. m. Stann. Sulph.
Swelling, Agar. Aur. Bry. Bell. ****Calc.*** °Chel. ? Merc. Petr. Ran. °Ruta. ? Sassap. Sil. Stann.
Ulceration, Calc. Phos.

Cataract.

Eyes, °Amm. Cann. °Dig. °Magn. c. °Phosph. °***Puls.*** °Sil. °***Sulph.***

Cerumen.

Blood-red, Con.
Decayed paper, like, Con.
Fluid, Amm. m. ***Con.*** Jod. ***Kal.*** Lach. ***Merc.*** Mosch. Selen. ***Sil.***
Hard, Lach. Selen.
Deficient, °***Calc.*** °***Carb. veg.*** °***Galv.***
Flour-pap, like, Lach.
Increased, Agar. Amm. m. Calc. ***Con.*** Hep. Selen. Sep. Sil. Thuj. Zinc. ox.
Purulent, Sep.
Yellow, Kal. Lach.

Chancre and the like.

Mouth, ulcers, °Lach. **Lyc.* **Merc.* °*Nitr. ac.* °*Thuj.*

Sexual organs, ulcers, Hep. **Merc.* *Nitr. ac. °*Sep.* °Thuj.

Chilblains.

In general, Amb. *Ant.* °*Arn.* **Ars.* **Bell.* °*Bry.* **Carb. an.* °*Carb. veg.* Cham. Chin. *Croc.* °*Cycl.* °Gran. ? *Hep.* °*Hyos.* *Kal.* **Lyc.* *Magn. aust.* **Nitr. ac.* N. mosch. **N. vom.* **Petr.* °*Phosph.* °*Phos. ac.* **Puls.* **Rhus.* Stann. **Sulph.* °*Sulph. ac.* **Thuj.* Zinc.

—, sensation as of (itching, burning, redness,) *Agar.* Asar. Aur. Berb. Borax. Cocc. *Colch.* Magn. arct. Magn. c. Op. Rhab. Ruta. *Sep.* Spig. Staph.

Blue-red, Arn. Bell. Kal. °*Puls.*

Burning, **N. vom.* °*Puls.* Spig.

Cracked, °N. vom. °*Petr.*

Inflamed, °Ars. Bell. Cham. Hep. Lyc. °*Nitr. ac.* Phosph. °*Puls.* Rhus. Staph. °*Sulph.*

Itching, *Agar.* Asar. Aur. *Berb.* Borax. Cocc. *Colch.* Croc. **Lyc.* Magn. arct. **Nitr. ac.* °*N. vom.* Spig. **Sulph.*

Red, and redness as of, *Agar.* Amb. *Ant.* °*Arn.* **Ars.* Asar. Aur. **Bell.* *Berb.* Borax. °*Bry.* **Carb. an.* °Carb. veg. *Cham.* Chin. Cocc. *Colch.* Croc. °*Cycl.* *Hep.* °*Hyos.* Kal. *Lyc.* Magn. arct. Magn. aust. **Nitr. ac.* N. mosch. **N. vom.* Op. **Petr.* °*Phosph.* °*Phos. ac.* **Puls.*

Rhab. *Rhus. Ruta. Sep. Spig. Stann. *Staph.* **Sulph.* °*Sulph. ac.* **Thuj.* Zinc.

Painful, Arn. Bell. Chin. Hep. Lyc. Magn. c. °*Nitr. ac.* N. vom. °*Petr.* Phosph. Phos. ac. °*Puls.* Sep.

Stinging, Magn. aust.

Titillating, Arn. *Colch. Magn. aust.* N. vom. °*Rhus.* Sep.

Hands, Nitr. ac. *Stann. Zinc.*

—. fingers, Carb. an. *Lyc.* °*Petr.* °*Puls.* **Sulph.* Sulph. ac.

Feet and toes, *Agar. *Ant.* Hep. Kal. *Nitr. ac.* **N. vom. Phosph.* Rhus. °*Sulph.* °*Thuj.*

CHILBLAINS LIKE, ITCHING AS OF CHILBLAINS, OR AS IF FROZEN.

Ears, Agar. Colch.

Nose, Zinc.

Hands, itching and redness, **Agar. Berb.* Borax. *Lyc.* Magn. arct. **N. vom.* Spig. **Sulph.*

Feet and toes, itching, redness and pain, **Agar. Alum. Amm.* Asar. Berb. Borax. Bry. Cann. Carb. an. Carb. veg. Caust. Chin. *Cocc. Colch. Kal. Lach.* Lyc. Magn. aust. *Nitr. ac. N. mosch.* **N. vom.* Petr. Phosph. **Puls.* Rhab. *Sabin. Staph. Zinc.*

CHIN, REGION OF THE.

Aneurysm by anastomosis, Plat.

Blisters, vesicles, Hep. Natr. Sassap.

Blue-red, Plat.

Blotches, Bry. Carb. an. Euphorb. Hep. Magn. m. Oleand.

Boils, Hep. Nitr. ac. Sil.

Burning, Anac. Ant. Berb. Bov. Canth. Caust. Magn. c. Mang. Merc. Ol. an. Rhus. Spig. Spong.

Burns, that which, Bell. Canth. Hep. Rhus.

Cutting, Caust. Rhus. Stann.

Eruptions, Agn. Alum. Amb. Amm. Anac. Ant. Bell. Borax. *Bov. Calc. Canth. Caust. *Chel.* Cic. Clem. Con. Dig. Dulc. **Graph. Hep.* Hyos. Kal. °*Lach. Lyc.* Magn. arct. Magn. aust. Magn. c. Merc. Mez. Natr. Natr. m. Nitr. ac. N. mosch. N. vom. Oleand. *Par.* Phosph. Phos. ac. Plat. Puls. **Rhus.* Sabin. Sassap. Sep. **Sil.* Spig. Spong. Squill. Stront. Sulph. Tarax. Thuj. *Veratr.* Verb. Zinc.

Granular, Ant.

Hardness, hard, Staph.

Herpes, Bov. Chel. Natr. m. N. vom. °*Sil.*

Itching, Alum. Amm. Berb. Calc. Con. Dig. Grat. Hydroc. *Kal.* Laur. *Lyc.* Magn. aust. Magn. c. Meph. Natr. Natr. m. Oleand. Ol. an. Op. Phosph. Plat. Sassap. Spig. Squill. *Stront.* Sulph. Tarax. Thuj. *Zinc.*

—, of eruptions, Bell. Dulc. Lyc. Natr. Natr. m. N. vom. Par. Sassap. Sep. Thuj. Zinc.

Inflammation, Caust.

Painfulness, Mang. N. mosch.

Pain as if ulcerated, Euphorb. Mang. Spong.

Pimples, Alum. Amb. Anac. Ant. Bell. Berb. Calc. Canth. Caust. Cic. Clem. Con. Dros. Dulc. Hep. Hyos. Laur. Lyc. Magn. art. Magn. aust. Natr. Natr. s. Nitr. ac. N. mosch.

N. vom. Oleand. Par. Rhus. Sabin. Sassap. Sep, Sil. Spig. Spong. Sulph. Thuj. Veratr. Verb. Zinc.
Pock-shaped, Hyos.
Pustules, Bell. Canth. Caust. Graph. Mang. Merc. Nitr. ac. N. mosch. Oleand. Rhus, Sabin. Sassap. *Zinc.*
Red skin, Canth. Gins. Zinc.
Red, that which is, Natr. Natr. m.
Scurfs, Sep.
As after shaving, Mang.
Smarting, Stront.
Smarting as if excoriated, Veratr.
Sore, Ant. Hep. Magn. aust. Mang. Veratr.
Spots, Natr. m. Sep. °*Sil.*
Stinging, Bell. Canth. Sil. Stann.
Suppuration, Anac.
Swelling, Carb. veg. Caust. Rhus. Spig. Staph.
Tensive, that which is, Natr. s. Plat. Verb.
Ulcers, Hep. Merc.
Ulceration, Natr. m. Sabin. Sep.

Choky sensation.

Glands, Amm. *Chin.* Ign. Magn. arct. N. vom. Plumb. *Puls. Spong.*

Cicatrices of old Ulcers and Wounds.

In general, affections of, Carb. veg. Crotal. Graph. Jod. **Lach.* Natr. m. °*Nitr. ac.* °N. vom. Oph. *Phosph. Sil.* Vip. torv.
—, cicatrized skin, *Sabin.*
Breaking again, Carb. veg. *Crotal.* **Lach.* Sil.
Bleeding, Lach. Oph. Phosph.

Brown, Lach.
Burning, Ars. Carb. veg. Graph. Lach.
Thin-skinned, Oph.
Red, Lach. **Merc.* Natr. m.
Painful, Carb. veg. Lach. Natr. m. °*Nitr. ac.* °*N. vom.*
—, during change of weather, Carb. veg. °*Nitr. ac.*
Sore, °N. vom.
Contractive-painful, Phosph.

Eyes, °*Euphr.* °*Sil.*
Lower limbs, cicatrized skin, Sabin.

Claret-red.

Spots, **Cocc.* **Sep.*
Dorsal region, Sep.

Close together, that which is.

Eruption, *Agar. Sep. Squill. Thuj.
Blisters, vesicles, Ran. Rhus. Veratr.
Pimples, Cham. Veratr.
Spots, Calc.

Face, pimples, Sep.
Dorsal region, eruptions, Squill. Thuj.
Hands, eruption, Rhus.

Clustered, grouped.

Blisters, vesicles, Rhus. v. Sulph.

Face, pimples and eruptions, Sep. Sulph.

Comedones.

Excrescences, Aur. Bry. Calc. Graph. °*Natr.* Natr. m. Nitr. ac. Plumb. Sabin. **Selen.* Sulph.

Face, Sabin. °Selen.

Conditions of Appearance, or Aggravation of the cutaneous Symptoms.

In the afternoon, Ant. Chel. Coloc. Laur. Magn. c. Natr. Rhus. Val.

In bed, Alum. Anac. Ang. Ant. Baryt. Bell. Bry. Calc. Camph. Carb. an. *Carb. veg.* Caust. Chin. Clem. Cocc. Coloc. Con. Cycl. Daph. Ign. Ipec. Kal. Kal. chl. Lam. Lyc. Magn. art. Magn. arct. **Magn. aust.* Magn. c. Magn. m. Merc. Mez. Mur. ac. Natr. m. **N. vom.* Phos. ac. *Plat.* Puls. Sassap. Seneg. Sep. Sil. Stann. Staph. Stram. Stront. Sulph. Tart. Teucr. *Zinc.*

—, improved in bed, Amm. m. Bry. Caust.

After abuse of Belladonna, °*Hep.* °Hyos.

From burns, s. Injuries.

During change of weather, Bry. Calc. *Carb. veg.* Colch. *Dulc.* Graph. Mang. Merc. °*Nitr. ac.* *Phosph.* Rhod. **Rhus.* Sil. Sulph. Verat.

In children, °*Acon.* Amm. °*Baryt.* °*Bell.* °Bry. °Carb. an. °*Carb. veg.* °*Calc.* Caust. °*Cham.* °*Chin.* Crotal. °*Graph.* °*Hep.* °*Ipec.* °Lach. °*Lyc.* °*Merc.* °N. vom. °*Puls.* °*Rhus.* °Ruta. °*Sep.* °*Sulph.* °Tart. °Viol. tr.

In cold air, **Daph.* °Nitr. ac. Phos. ac. Sassap.

When feeling cold, Spong.

During contact, Ant. Ars. Asa. **Bell.* Camph. Canth. Caust. Cham. *Chin.* Chinin. Clem. Cocc. Dig. Ferr. Graph. **Hep.* Kal. Lach. Magn. c. **Merc.* Mez. Natr. Nitr. ac. N. vom. Par. Phos. ac. Puls. °*Rhus.* Sassap. Seneg. Sep. Sil. Spig. Tab. Thuj. Vip. torv. Zinc.

—, improvement, Bry. Thuj. Zinc.

From contusion, s. INJURIES.

When coughing, Bell. Con. Lach. Lact. Puls.

After dancing, Borax.

In drunkards, Ant. Ars. *Calc. Carb. veg. Kreas.* Lach. °*Led.* N. vom. Rhus. Ruta. Veratr.

While dressing, N. vom.

After eating. Bry. Puls.

After emotions, Bry.

In the evening, Agn. *Alum.* **Amm. m.* Ang. *Ant. Ars.* Baryt. Bov. Bry. Camph. Cham. Chin. Cin. Clem. *Cocc. Coloc.* Con. Crotal. °*Cycl.* °*Daph.* Diad. Ferr. magn. Graph. °*Ign.* Ipec. *Kal.* Kreas. Laur. *Led.* Magn. arct. °*Magn. aust.* Magn. c. Magn. m. Mang. *Merc.* Merc. corr. Mez. Mur. ac. Natr. Nicc. Nitr. **N. vom.* Oleand. Op. Petr. Phosph. *Phos. ac. Plat.* Plumb. **Puls.* °*Ran.* °*Ran. sc.* °*Rhus.* Sabad. Sassap. Seneg. Sep. Sil. **Staph.* Stram. Stront. Sulph. Tab. Tarax. Thuj. *Zinc.*

In the evening, in bed, Alum. Anac. Bell. Bry. Calc. Carb. an. Carb. veg. Clem. Coloc. Con. *Cycl.* °Daph. **Ign.* Ipec. Kal. Kal. chl. Lyc. Magn. art. Magn. arct. *Magn. aust.* Mez. Natr.

m. *N. vom. Phos. ac. *Puls.* Sassap. Seneg. Sep. Stront. Sulph. Tarax. Tart. Zinc.

After a fall, s. INJURIES.

In the forenoon, Cycl. Lach.

When heated, Bry. Ign. °*Lyc.* Mang. Puls. Sabad.

While laughing, Bry. Hep.

While lying, Lam. Magn. arct. **Merc.*

On the side on which one is lying, Carb. veg. Chin. Con.

Improved after lying down, Amm. m. Nicc.

In lying-in females, °*Acon.* Ant. °*Arn.* °*Bell.* °*Bry.* °*Calc.* Carb. an. **Cham.* Chin. Con. Ferr. Hyos. **Ign.* **Ipec.* Kal. °*Natr. m.* °N. vom. °*Phosph.* °*Puls.* °*Rhus.* °*Sep.* °*Sulph.*

During decline of moon, *Dulc.*

—, new moon, Alum. *Amm.* Calc. *Caust. Cupr.* Lyc. Sabad. Sep. Sil.

—, full moon, *Alum. Calc. Cycl. Graph. Natr.* Sabad. **Sil.* Spong. °*Sulph.*

—, increase of moon, *Alum. Clem.* °*Daph.*

From abuse of mercury, s. MERCURIAL.

—, before midnight, Bry. °*Puls.*

—, after midnight, *Dulc.* Sabad. Sabin. Spong.

Early in the morning, Amb. Amm. Amm. m. Ant. Ars. Bov. Bry. Clem. Coloc. Cupr. Cycl. Daph. Hell. *Hep. Kal.* Kal. chl. Lach. Lam. Lyc. Magn. arct. Magn. aust. Magn. c. Magn. m. Mang. Merc. Merc. corr. N. vom. Petr. Puls. Rhus. Rhus v. Ruta. Sassap. Sep. Sil. *Spong.* Stann. *Staph.* Stram. Sulph. Teucr. Kal. Mang. Nicc.

During motion, Chin. Con. Graph. Hyos. Lach. Led. Nitr.

During motion, improved, Bry. Dros. Sil.
At night, **Amm. m.* Anthrok. Ant. Ars. Asa. *Baryt.* Bell. Bry. Calad. Cann. Carb. veg. Caust. *Cham.* Cin. *Cocc.* Con. *Dig. Dulc.* Euphr. Graph. Hep. Ign. Kal. Kal. chl. Kreas. Lyc. Magn. m. Mang. **Merc.* °*Mez.* N. vom. *Phosph.* Prun. **Puls.* Rhus. Rhus v. Sep. Sil. **Sulph.* *Thuj.* * *Veratr.* *Viol. tr.* *Zinc.*
At noon, Arn. Magn. arct.
In the open air, Graph. Ign. Rhus. Sulph.
—, improved, Calc.
From poison of glanders, °*Ars.* °Carb. veg. °Sil.
From poison of glanders, °*Ars.* Bell.? Calc.? *Merc.* °*Phos. ac.* Sil. Sulph.
In putrid fever, °*Ars.* °*Bry.* °*Rhus.*
In a recumbent posture, **Ign.*
During rest, Dros. Graph.
From riding on horseback, Ars. *Carb. veg.* Graph. °*Ruta.* °*Sulph. ac.*
After scratching, s. SCRATCHING.
After shaving, **Carb. an.*
From stings of insects, Ant. °*Bell.* °*Calad.*
While sitting, Chel. Crotal. Cycl. Lach. **Merc.*
From splinters, s. INJURIES.
In summer, °*Ant.* Baryt. Bell. Bry. **Calc. Carb. veg.* Cham. *Con. Dros.* °*Dulc.* °*Graph.* Hyos. Jod. *Kal.* Lach. Laur. **Lyc. Merc.* Mez. Natr. Nitr. ac. *N. mosch. Petr.* **Phosph.* Plumb. °*Puls.* °*Sep. Sil.* Stann. **Sulph.* Tart. Thuj.
From heat of sun, Acon. *Bell.* Camph. Clem. *Hyos. Sil.* Sulph.
During sweat, Camph. Led. Op. Par. Sabad.
—, after sweat, Bry. Op.
From uncleanliness, *Caps.* Chin. Puls. *Sulph.*

While undressing, Amm. m. °*Cocc.* Magn. c. Mez. N. vom. Oleand. °*Puls.* °*Rhus.* Sil. Stann.

On waking, Amb. Coloc. Magn. arct. Magn. aust. Rhus. Spong. Sulph.

While walking, Ign. **Merc.* Puls. Rhus. °*Ruta.* Sulph.

—, improved, Staph.

In warmth, Caust. Chin. Cocc. N. vom. Puls. Sassap. Sep. Stram. °*Sulph.* Teucr. Veratr.

While getting warm, Bov. Bry. Dros. Dulc. Ign. Led. Lyc. Magn. arct. Mang. Merc. Nitr. ac. Petr. Puls. Sabad. Sec. Seneg. Sil. Spig. Staph. Sulph. Veratr.

—, in bed, Alum. Ant. Bov. Calc. Calad. Cann. Carb. veg. Caust. Cham. Chin. Clem. *Cocc.* Dros. Graph. Jod. Kal. Led. Lyc. Magn. arct. Merc. Natr. m. °N. vom. Phosph. Phos. ac. °*Puls.* Rhus. Sabin. Sassap. Sec. Seneg. Spong. **Sulph.* Thuj. Veratr.

In wet weather, **Amm.* Ant. Aur. Borax. **Calc.* *Carb. an.* **Carb. veg.* Cham. *Chin.* Clem. Cupr. **Dulc.* Ferr. Hep. **Lach.* Laur. *Lyc.* Magn. c. **Mang.* **Merc.* Mur. ac. Natr. Nitr. ac. Petr. **Puls.* **Rhod.* **Rhus.* °*Ruta.* °*Sassap.* Seneg. Sep. Spig. Staph. *Stront.* **Sulph.* Sulph. ac. **Veratr.* Zinc.

After working in water, washing, &c., **Amm.* Amm. m. **Ant.* *Bell.* Borax. Bov. Bry. **Calc.* *Canth.* **Carb. veg.* Caust. *Cham.* **Clem.* Con. °*Dulc.* Kal. Lyc. Magn. c. **Merc.* Mez. Nitr. **Nitr. ac.* N. mosch. Phosph. **Puls.* °*Rhus.* Sassap. **Sep.* Sil. Spig. Staph. Stront. **Sulph.* Sulph. ac. Zinc.

Confluent.

Eruption, Agar. Ant. **Cic.* Hyos. Phos. ac. Val.
Blisters, vesicles, Alum. Phell. Rhus.
Pimples, Mur. ac. Phos. ac.
Pustules, **Cic.* *°Merc.* Tart.
Spots, *°Bell.* *°Cic.* *Hyos.* Phos. ac. *Val.*
Ulcers, Tart.

Face, Alum, *Cic.
Hands, eruptions, Cic.
Lower limbs, eruptions, Phos. ac.

Contracting Sensation.

In general, Acon. Alum. Amm. *Anac.* *Asar.* Bell. *Bism.* Bry. *Carb. veg.* **Chin.* Chinin. Cocc. Cupr. Ferr. *Graph.* Kal. Kreas. *Lyc.* Merc. Natr. *Natr. m.* Nitr. ac.. **N. vom.* Oleand. Par. Petr. Phosph. *Plat.* Plumb. Puls. *Ran.* *Ran. sc.* Rhod. **Rhus.* Ruta. Sabad. *°Selen.* Sep. Sil. Spig. *Stann.* *Stront.* **Sulph.* Sulph. ac. Zinc.

Scalp, *Carb. veg.* **Chin.* *Lyc.* Natr. m. Par. Plat. Rhus. Stann.
Eyebrows, skin of, Bry. Hell.
Glands, *Acon.* Alum. Arn. *Bell.* *Borax.* *Chin.* Cocc. Con. *Ign.* Jod. Lyc. *Mang.* *Nitr. ac.* N. vom. Phosph. *Plumb.* *Puls.* *Rhus.* Sep. *Sulph.* Sulph. ac.

Contraction of Muscles.

In general, **Amm.* **Amm. m.* Baryt. *°Caust.*

**Coloc.* Graph. °*Lach.* Lyc. °*Natr.* °*Natr. m.* N. vom. Puls. Rhus. Sep. °*Sulph.* Vip. torv.

Contraction, sensation of, *Amb.* **Amm.* **Amm. m.* Anac. *Ang. Arn. Ars. Aur. Baryt.* Bov. **Bry.* Calc. *Carb. an. Carb. veg.* **Caust.* Cic. **Coloc. Con.* Croc. Dig. Dros. *Euphorb.* Euphr. **Graph.* **Guaj. Hell.* Hep. Hyos. *Ign.* Kal. **Lach.* Led. *Lyc.* Magn. art. *Magn. c. Mez.* Mosch. **Natr.* **Natr. m.* Nitr. ac. **N. vom.* Petr. *Phosph.* Plumb. **Puls.* Ran. Rhab. **Rhus.* Sabin. Samb. **Sep.* Sil. Spig. Stann. **Sulph.* Sulph. ac. Veratr.

Arms, Bell.

—, elbows, Caust. Sassap. Sulph.

Hands, fingers, **Caust. Sulph.*

Lower limbs, Amm. m. °*Caust.* °*Graph.* °*Natr. m.* °*Ruta.*

—, contraction, sensation of, *Berb.* Carb. an. Magn. m. Merc.

—, hip, °*Lach.* Prun.

—, thigh, Amm. *Kreas. Lach.* N. vom. *Sabin. Spong.*

—, knee, Amm. m. *Graph.* °*Lach.* **Lyc.* Magn. arct. Magn. c. °*Natr. m.* Nitr. ac. N. vom. Ol. an. Phosph. Rhus. °*Ruta.* Samb. *Sulph. Veratr.*

—, calves, Caust. *Kal. Magn. art.* Natr. Natr. m. Rhus. *Sil.*

Feet, **Caust.* Plumb. Vip. torv.

—, sensation of contraction, Berb. *Carb. an.* In. dig. *Sep. Spig.* Sulph.

Feet, tarsal joints, *Carb. an.* **Caust.* Plumb. *Sep. Spig.* Vip. torv.
—, soles, Berb. Indig. *Spig.* Sulph.

Contraction of Skin.

Head, Carb. an.

Copper-coloured.

Eruption, Alum. °*Ars.* Calc. Cann. °*Carb. an.* Carb. veg. Corall. °Kreas. Led. *Mez.* Phosph. °*Rhus.* °Ruta. °*Veratr.*
Spots, Corall. °*Nitr. ac.* Phosph.

Hands, spots, °*Nitr.* ac.
Face, °Ars. Calc. Calc. ph. Cann. *Carb. an.* Carb. veg. °Kreas. °*Rhus.* °*Ruta.* °*Veratr.*

Corns, Pain as of Corns.

In general, Agar. *Alum.* Amb. °*Amm.* **Ant.* °*Arn.* Baryt. Borax. *Bov.* Bruc. Bry. **Calc.* Camph. *Carb. an.* Carb. veg. Caust. Chen. Cocc. Con. *Gran.* Graph. Hep. *Ign.* Jod. Kal. Lach. **Lyc.* Magn. art. *Magn. arct.* Magn. aust. Magn. m. *Meph. Natr. Natr. m.* Nitr. **Nitr. ac. N. vom. Petr. Phosph.* Phos. ac. Puls. Ran. Ran. sc. *Rhod.* Rhus. Ruta. **Sep.* **Sil.* Spig. Staph. **Sulph.* Sulph. ac. Thuj. Veratr.
Aching, Anac. **Ant.* Bry. Calc. Caust. Graph. Ign. °*Lyc.* Magn. arct. Magn. aust. Phosph. Phos. ac. **Sep.* °*Sil.* Staph. °*Sulph.*
Boring, *Borax.* Calc. *Caust.* Hep. Kal. *Natr.*

Natr. m. *Phosph.* Puls. °*Ran. sc.* Rhod. °*Sep.* °*Sil.* Spig. Thuj.

Burning, Alum. Amm. Bruc. **Bry.* Calc. Carb. veg. Caust. Chen. Graph. Hep. Ign. Kal. Lyc. Magn. art. Meph. Petr. Phosph. Phos. ac. Puls. Ran. sc. Rhus. **Sep.* Sil. Sil. Spig. **Sulph.* Thuj.

Horny, *Ant. Graph. Ran. Sulph.

Inflamed, Borax.? Calc.? Hep.? °*Lyc.* °*Puls.* °*Rhus.* **Sep.* °*Sil.* Staph.? **Sulph.*

Jerks in the corns, Cocc. °*Magn. arct.* Sep. °*Sulph.* °*Sulph. ac.*

Pain as if ulcerated, °*Amm.* °*Borax.* N. vom.

Painful, sensitive, Agar. Alum. Amm. **Ant.* °*Arn.* °*Baryt.* Bov. Bry. **Calc.* Camph. Carb. an. Carb. veg. Gran. Hep. **Ign.* Jod. Kal. *Lach. °*Lyc.* Magn. art. °*Magn. arct.* Magn. aust. Meph. Natr. Natr. m. **Nitr. ac.* °*N. vom.* Petr. Phosph. °*Puls.* Ran. Rhus. **Sep.* °*Sil.* Spig. °*Sulph.*

Stinging, Agar. *Alum.* Ant. Berb. Borax. Bov. **Bry.* °*Calc.* Carb. an. Carb. veg. Caust. Chen. Cocc. Graph. Hep. Ign. Kal. **Lyc.* °*Magn. arct.* Magn. m. *Natr. Natr. m.* Nitr. ac. *Petr.* Phosph. Phos. ac. °*Puls.* Ran. sc. *Rhod.* °*Rhus.* **Sep.* **Sil.*. **Sulph.* Sulph. ac. Thuj. Veratr.

Sore, Agar. Amb. Bry. Calc. Caust. Graph. °*Hep.* °*Ign. Lyc.* Magn. art. Magn. arct. Natr. m. Nitr. ac. Phosph.? Rhus. °*Sep.* °*Sil.* °*Sulph.* Veratr.

Tearing, °Arn. °Calc. *Cocc.* Ign. °*Lyc.* Magn. m. Rhus. °*Sil.* °*Sulph.* Sulph. ac. Thuj.

Corroded, as if, &c.

Ulcers, *Merc. Mercurial.*
Buccal cavity, Ars. Kal. Merc.

Covered Parts, on.

Eruption, Led. Thuj.

Cowpock-shaped.

Chest, eruption, Tart.
Dorsal region, eruption, Tart.

Cracked, that which cracks.

Vesicles, **Bry.* *Crotal.* *Lach.* Lam. Lupul. Nitr. Phosph. *Vip. torv.*
Pimples, Merc. ac.
Pustules, Rhus.
Chilblains, °N. vom. °*Petr.*
Swelling, Ars.

Buccal cavity, vesicles, Phosph.
Dorsal region, vesicles, Lach.
Hands, ridges, Graph.
Feet, vesicles, Lach. Lam. Selen.

Crampy-painful.

Blood-vessels, swelling of, Graph.

Crampy Sensation.

Bones, periosteum, Ang. Asa. *Aur.* Bell. Calc. *Euphr.* Ign. Lact. Mez. Petr. *Phos. ac.* Plat. Spig.

Glands, Amm. m. Anac. Ang. Bell. Bov. Calc. Carb. veg. Chin. Jod. Kal. Lyc. Magn. art. Magn. aust. Natr. Phos. ac. Plat. Sabad. Sep. Sil.

Crawling.

Head, Alum. Ant. Baryt. Ran. Rhus. Sil. Spig. Thuj.
Ears, Ratanh.
Dorsal region, axilla, Bry.
—, small of back, Alum. Tarax.
—, Back, Alum. Bov. Lach. Laur. Magn. s. *Natr.*
Arms, °*Bell.* °*Ign.* Lach.
Hands, Lach.
Lower limbs, Magn. art. *Sep.*
—, thighs, Berb.
—, knees, Ratanh.
—, legs, *Ol. an.* *Sep.* Tab. Zinc.
Feet, ankles, Bell.
—, heels, Par.
—, toes, Ars. Spig.
Glands, sensation of creeping in the, Bell. Calc. Laur. Sep. Spong. Sulph.

Creeping.

In general, Agn. Alum. Amm. *Arg.* Aur. Baryt. *Berb.* Borax. Bov. Calc. Cann. Caps. *Carb. veg.* *Caust.* Laur. *Led.* *Lyc.* Magn. aust. Magn. c. Magn. m. Mang. *Mur. ac.* *Natr.* Nitr. ac. N. vom. *Oleand.* *Phosph.* *Phos. ac.* *Plat.* *Ran.* Ran. sc. **Rhod.* **Rhus.* **Sabad.* *Sec.* *Sil.* *Spig.* *Spong.* **Staph.* **Sulph.* Zinc.

Ants, as of, s. FORMICATION.

Head, Alum. Cann. Chin. Kal. Kal. chl. Ran. Sil. Staph. Thuj.
Ears, Rhod.
Face, Magn. m.
Chest. Alum. Coloc. Magn. aust. Magn. m. Mang. Ran. sc.
Arms, Bell. Magn. aust.
—, forearms, Caust.
Hands, Arn.
Lower limbs, thighs, Berb. Natr.
—, knees, Merc.
Feet, Arn. Phosph.
—, soles, Magn. m.

CRUSTA LACTEA.

In general, °*Ars.* °Baryt.? Bell.? *Calc.?* Carb. veg.? *Cic.?* Dulc.? Lyc.? °*Merc.* Natr. m.? Phosph.? Phos. ac.? °*Rhus.* Sassap.? Sep.? °*Sulph.* Viol. tr.

CUTTING.

In the skin in general, **Bell.* **Calc.* Dros. Graph. Ign. Lyc. **Mur. ac.* **Natr.* Phos. ac. Rhus. Sep. Sil. Sulph. ac. **Viol. tr.*

Scalp, Clem.
Chin, Caust. Rhus. Stann.
Bones, Anac. Dig. Sabad.

Glands, Arg. Bell. Calc. Con. Graph. Ign. Lyc. Natr. Phos. ac. Sep. Sil. Staph. Sulph.

Cuts, which.

Bloodvessels, swelling of, Carb. an. Plat.
Eruption, Lyc.
Blisters, vesicles, Graph.
Pimples, Rhus.
Swelling, Kal. Stann.
Ulcers, **Bell.* °*Calc.* *Dros.* Graph. Ign. *Lyc.* Mur. ac. *Natr.* Phos. ac. Rhus. Sep.. *Sil.* Sulph. ac.

Lips, blisters, Graph. Lyc.
Feet, chilblains, Kal.

Dampness, Humour.

In general, Acon. Aloë. *Alum.* Amm. Ars. Baryt. Bell. °*Bov.* °*Bry.* *Calc.* *Carb. an.* *Carb. veg.* *Caust.* Chinin. *Cic.* *Clem.* *Con.* °*Dulc.* *Graph.* Grat. Hell. *Hep.* Heracl. *Kal.* °*Kreos.* *Lach.* *Led.* °*Lyc.* Magn. arct. °*Merc.* Natr. *Natr. m.* Nitr. *Nitr. ac.* *Oleand.* *Petr.* Phosph. °*Phos. ac.* Plumb. Raph. Ran. *Rhus.* *Ruta.* Sabin. *Selen.* °*Sep.* *Sil.* *Squill.* *Staph.* Sulph. Sulph. ac. Tab. Tarax. Thuj. *Viol. tr.* Vip. red. Vip. torv.

Ears, **Calc.* °*Lyc.*
—, behind the ears, Amm. **Calc.* Carb. veg. Caust. °*Graph.* Kal. °*Lyc.* Nitr. ac. °*Oleand.* °*Petr.* Phosph. Sil.
—, margins of ears, *Sil.*
Anus, Amm. Calc. Carb. an. *Carb. veg.* *Caust.*

Led. Natr. m. *Nitr. ac.* Rhod. Sil. Sulph. Zinc.

Sexual parts, Calc. *Cann.* Carb. veg. *Hep. Lyc.* Natr. m. Nitr. ac. **Petr. Sep. Staph.* °Sulph. **Thuj.*

—, glans, *Cann.* Cinn. *Lyc.* **Merc.* Mez. Natr. m. Nitr. ac. *Sep.* Staph. Thuj.

—, scrotum, Carb. veg. **Petr.* °Sulph.

—, pudendum and thighs, between, Calc. *Hep.*

—, mons veneris, Sulph.

—, prepuce, Nitr. ac.

Dorsal region, axilla, Carb. veg.

—, axillary glands, Sulph.

—, scapula, Lach.

—, os sacrum, Graph. Led.

Lower limbs, between thighs, *Hep.* °*Sulph.*

—, calves, Tarax.

Feet, Mez. Selen.

Darting, darting pain.

Bones, periosteum, Anac. **Asa.* Aur. Bell. °*Calc.* Caust. **Chin.* Clem. Colch. Lyc. Merc. *Natr. m.* N. vom. Petr. Phosph. °*Puls.* Rhod. Rhus. Sep. Sil. Sulph. ac. Val.

Nails, Calc. Caust. Graph. Magn. aust. Merc. Natr. m. N. vom. Puls. Rhus. Sil.

Glands, Arn. *Asa.* Aur. *Bell.* Bry. *Calc. Caps. Caust.* Chin. *Clem.* Graph. Lyc. Men. Merc. Natr. *Natr. m.* Nitr. ac. *N. vom.* Petr. *Puls. Rhus.* Sep. Sil. *Sulph.*

DARTING, PAINFUL, WHICH IS.

Eruption, Asa. Calc. *Caust.* Cham. Chin. Cupr. Lyc. *Puls. Rhus.* Sep. Sil. *Staph.* Vip. torv.
Ulcers, °*Asa.* Bell. °*Calc.* *Caust.* Cham. Chin. Cupr. Lyc. Merc. Natr. °*Natr. m.* Nitr. ac. N. vom. °*Puls.* °*Rhus.* Sep. °*Sil.* Staph. Sulph.
Scurfs, crusts, Staph.
Nails, Calc. Caust. Graph. Magn. aust. Merc. Natr. m. N. vom. Puls. Rhus. Sil.

Lower limbs, ulcers, Natr.

DEEP, WHICH IS.

Rhagades, Mang. Merc.
Blisters, vesicles, Lach.
Impressions (from instruments), Bov. Veratr.
Ulcers, *Ant.* Ars. *Asa. Aur.* °*Bell. Bov.* °*Calc. Carb. veg.* Caust. Chel. Clem. °*Con.* Dros. *Hep.* Kreas. **Lach.* °*Lyc.* **Merc. Mur. ac.* Natr. Natr. m. **Nitr. ac. Petr. Phos. ac.* °*Puls.* Rhus. Ruta. Sabin. Selen. *Sep.* °*Sil.* Staph. °*Sulph.* Thuj.

DIGGING UP, WHICH IS.

Ulcers, Asa. Bell. Bry. Calc. Caust. Chin. Natr. Phosph. Ruta. *Sep.* Stront. Sulph.
Erysipelas, Euphorb.

DIGGING UP SENSATION.

Bones, periosteum, Asa. Calc. *Carb. an. Cocc.*

Diad. Dulc. Mang. Natr. Rhod. *Ruta.* Sep. Spig. *Thuj.*
Glands, Acon. Amm. m. *Arn.* Asa. *Bell.* Bov. Bry. Calc. *Dulc.* Kal. Natr. *Phosph.* Plat. *Rhod. Rhus.* Ruta. Sep. *Spig.* Stann.

Discharges, Expectorations and Secretions of every kind, according to their quality.

Albuminous, Amm. m. Borax. Bov. Jatroph. Mez. Petr. Plat.
Of bad taste or smell, Cop. Dros. Puls.
Bitter, Arn. Ars. Carb. veg. Cist. Dros. *Merc.* Nitr. ac. Phos. ac. **Puls.*
Bluish, Amb. Ars. Cupr. ac.
Bloody, s. Hæmorrhage.
With bloody points, Amm. c. Laur.
With bloody mucus, °Acon. Alum. Amm. m. Ars. *Asar. Baryt.* **Bell. Canth.* Caps. *Carb. veg.* Caust. Chen. °*Chin.* Cocc. Con. Cop. Evon. Ferr. Graph. Hep. *Jod. Kal. Kal. chl. Led. Lyc. **Merc.* Mez. Murex. Natr. m. Nitr. N. mosch. **N. vom.* Op. Par. Petr. Phosph. **Puls. Sep. Sil.* Sulph. Sulph. ac. Thuj. Veratr. Vip. torv. Zinc.
Blood-streaked, **Ars.* Borax. **Chin.* °Daph. Ferr. Lach. Magn. c. Magn. m. Sabin. *Sep.*
Brownish, Amm. m. *Ars. **Bell.* Bism. Borax. Carb. veg. Grat. Nitr. ac. Sulph.
Burning, Alum. Amm. Amm. m. **Ars.* Calad. °*Calc.* °*Carb. an.* Cast. Chin. Cin. *Con. Kal. hdr.* Magn. art. Magn. s. Mez. Puls. **Sulph.* Sulph. ac.

Cheese, smelling like old, Calc. °*Hep.* Merc. Sulph.

Cheesy, Merc.

Like old catarrhal mucus, **Bell.*

Copious, Acon. *Alum.* **Amm.* *Arg.* *Ars.* *Asa.* Bry. *Calc.* Canth. Cast. Caust. Chin. Cic. °Daph. °Dulc. Ferr. **Graph.* *Guaj.* Jod. Kal. Kreas. °*Lach.* Laur. Lyc. Magn. m. Magn. s. Mang. **Merc.* *Mez.* Natr. **Natr. m.* Nicc. Nitr. ac. **Phosph.* Phos. ac. **Puls.* Ran. *Rhus.* Ruta. *Samb.* Sabin. °*Sassap.* **Sep.* *Sil.* Squill. Staph. **Sulph.* Thuj.

Corrosive, **Alum.* **Amm.* **Amm. m.* Anac. Ant. **Ars.* **Borax.* Bov. Calc. Cann. Canth. Carb. an. *Carb. veg.* *Cham.* Chin. *Con.* Euphorb. **Ferr.* Hep. *Ign.* *Jod.* Kal. Kal. hdr. *Kreas.* *Lach.* Lyc. Magn. arct. Magn. c. *Magn. m.* Mang. **Merc.* Mez. Mur. ac. **Natr. m.* *Nitr. ac.* °*N. vom.* **Phosph.* Phos. ac. Prun. **Puls.* *Ran.* °Ruta. **Sep.* **Sil.* *Spig.* *Squill.* **Sulph.* *Sulph. ac.* Thuj.

Fetid, Caps. Magn. c. Nitr. ac. **N. vom.* *Sabin.*

Of fetid smell or taste, °Ars. Bell. °*Chel.* Cupr. Ferr. Graph. Kreas. Merc. Mur. ac. °*Natr.* Nitr. ac. °*Puls.* Sep. Sil. °*Stann.*

—, like putrid eggs. Con.

Flesh-coloured, *Alum.* °*Cocc.* Kreas. Merc. Nitr. ac. Sabin. *Tab.*

Flocculent, Agar. Amb. *Merc.* Sep. **Sulph.*

Frothy, °Ars. *Chen.* Ferr. Op. Sec. Sulph. ac.

Gelatinous, Arg. Berb. Chinin. Hell. Laur. Rhus. Selen.

Globular, Sil. Thuj.

Gray, *Amb.* Anac. *Arg.* Ars. Carb. an. Caust.

Chin. Cop. Kreas. Lach. Magn. m. Merc. Sep. *Sil.* Thuj.

Greasy, Magn. c.

Green, greenish, Ars. Asa. Aur. Borax. **Carb. veg.* Caust. Colch. °*Dros.* Ferr. Hyos. Kal. Kreas. Lach. °Led. **Lyc.* Magn. aust. *Magn. c.* Mang. **Merc.* Murex. Natr. Natr. m. Nitr. ac. N. vom. *Par.* **Phosph.* °*Puls.* Rhus. Sabad. *Sep.* Sil. **Stann.* **Sulph.* °Thuj.

Herring-brine, smelling of, Graph.

Inodorous and insipid, Amm. m. *Calc.* Carb. an. Corall. Kreas.

Lumpy, Kal. Kreas. Phosph. Sabad. Sabin. Stann.

Of metallic taste, Calc. Cupr. Ipec. N. vom. Rhus.

Milky, Electr. Natr. m.

Like milk, **Calc.* Carb. veg. Con. Ferr. Lyc. Phosph. **Puls.* Sabin. Sep. °*Sil.* Sulph. ac.

Of thick mucus, °Acon. Agar. *Alum.* Amm. m. Ant. Arg. Ars. *Baryt.* Berb. *Borax.* Calc. Carb. an. Carb. veg. Cast. Con. Cop. Electr. Graph. Ipec. Jod. Kal. hdr. °Kreas. Lam. Lyc. Magn. arct. *Magn. m. Magn. s.* Murex. Mur. ac. *Natr. Natr. m.* Nicc. Nitr. ac. Ol. an. Op. Par. Puls. °Ruta. Sabad. Samb. Sassap. Scroph. Sec. Selen. Seneg. *Sil.* Staph. **Sulph.* Tong. Zinc. Zing.

Of thin mucus, Borax. Caps. Carb. veg. Colch. Electr. *Graph.* Ferr. Kal. hdr. Laur. Lyc. *Magn. c.* Mez. Natr. m. Nitr. N. vom. Ol. an. **Puls.* *Rhus. Seneg. Stann. Staph. Sulph. ac. Tereb.

Of musty smell or taste, Borax. Carb. veg.

Purulent, Cop. Ign. Merc. Sep. (Comp. SUPPURATION.)

Reddish, Asar. Borax. °Bry. Graph. Par. Phosph. Rhus. Sil. °Squill. Sulph.

Ropy, Asa. Carb. veg. Graph. Magn. aust. Magn. c.

Salt, Alum. *Amb.* **Ars.* °*Baryt.* Calc. Chin. Dros. *Graph.* **Lyc.* Magn. c. Magn. m. *Merc.* **Natr.* N. vom. *Petr.* °*Phosph.* Puls. Samb. **Sep. Sil.* Stann. Staph. Sulph. Zinc.

Slimy, Acon. Agar. Agn. *Alum.* Amb. Amm. c. Amm. m. Ang. Ant. Arg. Arn. Ars. Arum. Asa. **Asar.* Aur. Baryt. **Bell.* Bism. *Borax.* Bov. Bry. **Calc.* Camph. Cann. Canth. Caps. Carb. an. **Carb. veg.* **Caust.* *Cham.* Chel. *Chen.* **Chin.* Cin. Cocc. Coff. **Colch.* Coloc. *Con.* Cop. Croc. *Cupr.* Dig. Dros. *Dulc. Euphorb.* Euphr. Ferr. Galv. Grat. **Graph.* Guaj. Hell. *Hep.* Hyos. Ign. Ipec. **Jod.* **Kal.* *Kal. chl. *Kreas.* **Lach.* Lact. Laur. *Lyc.* Magn. art. Magn. arct. Magn. aust. Magn. c. *Magn. m.* **Merc.* **Mez.* Mur. ac. **Natr.* *Natr. m.* Natr. s. Nicc. Nitr. *Nitr. ac.* *N. mosch.* **N. vom.* Oleand. *Par.* **Petr.* **Phosph.* Phos. ac. *Phell.* Plat. Plumb. **Puls.* Ran. Raph. Ratanh. Rhab. Rhod. **Rhus.* Ruta. Sabad. Sabin. Samb. *Sassap.* Sec. Selen. Seneg. **Sep.* Sil. *Spig.* Spong. **Squill.* **Stann.* Staph. **Sulph.* Sulph. ac. **Tart.* Tong. *Thuj.* Val. Veratr. *Zinc.*

Smarting, Ant. Ars. *Cham.* °*Con.* Ferr. Ipec. °Lach. Merc. °*Phosph.* Sil. Sulph.

Sour smelling or tasting, Calc. Graph. Hep. Kal.

Lam. Magn. m. Merc. Natr. Nitr. N. vom. *Plumb.* Sep. Sulph. Tarax.

Like starch, °Sabin.

Of sweetish smell or taste, Asar. Lach. Magn. c. Merc. corr.

Tenacious, Acon. Agn. *Alum.* Amm. m. Anac. *Ant.* °*Ars.* Baryt.**Bell.**Bov.* Bry. Calc. °*Cann.* Canth. Carb. veg. Caust. **Cham.* Chin. *Chinin.* **Cist.* Cocc. Colch. Con. Dulc. Euphr. Graph. Jod. Kal. Lach. Lact. Laur. Lob. Magn. arct. *Magn. c.* Magn. m. **Merc.* °*Mez.* Natr. N. vom. °*Par.* Ol. an. °*Phosph.* Phos. ac. Plumb. Puls. *Ran.* Raph. Rhus. Sabad. Sabin.°*Samb.* Scroph. *Seneg.* Sep. Spig. Spong. Squill.**Stann.* Staph. *Tab.* Tart. Tong. Veratr. Zinc.

Viscous, Carb. an. Carb. veg. Hep. Phosph. °*Phos. ac.* Plat. **Sulph.*

Transparent, Alum. Cast. Crotal. Ferr. mur. Graph. Kal. hdr. Magn. s. Mang. Natr. m. Phosph. Puls. Sabad. *Sep.* **Sil.* **Stann.* Sulph. ac.

Traversed by threads, Arum.

Tuberculous, Magn. c.

Vesicular, Phosph.

Yellow, yellowish, *Acon.* Agn. *Alum.* Amb. Amm. Amm. m. Anac. Ang. **Ant.* Arg. *Ars.* Aur. Baryt. **Bell.* *Berb.* Bov. **Bry.* **Calc.* °*Cann.* *Canth.* Caps. *Carb. an.* **Carb. veg.* Cast. Caust. *Cham.* *Cic.* Clem. Con. Corall. Croc.°*Daph.* °*Dros.* Dulc. *Eugen.* Gran. *Graph.* *Hep.* *Jod.* *Kal.* **Kreos.* Lach. **Lyc.* Magn. c. Magn. m. Magn. s. Mang. Merc. Mez. Mur. ac. **Natr.* *Natr. m.* Nitr. **Nitr. ac.* **N. vom.* **Phosph.* Phos. ac. Prun. **Puls.* Rhus. Ruta.

Sabad. Sabin. Sec. *Selen.* Seneg. **Sep.* **Sil.* *Spig.* **Stann.* Staph. **Sulph.* Sulph. ac. °*Thuj.* Veratr. Viol. tr.

Watery, *Agar.* Alum. Amb. *Amm. Amm. m.* Ant. Arg. *Ars.* Asar. Bell. *Bov.* Calc. Cann. *Carb. an.* **Carb. veg.* Cast. **Cham. Chin.* Clem. Coff. Con. **Graph. Guaj.* Ign. Jod. Kal. hdr. Kreas. **Lach. Magn. arct. Magn. c.* **Magn. m.* Men. **Merc. Mez.* Murex. *Mur. ac.* Nicc. Nitr. *N. vom.* Par. Phosph. *Plumb. Puls.* Ran. Rhus. Seneg. *Sep. Sil. Squill.* Stann. Staph. **Sulph.* Sulph. ac. Thuj.

White, Amb. °Asar. **Bell.* Borax. Bov. **Calc.* Canth. *Carb. veg.* Caust. °Colch. *Con.* Ferr. Graph. Grat. Hell. Kreas. Lyc. Magn. arct. Magn. c. *Merc.* Natr. m. Nitr. N. vom. Ol. an. *Phosph.* Prun. **Puls.* Raph. Ratanh. Sabin. Sep. **Sil.* Sulph. ac. Tab. Tart.

Ears, Alum. Amm. m. Anac. *Asa.* Aur. Bell. Bry. Calc.°*Carb. an.* °*Carb. veg.* Caust. °*Cham.* °*Cist.* °*Colch.* Kal. *Lyc.* °*Men.* **Merc.* Mosch. *Natr. m. Nitr. ac.* Petr. Puls. Sep. *Sil. Sulph.* Zinc.

—, brown, Anac. °*Carb. veg.*

—, yellow, Merc. Phosph.

—, slimy, Bar. m. Con. Magn. arct. Nitr. ac.

—, fetid, Aur. Bov. °*Carb. veg.* Caust. Hep. Hyos. **Merc.* Zinc.

—, watery, Galv. *Sep.*

Discoloration, dirty colour.

Of the skin in general, Ant. Ars. Bry. Ferr. Jod. Merc. Phosph. Plumb. Sec. Vip. torv.

Nails, *Ant.* Ars. °*Graph.* Mur. ac. °*Nitr. ac.* Sil. Sulph.

Discoloured, dirty, which is.

Spots, Berb. *Sabin.* Sec.
Swelling, Crotal.
Ulcers, **Lach.* **Merc.* **Nitr. ac.* N. mosch. °*Sabin.* °*Thuj.*

Distended, Sensation as if.

Mammæ and nipples, Zinc.

Dorsal Region, Axilla, Neck, small of Back, Nape of Neck, and Scapulæ.

Abscess, axilla, Petr.
—, nape of neck, Sil.
—, neck, Hyos.
—, back, Lach.
—, loins, °Sil. °Staph.
Aching eruptions, Merc.
—, swelling, °Merc.
Acne of drunkards, °Led.
Back, *Agar.* Alum. Amm. m. Anac. *Ant.* Baryt. Berb. *Calc. Caust.* Daph. Eugen. Graph. Guaj. Jod. Kal. °Lach. Laur. Lyc. Magn. aust. Magn. m. Magn. s. Merc. Mill. Mur. ac. *Natr.* Natr. m. Natr. s. Nicc. *Nitr. ac.* N. vom. Ol. an. Phosph. *Phos. ac.* Seneg. Sep. Sil. Spig. Therid. Thuj. Zinc.
—, scapular region, Alum. Arn. Baryt. Calc.

Crotal. Laur. Merc. Oleand. Phell. Ratanh. Ruta. Seneg. Sil. Stront. Therid. Zinc.
Back, os sacrum, Agar. Alum. Borax. Bov. Graph. Laur. Led. Par. Plumb.
Blisters, vesicles, neck, Alum. Magn. c. Vip. red.
—, nape of neck, Caust. °Graph. Natr. c.
—, scapulæ, Amm. Ant. Caust. Cic. Lach. Vip. red.
Blotches, Lach.
Blotches, axilla, Petr.
—, neck, Graph. Natr. m. Sassap. Sec.
—, nape of neck, °Sil.
—, back, Lach. Mez.
—, axilla, Bry. Mez.
—, neck, Electr. Sec. Spong.
—, small of back, Lyc. Sassap. Stann.
—, loins, Croton.
—, nape of neck, Lact.
—, back, Acon. Baryt. Caust. Electr. Evon. Graph. Natr. Sec.
—, scapular region, Anac. Arg. Lach. Magn. arct. Mez. Sil.
—, os sacrum, Lyc.
Blotches, axilla, Nitr. ac. Phosph.
—, neck, Amm. °Lach. Lyc. Mur. ac. Nicc. Phosph. Phos. ac.
—, small of back, Nicc.
—, nape of neck, Ant. Carb. an. Caust. Nicc. Zinc.
—, back, Caust.
—, scapular region, Amm. Squill.
Bloodvessels, swelling of, neck, Bell. Thuj.
Blue spots, neck, Phell.

Boils, axilla, Borax. Lyc. °*Phos. ac.*
—, neck, Magn. c. Natr. m. Sep.
—, nates, Agar.
—, small of back, Aeth. Thuj.
—, nape of neck, Electr. Nitr. ac. Phosph.
—, back, Caust. Electr. Mur. ac. Sulph. ac. Zinc.
—, scapulæ, Amm. Bell. Led. Lyc. Nitr. ac. Zinc.
Bones, affections of, °*Calc.* °*Puls.* °*Rhus.* °*Sil.* °Staph. **Sulph.*
—, swelling, °Calc. °Puls. °Rhus. °Sil. Sulph.
—, curvature, °Calc. °Lyc. °Puls. °Rhus. °Sil. °Staph.? **Sulph.*
Brown spots, Thuj.
Burning, axilla, Carb. veg. Caust. Kal. Natr. m. Sep. Spig. Zinc.
—, neck, Caust. Grat. Nicc. Ol. an. Phell. Stront. Tab.
—, small of back, Aeth. Amm. Asar. Berb. Borax. Kal. Lach. Magn. aust. Natr. Phosph. Phos. ac. Rhus. Stann. Sulph. Sulph. ac.
—, loins, Aeth. Baryt. Berb. Nitr. ac.
—, nape of neck, Amm. Calc. Ign. Merc. Natr. Nitr. Ol. an.
—, back, Amm. Arn. Bism. Bry. Calc. °*Carb. an.* *Carb.* Lyc. Magn. m. Merc. Mur. ac. Natr. *Nitr. ac.* N. vom. Oph. Raph. Seneg. Sil. *Sulph.* Tart. Zinc.
—, vertebræ, Asa. Tart.
—, scapulæ, Alum. Amb. Baryt. Bry. Cann. Carb. veg. Carb. Electr. Galv. Jod. Kal. Laur. Lyc. Magn. m. Merc. Natr. Natr. m. Seneg. Sil. Sulph. Tab. Teucr. Veratr. Zinc.
Burning eruptions, Cinn.
—, blotches, Lach.

Burning, pimples, Cinn. Lyc. Magn. aust. Phosph. Ratanh. Squill.
—, spots, Thuj.
—, swelling, °Baryt. Phosph.
Callosities, neck, Rhus v.
Claret-coloured spots, Sep.
Close-standing eruptions, Squill. Thuj.
Colourless eruption, Ars.
Creeping, axilla, Bry.
—, small of back, Alum. Tarax.
—, back, Alum. Bov. Lach. Laur. Magn. s. *Natr.*
Cow-pox, like, Tart.
Dampness, axilla, Carb. veg.
—, axillary glands, Sulph.
—, scapula, Lach.
—, os sacrum, Graph. Led.
Dry eruption, Evon.
Eczema, Ant. Sulph.
Eruption, neck, Ant. *Ars.* Bry. *Cinn.* *Lyc. Magn. aust. *Staph.* Tart.
—, loins, Clem. Rhus.
—, nape of neck, Bry. Carb. an. Carb. veg. Caust. Cham. Clem. Nitr. °Petr. °Sec.
—, back, Alum. Baryt. Bry. °Carb. veg. Evon. Lach. Led. Merc. Mercurial. Natr. m. °Sep. Squill.
—, scapulæ, Ant. Caust. Lach. Phos. ac.
—, shoulders, Ars.
Erysipelas, Cist. °Graph. °Merc. °Rhus.
Erysipelas, vesicular, °Graph. °Merc. °*Rhus.*
Flea-bite, itching as of, Alum. Laur. Squill.
Formication, neck, Electr. Sec.
—, back, Evon. Graph. *Natr.* Sassap.
Glandular indurations, °Ign. *Nitr. ac.* Phosph.

Glands, diseases of, in general, Amm. Amm. m. Ars. Asar. Baryt. **Bell.* Calc. Calend. °*Carb. an.* Clem. Coloc. Cupr. *Hep.* Jod. *Kal. Lyc. Natr. m.* **Nitr. ac. Phosph.* Phos. ac. Prun. *Rhus. Sep.* **Sil.* °Staph. **Sulph.* Sulph. ac.
—, neck, Alum. °*Amm. Arn.* Bar. m. **Bell.** *Calc.* Caps. **Carb. an.* Carb. veg. *Caust.* Cinn. °*Cist.* Cupr. °Electr. *Ferr. Graph.* Hell. Ign. *Kal.* °Kreas. °*Lach.* **Lyc. Magn. m.* **Merc. Natr.* Natr. m. **Nitr. ac.* °Phosph. Puls. Selen. **Sil. Spig. Spong.* °Staph.? **Sulph.* Tart. Viol. tr.
—, nape of neck, Baryt. Calc. °Hell. °Jod. °Mur. ac. °Petr. °Phosph. **Sil.* °Staph.? **Sulph.*
Gnawing, Agar. Alum. Anac. Berb. Dig. Guaj. Spig.
—, axilla, Mez.
—, neck, Magn. m.
—, hips, Amm.
—, small of back, Amm. Canth. Magn. m. Nicc. Phosph. Stront. Sulph.
—, loins, Phos. ac.
—, back, Bell. Hell. Magn. aust. Magn. m.
—, scapulæ, Alum. Natr.
—, os sacrum, Alum. Kal.
Goïtre, °Amm. °*Calc.* Con. **Jod.* Kal. hdr. °*Lyc. Natr.* Natr. m. Plat. °*Spong.*
—, pressing outward, Spong.
—, pressing, Natr.
—, sensitive, Kal. hdr.
—, hard, Spong.
—, titillating, Plat.
—, as if alive inside, Spong.
—, beating, Jod. Lyc.
—, painful, Jod. Plat.

Goïtre, tensive, Jod.
—, indurated, **Jod.* Spong.
—, soft, Kal. hdr.
—, jerking, Lyc.
—, constrictive, Jod.
Hard, blotches, Ant. Phosph. Zinc.
—, swelling, Amm. m. °*Calc.* °*Carb. an. Kal.* °Lyc. °Sil. Spig. °Spong.

Hepatic spots, back, Sulph.
—, shoulders, Ant.

Herpes, axilla, °Carb. an. °Lyc. °Sep.
—, neck, Lach.
—, nape of neck, Caust. °Lyc. °Petr. °Sep. Sulph.
Herpetic spot, Hyos. Sep.

Spots, neck, Ars. Bell. Bry. Carb. veg. Cinn. Cocc. Jod. Lyc. Nitr. Phell. Sep. Stann. Vip. torv.
—, axilla, Thuj.
—, hips, Sep.
—, small of back, Sep.
—, nape of neck, Carb. veg. Hyos.
—, back, Lyc. °Sep. Sulph. Zinc.
—, scapula, Calc. Cist. Lach.
Humid, eruptions, Clem.
—, herpes, Caust. °Sep.
—, spots, Lach.
—, swelling, Sulph.
Inflamed, blotches, Amm. m.
Inflammation, axillary glands, Magn. aust. Nitr. ac.
—, cervical glands, *Sulph.*

Inflammatory swelling, °Merc. °Sil. Sulph.

Itching, axilla, Anac. *Asar.* Carb. an. Carb. veg. Dig. Grat. Kal. Nitr. ac. *Phosph.* Sep. *Spig.* Spong.

—, neck, *Alum.* Anac. Ant. Calc. Carb. veg. Cin. Mez. Nicc. Nitr. ac. *Puls.* Rhus. Squill. Stront. Sulph. Tab. Teucr. Thuj.

—, small of back, Berb. Grat. Kal. Magn. m. Merc. Natr. m. Phell.

—, lumbar region, Alum. Dig. Puls.

—, nape of neck, Alum. Amm. m. Berb. Carb. veg. Mez. Nitr. ac. Ol. an. Phell. *Sep.* Staph. Therid.

Itching, eruption, Caust. Cin. Led. °Sep.

—, blisters, Natr.

—, pimples, Baryt. Calc. °Carb. veg. Cinn. Clem. Kal. Led. Magn. art. Magn. aust. Mill. Natr. m. Phosph. Puls. Selen. Sil. Squill. Staph.

—, herpes, Caust.

—, spots, Carb. veg. Cinn. °Sep. Zinc.

—, swelling, Sulph.

—, blotches, Lyc.

Lupia, nape of neck, °Baryt.

Moles, axilla, Thuj.

Nettlerash, Sil.

Pain as if sore, neck, Bry.

—, cervical vertebræ, °Con.

—, vertebræ, °Con. Dig. Sep.

—, small of back, Cast. Caust. **Natr.*

—, nape of neck, Bry. Dig. Phos. ac. Sep.

—, back, Cast. Thuj.

—, scapulæ, Coloc. Lach. Plat.

Painful as if sore, pocks, Natr.

—, pimples, Bell. Clem. Magn. art. Mez. Spig.

Pain as if strained by lifting, Bell. **Calc.* Canth. *Caust.* Cocc. Kal. Mur. ac. *N. vom.* Oleand. °*Rhus.* Stann. Staph. Val.

Pain as if sprained, **Calc.* N. vom. *Puls.*

—, neck, Cinn. Sassap.

—, small of back, Agar. Lach. Magn. aust. Ol. an. Petr. Rhod. Sep. *Sulph.*

—, nape of neck, Agar. Nicc. Nitr. Sulph. Tong.

—, back, Agar. Bell. Con. Lyc. *Petr. Sulph.*

—, scapular region, Baryt. Kal. Petr. Plumb. *Rhod.* Sulph.

Pain as if dislocated, Natr. m. Sulph.

Pain as if ulcerated, axillary glands, Prun.

—, lumbar vertebræ, Kreas.

—, nape of neck, Puls.

—, dorsal spine, Carb. an.

—, scapulæ, Oleand. Cist.

—, swollen parts, Baryt. Calc.

Painful, eruption, Clem. °*Lyc.* Magn. aust.

—, blisters, Cic.

—, pimples, Ant. Arn. Puls. Spong. Squill.

—, swelling. Amm. Arn. **Bell.* Carb. veg. Cupr. Kal. Lach. Lyc. Magn. m. Natr. **Nitr. ac.* N. vom. Rhus. Sassap. Spig. Spong. Sulph.

—, blotches, °Lach. Phos. ac. Zinc.

Painless, eruption, Nitr.

—, swelling, Sep.

—, indurations (glandular), °Ign.

Peeling off, eruption, Phell.

Petechiæ, neck, Phell.

Pimples, axilla, Phosph.

—, neck, Ant. Aur. Berb. Bov. *Cinn.* Clem. Gins. Hep. Magn. arct. Magn. c. Mez. Nitr.

Phell. Phos. ac. *Puls.* Spig. Spong. *Squill.* Staph. Sulph. *Thuj.*
Pimples, small of the back, Calc. Tab.
—, loins, Cham. Chin.
—, nape of neck, Arn. Bar. m. Bell. Berb. Borax. Calc. °Carb. veg. Hep. Kal. Lyc. Magn. aust. Magn. c. Natr. Nitr. *Sil.* Staph.
—, back, Alum. Berb. Calc. °Carb. veg. Cocc. Con. Dig. Jod. Led. Magn. m. Meph. Mill. *Natr. m.* Phos. ac. Puls. Sassap. *Selen. Squill.* Sulph. Tab. Zinc.
—, scapulæ, Ant. Bell. Berb. Crotal. Kal. chl. Lyc. Magn. m. Mosch. *Puls.* Ratanh. Squill.
Pocks, neck, Hydroc.
—, nape of neck, Natr.
—, dorsum, *Tart.* Zinc.
Pustules, neck, Ant. Aur. °Clem. *Squill.* Tart.
—, small of back, Calc. Natr.
—, nape of neck, Bell. Natr. Nitr.
—, back, °Dulc. Evon.
—, scapulæ, Cocc. Magn.
Raised, eruption, Mez. Val.
Rash, neck, Amm. Bry. Galv.
—, nape of neck, Ant. Caust. Mez. °Sec.
—, back, Merc. Mez. Stram.
—, scapula, Ant. Caust.
Redness, neck, Bell. Jod. Veratr.
Red, eruption, Ant. Bry.
—, blisters, Ant. Cic.
—, pimples, Ant. Bell. Led. Mez. Phos. ac. Spig. *Squill. Thuj.*
—, swelling, Amm. m. Baryt.
—, blotches, °Lach. Mur. ac.

Red, spots, Ant. Bell. Carb. veg. Cist. Cocc. Lach. Sep. Stann. Vip. torv.
Sarcoma, nape of neck, Baryt.
Scarlet-spots, **Bell.* Galv.
Scurfs, Graph. Natr. m.
—, axilla, Natr. m.
—, nape of neck, Bell.
Soreness, axilla, Arg. Carb. veg. Mez. Teucr. Zinc.
Smarting, axilla, Ruta.
—, neck, Magn. c. Nitr.
—, small of back, Canth. Phell.
—, nape of neck, Grat. Kal. hdr. Magn. c. Nitr. Ol. an.
—, back, Magn. aust. Mur. ac. Natr.
—, scapulæ, Stront.
Smarts, which, Ars. Bry.
Stinging, tumour, Petr.
—, blisters, Amm.
—, pimples, Arn. Bell. Squill.
—, swelling, Carb. an. Electr. °Merc.
—, tubercles, Squill.
Suppurations, axilla, Petr.
—, axillary glands, °Calc. Coloc. *Hep. Sep.* °*Sil.*
—, neck, Hyos. °Ipec.
—, cervical glands, °Cist.
—, nape of neck, °Sil.
—, lumbar region, °Sil. *Staph.
Swelling, axilla, Baryt.
—, axillary glands, Amm. *Amm. m.* Ars. **Bell.* Clem. Coloc. *Kal.* *Lyc. *Natr. m.* **Nitr. ac.* **Phosph.* Phos. ac. Prun. *Rhus. Sep.* **Sil.* °Staph.? **Sulph.*
—, neck, Ars. **Bell.* Bov. Calc. Canth. Cic. Con.

Croc. Crotal. Hyos. °Kal. °Lach. °Lyc. Magn. art. Mang. *Natr.* Nitr. ac. N. vom. Par. Puls. *Sassap.* Sil. Sulph. Tart. Vip. red. *Vip. torv.*

Swelling, cervical glands, Alum. °Amm. Arn. Bar. m. **Bell.* **Calc.* **Carb. an.* Carb. veg. Caust. Cinn. °Cist. Cupr. °Electr. *Ferr. Graph.* Hell. Ign. *Kal.* °Kreos. °*Lach.* **Lyc. Magn. m.* **Merc. Natr.* **Nitr. ac.* °Phosph. **Sil. Spig. Spong.* °Staph.? Sulph. Tart. Viol. tr.

—, lumbar region, Berb. Lyc. °Sil. °Staph.

—, nape of neck, Baryt. **Bell.* Calc. Puls. Sep.

—, posterior cervical glands, **Baryt.** *Calc.*° *Hell.* °Jod. Mur. ac. °Petr. °Phosph. °*Sil.* °Staph. ? **Sulph.*

—, back, °Sil. °Staph.

—, dorsal vertebræ, °Puls. °Sil.

—, thyroid cartilage, Sil. *Sulph.*

Tearing, tumour, Petr.

Tensive, swelling, Bov. Graph. Magn. m. Mang. Mur. ac.

—, tumours, swellings, Caust. Mur. ac.

Ulcers, throat, °Lach.

Vesicles, Vip. red.

Vesicles, breaking, Lach.

Yellow, blisters, Ant.

—, spots, Jod.

Wart-shaped pimples, Phell.

Drawing.

Mammæ and nipples, Kreas.

Bones, periosteum, Acon. Agar. Anac. Ang. Asa Atham. Aur. *Baryt.* Bry. **Carb. veg.* **Caust* *Chin.* Crotal. Cupr. Ign. Indig. Kal. Kreas

Lyc. Magn. arct. Mang. Men. Merc. Par. Phos. ac. Plumb. Rhod. *Sabin.* Samb. Seneg. Stann. Staph. Tereb. Thuj. Zinc. ox.
Glands, Alum. Ign. **Merc.* **Puls. Sil. Zinc.*

Drawing-painful.

Blisters, Clem.
Pimples, Con. Magn. m. Staph.
Swelling, Amm. M. Cham. Chin. Ferr. Kal. N. vom.
Ulcers, Clem. Graph. Mez. Nitr. N. vom. Staph. Sulph.
Blotches, Cham.

Face, Con. Magn. m. Staph.
Buccal cavity, blisters, Staph.
—, Ulcers, Calc.
Hands, swelling, Chin.
Feet, swelling, *Ferr.

Dropsical.

Swelling, °*Acon.* Anthrok. **Ant.* **Ars.* **Aur.* °*Bar. m.* °Bell. °*Bry.* Canth. Chel. **Chin.* °Chinin.? °*Colch.* Coloc. Con. Crotal. °*Dig.* °*Dulc.* Euphorb, °*Ferr.* Guaj. **Hell.* Hyos. *Jod.* **Kal.* Lach. °*Led.* **Lyc.* **Merc.* Oph. Mez. Mur. ac. Natr. Nitr. Nitr. ac. Oleand. *Op.* °*Phosph.* *Plumb.* °*Puls.* °*Rhod.* °*Rhus.* °*Ruta.* °*Sabin.* °*Samb.* Sassap. Sec. Seneg. Sep. Sil. **Squill.* °*Stram.* **Sulph.* Tereb. Veratr.

Lower limbs, knee, swelling, °Jod.? °*Sulph.*
—, thigh, *Jod. Merc.*

Feet, swelling, °*Ferr.* Hep. *Jod.* Kreas. °*Led.* °*Puls.* *Rhod.* *Samb.* *Sec.*

DRUNKARDS, AS IN.

Pimples, Kreas. °Led.

Nose, °Lach.
Face, °Kreas. °Lach. °Led.
Dorsal region, pimples, °Led.

DRY, WHICH IS.

Eruption, Alum. Ars. **Baryt.* Bov. *Bry. **Calc.* Carb. veg. Caust. Clem. Cocc. *Cupr.* *Dulc.* Evon. *Graph.* Heracl. Hyos. Kreas. Led. Lyc. Magn. c. **Merc.* **Mez.* Natr. Natr. m. Par. *Petr.* *Phosph.* Phos. ac. Rhus. Sassap. **Sep.* **Sil.* Stann. **Staph.* Sulph. Teucr. Val. **Veratr.* *Viol. tr.* Zinc.
Blisters, Rhus.
Pimples, Bov. Kreas.
Pustules, Evon. °*Merc.*
Figwarts, °*Sassap.* °*Sulph.*
—, after mercurial treatment, °*Sassap.* °*Sulph.*
Herpes, Amm. m. °Clem. °Dulc. Kal. hdr. °Kreas. **Led.* Merc. Nicc. °Phosph. °Phos. ac. °Sulph. Tax. °Veratr.
Spots, Baryt. Kal. hdr.
Scurfs, crusts, Ars. **Aur.* **Aur. m.* °*Baryt.* °*Calc.* Chinin. Graph. Lach. Led. Merc. °*Sulph.* Thuj.
Itch, Ars.? °*Calc.?* °*Carb. veg.* °*Caust.* Cupr.? °*Dulc.?* Graph.? °*Lach.* Led.? °*Merc.?* °*Natr.* °Petr.? Phos. ac.? °*Sep.* °*Sil.?* °Staph.? °*Sulph.* Val.? °*Veratr.*

Head, °*Baryt.* °Calc. Merc. °Mez.
Face, Amm. m. Baryt. Kal. hdr. Kreos. °Led.
Chest. eruption, Heracl.
Dorsal region, eruption, Evon.
Hands, eruptions, &c., Bov. Lyc. Veratr.

Dry skin.

In general, **Acon.* Alum. °Amb. ***Amm.*** Ant. Arg. *Arn.* **Ars.* Asa. Baryt. **Bell.* Bism. Borax. **Bry.* **Calc.* Camph. *Cann.* Canth. Carb. an. Carb. veg. Caust. **Cham.* **Chin.* Clem. Cocc. **Coff.* **Colch.* Coloc. Con. **Dulc.* Ferr. *Graph. Haemat. Hell. Hep. Hydroc. **Hyos.* Ign. **Jod.* *Ipec.* **Kal.* Kreos. Lach. Laur. *Led.* **Lyc.* Magn. art. Magn. aust. Magn. c. Mang. *Merc.* Mez. Murex. Mur. ac. **Natr.* Natr. m. Nitr. **Nitr. ac.* **N. mosch.* N. vom. *Oleand.* *Op.* Par. **Phosph.* *Phos. ac.* *Plat.* Plumb. *Puls.* Ran. Ran. sc. *Rhus.* Ruta. Sabad. Samb. *Sec.* *Seneg.* Sep. *Sil.* *Spig.* *Spong.* Squill. *Staph.* Stram. Stront. **Sulph.* Sulph. ac. Tart. Teucr. Val. *Verb.* *Viol. od.* Viol. tr.
Parched skin, **Calc.* *Hyos. *Jod. Kal. Magn. c. Natr. Sec.
Parchment-like dryness, **Ars.* *Chin.* Dulc. Kal. Led. **Lyc.* Phosph. °*Sil.* Squill.
Break, liable to, **Hyos.* Natr. Sec. (Comp.: Cracked.)

Ears, Graph. Nitr. ac. Petr.
—, Dryness, feeling of, Bell. Graph. Lach. Nitr. ac. Petr. Phosph.
Hands, *Anac.* *Baryt.* Bism. Ferr. magn. *Hep.*

Lach. **Lyc.* *Natr.* *Natr. m.* Phosph. *Phos. ac.* *Sabad.* *Sulph.* Tax. *Thuj.*
—, finger, Anac. *Sil.* Tart.

Dwindling.

Mammæ and nipples, *Con.* *Jod.* Nitr. ac.

Ears and Region of Ears.

Blotches, in front of ear, Bry.
—, behind the ears, Bry. **Calc.* Carb. an. Caus Staph.
—, on the ear, Spong.
Blisters, vesicles, Alum. Chin.
Pimples, Agar. Amm. m. Berb. Cic. Kal. Kree Magn. art. Mur. ac. Natr. m. Petr. Phosp Sabad. Selen. Spong. Staph. Verbasc.
Bleeding, Bry. Caust. Cic. Galv. °*Graph.* *Me* Oph. Petr. Phosph. °*Rhus.* Sep.
Boils, Sil. Sulph.
Bone-pains, Baryt. Indig. Kal. Lach. Ra Ratanh. Sil. Staph.
Burning, Acon. *Agar.* Amm. m. Ang. A Arn. Ars. Bry. Calc. Canth. Caps. Carb. Carb. veg. Caust. Chel. Clem. Dros. Gr Ign. *Kreos.* *Laur.* Magn. c. Magn. m. M Natr. m. Oleand. *Ol. an.* Sabad. *Sabin.* S Spong. Zinc.
Burning eruptions, Mosch. Puls. Sassap.
—, herpes, Merc.
—, swelling, Natr. m. Phos. ac.
—, scurfs, Merc.
Caries, °*Aur.* °*Nitr. ac.* °*Sil.* °Asa.? °Sta
Cerumen, blood-red, Con.

Cerumen, purulent, Sep.
—, like decayed paper, Con.
—, fluid, Amm. m. *Con.* Jod. *Kal.* Lach. *Merc.* Mosch. Selen. *Sil.*
—, yellow, Kal. Lach.
—, hard, Lach. Selen.
—, deficient, °*Calc.* °*Carb. veg.* °*Galv.*
—, flour-pap, like, Lach.
—, increased, Agar. Amm. m. Calc. *Con.* Hep. Selen. Sep. Sil. Thuj. Zinc. ox.
Creeping, Rhod.
Crawling, Ratanh.
Dampness, °*Calc.* °*Lyc.*
—, behind the ears, Amm. **Calc.* Carb. veg. Caust. °*Graph.* Kal. °*Lyc.* Nitr. ac. °*Oleand.* °*Petr.* Phosph. Sil.
—, margins of ears, *Sil.*
Discharge, Alum. Amm. m. Anac. *Asa.* Aur. Bell. Bry. Calc. °*Carb. an.* °*Carb. veg.* Caust. °*Cham.* °*Cist.* °*Colch.* Kal. *Lyc.* °*Men.* **Merc.* Mosch. *Natr. m. Nitr. ac.* Petr. Puls. Sep. *Sil. Sulph.* Zinc.
—, brown, Anac. °*Carb. veg.*
—, yellow, Merc. Phosph.
—, slimy, Bar. m. Con. Magn. arct. Nitr. ac.
—, fetid, Aur. Bov. *Carb. veg.* Caust. Hep Hyos. **Merc.* Zinc.
Erysipelas, Lach. Meph.
—, watery, Galv. *Sep.*
Eruption, Amm. m. Ant. Agar. **Baryt.* Bov. **Calc.* Chin. **Cic.* Kal. Mez. Mosch. Mur. ac. Natr. m. Petr. Phosph. Puls. Sep. Sil. Spong. Staph. **Sulph.*
—, lobules, Sassap. Teucr.

Eruptions, behind the ears, Ant. **Baryt.* **Calc.* Canth. Chin. **Cic.* Graph. *Hep.* Mez. Oleand. **Puls.* Sabad. Selen. Sil. °*Staph.*
—, in front of the ears, **Cic.*
Excrescences, spongy, Merc.
Fetid, which is, ear, °Aur. °Bov. °Carb. veg. Caust. °Cist. °Graph. °Hep. Hyos. Merc. Zinc.
—, behind the ear, herpes, °Oleand.
Dryness, Graph. Nitr. ac. Petr.
—, sensation of dryness, Bell. Graph. Lach. Nitr. ac. Petr. Phosph.
Soreness, behind the ears, Anac. °*Graph.* Kal. °*Lach.* **Merc.* Nitr. ac. Petr.
Pain as if sore, Borax. Caust. Cic. Galv. Lyc. Magn. c. Phos. ac. Sep.
Frozen, as if, (itching, redness), Agar. Colch.
Fungous excrescences, Merc.
Glands, affections of, **Amm.* Baryt. **Bell.* **Calc.* Carb. an. °*Carb. veg.* **Cham.* Cocc. °*Con.* Dig. **Ign.* **Kal.* **Merc.* Nitr. ac. °N. vom.? **Rhus.* Sabad. **Sil.*
Gnawing, Arg. Dros. Indig. Kal. Kal. hdr. Mur. ac. Plat. Sulph.
Herpes exedens, *Merc.*
Humid eruptions, Bov. Calc. Lyc. Mez.
—, herpes, Amm. m. Kreas. Merc. Oleand.
Inflammation, external, **Acon.* **Bell.* *Borax.* Bry. *Calc.* Canth. **Cham.* °*Hep.* Kal. Kreos. °*Lyc.* Magn. aust. Magn. c. *Merc.* Nitr. °*N. vom.* °*Phos. ac.* **Puls.* °*Sil.* Spong.
—, internal, °*Acon.* Bell. *Borax.* Bry. Calc Canth. *Hep.* °*Merc.* **Puls.*
—, lobules, Nitr.
—, parotid glands, **Amm.* **Bell.* °Calc. °*Carl*

veg. °*Cham.* °*Kal.* °*Merc.* °*N. vom.* °*Rhus.* Sassap.

Inflammation, external, margins, Sil.

Inflamed scurfs, Lyc.

Herpes, Amm. m. Caust. *Graph.* Kreas. Magn. m. °*Oleand.* °*Sep.* Teucr.

—, behind the ears, Amm. m. °Graph. °*Oleand.* °*Sep.*

—, lobules, Caust. °*Sep.* Teucr.

—, in front of ear, °Oleand.

Itching, Aeth. *Agar.* *Alum.* Amb. **Amm.* Amm. m. °*Anac.* *Arg.* *Baryt.* Bell. Berb. Borax. *Bov.* *Caps.* Carb. veg. Cast. Caust. *Con.* Cupr. Ferr. magn. Gran. Graph. Hep. *Ign.* *Kal.* Kal. hdr. Kreos. Lach. *Laur.* *Lyc.* *Magn. art.* Magn. m. Mang. Men. Meph. Merc. Mez. Mill. Mosch. Mur. ac. Natr. m. Nitr. Nitr. ac. *N. vom.* Ol. an. Petr. Phell. *Phosph.* Phos. ac. *Puls.* Ratanh. Raph. Rab. Rhod. *Rhus.* Sabad. *Sassap.* *Sep.* *Sil.* *Spig.* Stann. **Sulph.* Tong. Veratr. Zinc.

Itching, externally, Agar. Carb. veg. Con. Hep. Kal. Sil. Spig. Sulph.

—, meatus auditorius, Alum. Caust. Ign. Nitr. Sassap.

—, lobules, Alum. Caust. Kal. Laur. Natr. m. Phos. ac. Sabad.

—, internally, Anac. Caps. Puls. Ratanh. Rhab. Ruta. Samb. Sep.

—, behind the ears, Agar. Alum. Carb. veg. Graph. Mosch. Natr. m. Nitr. ac. Therid.

tching eruption, Mosch. Mez. Natr. m. Petr. Sassap.

– pimples, Amm. m. Magn. arct. Mur. ac.

Itching herpes, Merc.
— scurfs, Sassap.
Lupia, lobule, °Nitr. ac.
Numbness, °*Mur. ac.*
Pain, contusive, Arn. Cic. Ruta.
Pain as if ulcerated, Anac. Calc. Ferr. Kal. Magn. c. Mang. Mur. ac.
Scurfs, Bov. °*Graph.* °*Hep.* Jod. °*Lach.* °*Lyc.* Mur. ac. °*Puls.* Sassap. Spong.
—, behind the ears, °*Graph.* °*Hep.* °*Lyc.* °Puls. °*Staph.*
Polypus, °*Calc.*
Pus, discharge of, Alum. Amm. °*Asa.* °*Aur.* Bell. **Borax.* °*Bov.* °*Calc.* °*Carb. veg.* Caust. °*Cist.* °*Graph.* **Hep.* Kal. Lyc. **Merc.* Petr. **Puls.* °*Rhus.* Sep. **Sulph.* Zinc.
Redness, Agar. *Alum. Ant. Camph.* Carb. veg. *Chin.* Electr. Evon. Galv. Graph. *Hep. Ign.* Kal. Kreas. *Magn. c.* Meph. *Merc.* Natr. m. Nitr. ac. Petr. Phosph. Plat. *Puls.* Sep. Sil. Sulph. *Tab.*
Red herpes, Oleand.
Roughness, Phosph.
—, before the ear, Oleand.
Scaly pimples, Merc.
— herpes, Teucr.
Scurfy eruption, Puls.
Smarting, Grat. Lach. Lyc. Ol. an.
Smarting eruptions, Mez. Petr. Puls.
Suppurating eruptions, Cycl. Kal. Sep.
— abscess, Merc.
— pimples, Amm. m.
— tympanum, °Amm. °Carb. veg.
— parotid gland, Sassap.

Swelling of bones, °Carb. an. °Puls.
—, behind the ear, periosteum, °Carb. an.
Swelling, ear, Alum. °*Anac.* Ant. Baryt. Borax. *Calc.* Caust. Cist. Electr. Graph. *Kal.* Kreas. °*Lyc.* Merc. Natr. m. Nitr. Nitr. ac. Phos. ac. **Puls.* **Rhus.* *Sep.* °*Sil.* Spong. Zinc.
—, behind the ears, Bry. Calc. Caps. Carb. an. Tab.
—, internal meatus, *Calc.* Caust. Cist. Electr. Graph. *Kal.* Natr. m. *Sep.*
—, in front of ears, Anac. Bry.
—, parotid glands, Amm. Baryt. **Bell.* **Calc.* Carb. an. **Carb. veg.* **Cham.* Cocc. °*Con.* Dig. Graph. *Ign.* **Kal.* **Merc.* Nitr. ac. °N. vom.? *Puls.* **Rhus.* Sep. **Sil.* Sulph.
Titillation, Alum. *Amb.* Amm. Ant. Ars. Baryt. Calc. Caps. Carb. veg. Caust. Chin. *Colch.* Coloc. Dros. Kal. Laur. Mill. N. vom. *Plat.* Phell. Ratanh. Rhus. Sabad. *Samb.* Sep. Spig. Sulph. Sulph. ac. Thuj. Tong. Veratr. Zinc.
Tubercles, blotches, Berb. Dros. Lach. Merc. Nicc. Nitr. ac. Phos. ac. Spong. Staph.
Ulcers, ear, Bov. Camph. Kal.
Ulcerated eruptions, ulceration, Alum. **Amm.* Bov. Bry. Camph. Galv. Gran. Graph. Kal. Lyc. **Merc.* °*Puls.* °*Ruta.* Spong. Stann.
—, Herpes, *Merc.*
Yellow scurfs, Jod.

Ecchymosis.

In general, *Arn. °Bry. °Calc. Cham. Chin. °*Con.* Crotal. Dulc. Electr. Euphr. Ferr. °*Hep.* Lach. Laur. Natr. Natr. m. **N. vom.*

Par. Plumb. °*Puls.* Rhus. °*Ruta.* Sec. **Sulph.* **Sulph. ac.*
Ecchymosed, sensation as if, Arn. Chin. Calc. Ferr. N. vom. Par. Ruta. Sec. Sulph. ac.

Eyes, °*Arn.* °*Bell.* °Calc. Cham. Crotal. **N. vom.* Plumb. Ruta. °*Seneg.*
Eyelids, °*Arn.*
Mouth, Con.

Eczema.

Dorsal region, Ant. Sulph.
Arms, Mez. Phosph. *Sil.*
Hands, Mez. Phosph.
—, fingers, *Sil.*

Eruption in General.

In general, **Acon.* *Agar. Agn. Alum. Amb. **Amm.* Amm. m. Anac. Ang. **Ant.* Arg. Arn. **Ars.* Asa. Asar. Aur. Aur. m. **Baryt.* Bar. m. **Bell.* Berb. Bism. *Borax.* **Bov.* **Bry.* Calad. **Calc.* Camph. Cann. Canth. Caps. **Carb. an.* **Carb. veg.* **Caust.* **Cham.* Chel. Chin. **Cic.* Cin. Cinn. **Clem.* Cocc. Coff. Colch. Coloc. **Con.* **Cop.* Corall. Croc. Cupr. **Cycl.* Daph. Diad. **Dig.* **Dulc.* Electr. *Euphorb.* Euphr. Evon. **Graph.* Grat. *Guaj.* **Hell.***Hep.* Heracl. Hyos. Jatroph. **Ign.* *Jod.* Ipec. **Kal.* Kal. chl. **Kreas.* **Lach.* Laur. **Lyc.* Magn. art. Magn. arct. Magn. aust. Magn. c. Magn. m. Magn. s. *Mang.* Men. **Merc.* *Mercurial.* *Mez.*

Mosch. Mur. ac. Natr. **Natr. m.* Natr. s. Nitr. **Nitr. ac.* N. mosch. N. vom. **Oleand.* Op. *Oph.* Par. **Petr.* **Phosph.* **Phos. ac.* Plat. **Puls.* *Ran.* *Ran. sc.* Rhab. Rhod. **Rhus.* Ruta. **Sabad.* Sabin. Samb. **Sassap.* Sec. Selen. Seneg. **Sep.* **Sil.* Spig. Spong. Squill. Stann. **Staph.* Stram. Stront. **Sulph.* Sulph. ac. Tarax. **Tart.* Tereb. Teucr. **Thuj.* Val. Veratr. Verb. **Viol. tr.* Vip. red. Vip. torv. Zinc.

Blackish, Ant. **Ars.* Asa. **Bell.* **Bry.* Chinin. (Con.) *Crotal.* Electr. *Lach.* °Mur. ac. °Nitr. ac. *Oph.* **Rhus.* *Sec.* Sep. °*Sil.* Spig. Vip. red.

Bleeding, Merc. Par. (Comp: BLEEDS, THAT WHICH.)

Brownish, Cann. *Nitr. ac.* Phosph. Phos. ac.

Burning, Agar. Alum. Amb. Amm. Amm. m. Anac. Ant. Arg. **Ars.* Aur. Baryt. *Bell.* Bov. *Bry.* Calad. *Calc.* Cann. Canth. Caps. *Carb. an.* *Carb. veg.* *Caust.* Chin. Cic. Cinn. Clem. Cocc. Coff. Colch. *Con.* Dulc. Euphorb. Guaj. Hell. *Hep.* Heracl. Ign. Kal. Kreas. Lach. Laur. Led. Lyc. Magn. art. Magn. arct. Magn. aust. Mang. **Merc.* *Mercurial.* Mez. Mosch. Natr. Natr. m. Nitr. Nitr. ac. *N. vom.* Oleand. Par. Petr. Phosph. Phos. ac. Plat. Plumb. *Puls.* Ran. Ratanh. **Rhus.* Sabad. Sassap. Seneg. Senn. Sep. *Sil.* Spig. Spong. Squill. Stann. Staph. Stram. Stront. **Sulph.* Teucr. Thuj. Veratr. Viol. od. *Viol. tr.* Zinc.

Close together, *Agar. Sep. Squill. Thuj.

Confluent, Agar. Ant. **Cic.* Hyos. Phos. ac. Val.

Coppery, Alum. °*Ars.* Calc. Cann. °*Carb. an.* Carb. veg. Corall. °*Kreas.* Led. *Mez.* Phosph. °*Rhus.* °Ruta. °Veratr.
On covered parts, Led. Thuj.
Cutting, Lyc.
Dry, Alum. Ars. **Baryt. Bov.* *Bry. **Calc.* Carb. veg. Caust. Clem. Cocc. *Cupr. Dulc.* Evon. *Graph.* Heracl. Hyos. Kreas. Led. Lyc. Magn. c. **Merc.* **Mez.* Natr. Natr. m. Par. *Petr. Phosph.* Phos. ac. Rhus. Sassap. **Sep.* **Sil.* Stann. **Staph.* Sulph. Teucr. Val. **Veratr. Viol. tr.* Zinc.
Excoriated, as if, Graph.
Fine, Agar. Alum. *Ars.* Bell. Bry. **Carb. veg.* Caust. Clem. Cocc. Con. Dulc. Graph. Hep. Jod. Ipec. Kreas. Led. Merc. Mez. Natr. m. Nitr. ac. N. vom. Par. Phosph. Phos. ac. Puls. Rhus. Sassap. Sulph. Val. Zinc.
Fiery-red, **Acon.* Bell. Stram. °*Sulph.*
Flat, *Amm.* Ang. *Ant. Ars. Asa. Bell.* Carb. an. Euphorb. *Lach. Lyc.* Merc. *Natr.* Nitr. ac. Petr. Phosph. *Phos. ac.* Puls. Ran. *Selen. Sep. Sil.* Staph. Sulph. Tart. Thuj.
Furfuraceous, Agar.
Granular, Amm. **Ars.* °*Carb. veg.* Graph. *Hep.* Natr. m. Phosph. Tab. Zinc.
Grape-shaped, Agar. **Calc.* Rhus. Staph. Veratr.
On hairy parts of the body, Kal. Lyc. *Merc. Natr. m.* Nitr. ac. Phos. ac. *Rhus.*
Hard, Ant. Aur. Mez. Ran. Rhus. Spig. Val.
Herpetic, Amm. *Anac.* Ipec. **Rhus.* Sep.
Horny, **Ant. Ran.*
Humid, Alum. Ars. Baryt. Bell. *Bov.* Bry. **Calc.* Carb. an. **Carb. veg.* Caust. **Cic.* **Clem.*

Con. Daph. Dulc. **Graph.* °*Grat.?* Hell. Hep. Heracl. **Kal.* Kreas. Lach. Led. **Lyc.* **Merc.* **Mez.* *Natr.* Natr. m. Nitr. ac. Oleand. Petr. Phosph. Phos. ac. **Rhus.* Ruta. Sabin. *Selen.* **Sep.* Sil. Squill. **Staph.* **Sulph.* Sulph. ac. Tarax. Thuj. Viol. tr.

Inflamed, Ars. Calc.

Itching, **Acon.* **Agar.* Agn. Alum. Amb. **Amm.* Amm. m. Anac. **Ant.* Arg. Arn. **Ars.* Asa. Baryt. Bell. Bov. **Bry.* *Calad.* **Calc.* Canth. Caps. Carb. an. Carb. veg. **Caust.* Cham. Chel. Cic. Cin. **Clem.* Cocc. Coff. Con. Cupr. Dig. Dulc. Graph. Hep. Heracl. *Ign.* Ipec. **Kal.* Kreas. *Lach.* Laur. *Led.* Lyc. Magn. art. Magn. arct. Magn. aust. Magn. c. Magn. m. Mang. **Merc.* Mercurial. **Mez.* Natr. Natr. m. Nitr. **Nitr. ac.* N. vom. **Oleand.* *Par.* Petr. Phosph. Phos. ac. Plumb. Puls. *Ran.* Ran. sc. **Rhus.* Sabad. Sabin. Sassap. *Selen.* **Sep.* *Sil.* Spig. Spong. *Squill.* Stann. **Staph.* Stram. Stront. **Sulph.* Tarax. Tart. Tax. Teucr. Thuj. Val. **Veratr.* *Viol. tr.* Zinc.

Itch-like, **Merc.* Sabad.

Marbled, Phosph.

Miliary, **Agar.* Amm. Ars. Cocc. Kreas. *Led.* N. vom. Par. Val.

Like nettlerash, °*Acon.* Amm. Amm. m. *Ant.* Anthroc. **Ars.* Baryt. *Bell.* **Bry.* **Calc.* Carb. an. **Carb. veg.* **Caust.* Chin. Cic. Cocc. **Con.* Cop. **Dulc.* Frag. Graph. **Hep.* °*Ign.* Ipec. Kal. Kreas. Lach. Led. *Lyc.* Magn. c. Merc. *Mez.* Natr. *Natr. m.* Nitr. ac. N. vom. °*Petr.* Phosph. Phos. ac. *Puls.* **Rhus.* Ruta.

Sec. Selen. *Sep.* Sil. Staph. Stram. *Sulph.* Tart. Thuj. °Urtic. Val. *Veratr.* Zinc.

Obstinate, incurable, Alum. **Amm.* **Baryt.* **Borax.* **Calc.* Carb. veg. Caust. *Cham.* Chel. *Clem.* *Con.* Croc. **Euphorb.* **Graph.* Hell. **Hep.* Kal. Lach. Lyc. Magn. c. Mang. Merc. Mur. ac. *Natr.* *Nitr. ac.* N. vom. Oleand. Par. **Petr.* Phosph. Phos. ac. Plumb. *Rhus.* Sep. **Sil.* Squill. Staph. **Sulph.* Tarax. *Viol. tr.* °*Zinc.*

Painful, *Agar.* Amb. *Ant.* Arg. *Arn.* **Ars.* *Asa.* Aur. Baryt. *Bell.* Calc. Cann. Canth. Caps. *Chin.* *Clem.* Cocc. *Con.* *Cupr.* *Dulc.* Guaj. *Hep.* Kal. Kal. chl. **Lach.* Led. **Lyc.* Magn-arct. Magn. aust. *Magn. c.* *Magn. m.* *Merc.* Natr. *N. vom.* Par. *Petr.* *Phosph. *Phos. ac.* *Puls.* Ran. Ran. sc. Rhus. Ruta. Selen. Seneg. *Sep.* *Sil.* *Spig.* Spong. Stram. Sulph. Tart. Thuj. Val. *Veratr.* Verb.

Painful as if ulcerated, Amm. Amm. m. Ant. Ars. Baryt. Caps. Caust. Con. Graph. Laur. Kal. Mang. Merc. Phosph. Puls. Rhus. Sep. Sil. Staph. Sulph. Tarax. Zinc.

Painless, *Amb.* *Anac.* Ant. Bell. Cham. *Cocc.* *Con.* Cycl. Dros. *Hell.* ***Hyos.*** Lach. Laur. *Lyc.* Nitr. *Oleand.* Phosph. *Phos. ac.* Puls. Rhus. Samb. *Sec.* Spig. Staph. *Stram.* *Sulph.* Tart.

Pale, colourless, Ars.

Peeling off, °*Acon.* °*Amm.* *Amm. m.* Ars. Aur **Bell.* Clem. Cupr. Dulc. Hell. Lach. **Led.* Magn. c. Merc. Mez. Oleand. Phell. °*Phosph.* Phos. ac. Puls. Ran. Sec. °*Sep.* °*Sil.* °*Staph.* Sulph. Teucr. Veratr.

Phagedænic, Alum. Amm. *Baryt. Borax. Calc.* Carb. veg. Caust. Cham. Chel. *Clem. Con.* Croc. *Graph.* Hell. *Hep.* Kal. Lach. Lyc. Magn. c. Mang. Merc. Mur. ac. *Natr. Nitr. ac.* N. vom. Oleand. Par. *Petr.* Phosph. Phos. ac. Plumb. *Rhus. Sep. Sil. Squill. Staph.* Sulph. Tarax. Viol. tr.

Purulent, **Ant.* Ars. Bell. **Cic.* Clem. Coccul. Con. Cycl. *Dulc.* Euphr. Hep. Kal. Led. *Lyc.* Magn. art. Magn. c. *Merc. Natr.* Natr. m. Petr. Plumb. Puls. **Rhus.* Samb. Sassap. Sec. *Sep.* Sil. Spig. *Staph.* Sulph. Tarax. Tart. Thuj. Veratr. Viol. od. Viol. tr. Zinc. (Comp.: PUSTULES, and HUMID.)

Raised, Ars. Asa. Calc. Caust. Dulc. Lach. Merc. Mez. N. vom. Oph. Op. Phosph. Sulph. Tab. Tax. Val.

Red, **Acon.* **Agar.* Agn. Alum. Amb. **Amm.* Amm. m. Ant. **Arn.* **Ars.* Aur. Baryt. *Bell.* Bov. Bry. Calad. *Calc.* Cann. Canth. Caps. Carb. an. Carb. veg. Caust. Cham. Chin. Cic. **Clem.* *Cocc.* Coff. **Con.* Croc. Croton. Cupr. *Cycl.* Dros. **Dulc.* *Graph.* Hep. Hyos. Jod. Ipec. **Kal.* Kreas. **Lach.* Led. Lyc. Magn. art. Magn. arct. *Magn. c.* Magn. m. **Merc.* Mez. Natr. Natr. m. Nitr. *Nitr. ac.* N. vom. Op. Par. Petr. **Phosph.* *Phos. ac.* Plumb. Puls. Rhod. *Rhus.* Ruta. *Sabad.* Sec. **Sep.* *Sil.* Spong. Stann. Staph. **Stram.* **Sulph.* **Sulph. ac.* Tab. Tart. Tax. Teucr. Val. Veratr. Vip. torv. Zinc. (Comp.: Coppery, ERYSIPELAS, and SCARLATINA.)

Like red spots, *Veratr.* Dig.

With red areolæ, Anac.

Rough, Anac. Phosph. Sep.
Sandy, Ars.
Sarcomatous, Ars.
Scaly, Agar. *Amm.* Amm. m. Anac. Ant. Ars. *Aur.* Bar. m. Bell. Cic. **Clem.* Cupr. Dulc. *Hep.* Hyos. Kal. *Led. Magn. c. Merc.* **Oleand.* **Phosph.* Plumb. Rhus. Sep. Staph. *Sulph.*
Scurfy, Ars. Electr. Mang. Phos. ac. Sep. (Comp.: SCURF.)
Shining through, Cin. *Merc.* Ran.
Smarting, Agn. Alum. Amm. Amm. m. Ant. Arn. Ars. Bell. Borax. Bov. Bry. Calc. Camph. Canth. Caps. Carb. an. Carb. veg. Caust. Cham. Chel. Chin. Cocc. *Colch.* Coloc. Con. Dros. *Euphorb.* Hell. *Ipec. Lach. Led.* Lyc. Magn. arct. Magn. aust. Magn. c. Mang. Merc. *Mez.* Mur. ac. Natr. Natr. m. N. vom. *Oleand.* Op. Petr. Phosph. Phos. ac. Plat. *Puls.* Ran. Ran. sc. Rhod. Selen. Sil. Spig. *Spong.* Stront. Sulph. Thuj. Veratr. Viol. tr.
Sore, as if excoriated, Acon. Agar. *Alum.* Amb. Ant. *Arg.* Ars. *Aur.* Baryt. *Bry. Calc.* Cann. Canth. Caps. Carb. an. Caust. Chel. Cin. *Cic.* Coff. *Colch. Dros.* Ferr. **Graph.* Hell. **Hep.* Ign. Kal. Lyc. Magn. art. Magn. aust. Magn. c. Mang. Merc. Mez. Natr. *Natr. m. Nitr. ac.* N. vom. Oleand. *Par. Petr.* Phosph. *Phos. ac. Puls.* Ran. **Rhus.* Rhus v. Ruta. Sabin. Sassap. Selen. *Sep.* Sil. *Spig.* Spong. *Squill.* Staph. *Sulph.* Tab. Teucr. Val. Veratr. Zinc.
Stinging, Acon. Alum. Amm. m. Anac. Ant. Arn. *Ars.* Asa. *Baryt. Bell.* Berb. Bov. Bry. Calc. Camph. Canth. Caps. Carb. veg. Caust. Cham. Chin. *Clem.* Cocc. Con. *Cycl.* Dig.

Dros. Graph Guaj. Hell. *Hep.* Ign. Kal. Kreas. *Led.* *Lyc. Magn. art. Magn. arct. Magn. c. *Merc.* Mez. **Mur. ac.* Natr. Natr. m. *Nitr. ac.* N. vom. Petr. Phosph. **Phos. ac.* *Plat.* *Puls.* *Ran.* Ran. sc. *Rhus.* Sabad. *Sabin.* Selen. *Sep.* **Sil.* Spong. Squill. **Staph.* Stront. *Sulph.* Thuj. Verb. *Viol. tr.* Zinc.

With swelling, Acon. Amm. Arn. Ars. **Bell.* *Bry.* *Calc.* *Canth.* Carb. veg. Caust. Chin. Cic. Clem. Con. Euphorb. Hep. **Kal.* Lyc. Magn. c. **Merc.* Natr. Natr. m. Nitr. ac. Petr. Phosph. Phos. ac. **Puls.* **Rhus.* Ruta. *Samb.* Sassap. *Sep.* Sil. *Stram.* **Sulph.* Thuj.

Tearing, Kal.

Tight, Alum. *Arn.* Baryt. Bell. Canth. Carb. an. **Caust.* Cocc. Con. Hep. Kal. Mez. Oleand. *Phosph.* Puls. **Rhus.* Sabin. Sep. Spong. Staph. *Stront.* Sulph. Tart. Thuj.

Twitching, painful, Asa. Calc. *Caust.* Cham. Chin. Cupr. Lyc. *Puls.* *Rhus.* Sep. Sil. *Staph.* Vip. torv.

Ulcerated, Ars. Caps. Carb. an. Chin. Squill. (Comp.: ULCERATION.)

As after vaccination, °Sulph.

Like varicella, °*Led.*

Whitish, Agar. Ant. **Ars.* Borax. Bov. Bry. Ipec. Merc. Phosph. *Puls.* Sulph. Tart. Thuj. Val. Zinc.

Yellowish, *Agar.* Ant. Ars. Aur. Bar. m. **Cic.* Croc. Cupr. *Euphorb.* Hell. Kreas. Led. Lyc. **Merc.* *Natr.* *Nitr. ac.* Par. Phos. ac. *Sep.* Val.

Like a zone, Ars. Bry. Cham. °*Graph.* °*Merc.* Natr. °*Puls.* °*Rhus.* Selen. *Sil.* Sulph.

Head, °*Baryt.* Bar. m. **Calc.* °*Carb. an.* Cic. °*Clem.* **Lyc.* **Merc.* **Oleand.* *Petr. *Rhus. Ruta.* Spig. *Staph.

Eyes, *Ars.* Calc. **Caust.* Con. °*Euphr.* Hell. *Hep.* Ign. **Kal. Merc.* Oleand. Par. Petr. Rhus. °*Selen.* Seneg. Sep. Sil. Spong. **Staph.* **Sulph.* Thuj.

Eyebrows, Clem. Cupr. Guaj. Kal. Par. Selen. Sil. Spong. Stann. Tarax.

Ears, Amm. m. Ant. Agar. **Baryt.* Bov. **Calc.* Chin. **Cic.* Kal. Mez. Mosch. Mur. ac. Natr. m. Petr. Phosph. Puls. Sep. Sil. Spong. Staph. **Sulph.*

—, lobes, Sassap. Teucr.

—, behind the ears, Ant. **Baryt.* **Calc.* Canth. Chin. **Cic.* Graph. *Hep.* Mez. Oleand. **Puls.* Sabad. Selen. Sil. °*Staph.*

—, in front of the ears, **Cic.*

Nose, in general, Calc. Carb. veg. Croton. Nicc. Sassap. Spong.

—, about the nose, Alum. Canth. Caps. Chin. Magn. arct. Natr. Rhus. Spig. Tarax.

—, on the nose, Ant. °*Aur.* Caust. Graph.

—, on the wings, Carb. veg. Con. Dulc. Euphr. Lam. Natr. Petr. Rhus. Sil. Thuj. Veratr.

—, in the nose, Ant. Arn. Canth. Carb. an. Cic. Cocc. Guaj. Lach. Magn. c. Nitr. Phell. Ran. Selen. **Sil.* Spig.

—, at the tip, Carb. an. Carb. veg. °*Caust.* Nitr. ac. Phos. ac. *Sep.* Sil. Spong.

—, in the corners, Anac. Dulc. Euphr. Mang. Plumb. Rhus. Thuj.

—, UNDER the nose, Arn. Baryt. Bov. Caps. Squill. Teucr.

Face in general, Agar. Agn. Alum. Amb. **Amm.* Amm. m. Ant. Arg. Arn. Ars. **Aur.* **Baryt.* Bell. Borax. Bov. Bry. **Calc.* Calend. Cann. Canth. Caps. Carb. an. **Carb. veg.* Caust. Cham. Chel. **Cic.* Clem. Cocc. **Con.* **Crotal.* Dig. **Dulc.* Electr. Euphorb. Ferr. magn. **Graph.* Hell. **Hep.* Hyos. °Ign. Kal. **Kreas.* Lach. Laur. Led. **Lyc.* Magn. arct. Magn. c. **Magn. m.* Magn. s. Mang. Merc. °Mur. ac. Natr. **Natr. m.* Nitr. **Nitr. ac.* N. vom. Oleand. Par. Petr. Phosph. **Phos. ac.* Puls. Rhus. Ruta. Sabad. Sabin. Sassap. Selen. **Sep.* Sil. Spong. Staph. Stront. **Sulph.* Sulph. ac. Tarax. Thuj. Veratr. Viol. tr. Zinc.

Lips and mouth, region of, **Ars.* Bov. **Calc.* Caps. Carb. veg. Cann. Chin. Chinin. Dig. Electr. Graph. °Hell. Hep. Ipec. Lach. Lyc. Mez. Mur. ac. *Natr.* Natr. m. Nicc. Nitr. ac. Petr. Phosph. *Phos. ac. Sep. Sil.* Spong. Squill. Sulph. Tab.

—, corners of mouth, Ant. **Bell.* **Calc.* Cann. Canth, Carb. veg. **Graph.* Hep. **Ign.* Magn. arct. **Merc.* Natr. °Nitr. ac. Petr. Rhod. Rhus. Sep. Tarax. °*Veratr.*

Chin, Agn. Alum. Amb. Amm. Anac. Ant. Bell. Borax. *Bov. Calc. Canth. Caust. *Chel.* Cic. Clem. Con. Dig. Dulc. **Graph.* *Hep.* Hyos. Kal. °*Lach.* *Lyc.* Magn. arct. Magn. aust. Magn. c. Merc. Mez. Natr. Natr. m. Nitr. ac. N. mosch. N. vom. Oleand. *Par.* Phosph. Phos. ac. Plat. Puls. **Rhus.* Sabin. Sassap. Sep. *Sil. Spig. Spong. Squill. Stront. Sulph. Tarax. Thuj. *Veratr.* Verb. Zinc.

Lower jaw, region of, Canth. °Graph. Par. Rhus. Veratr.
Abdomen and stomach, Bell. Bry. Merc.
Anal region, Calc. Carb. veg. Ipec. Lyc.
Sexual parts, N. vom. Rhus. °*Sep.* Sulph. Tart.
—, glans, Petr. Sep.
—, scrotum, Graph. Rhus.
—, mons veneris, Sil.
—, labia, N. vom. °*Sep.* Tart.
—, vagina, Sulph.
—, prepuce, Merc. Rhus.
Thoracic region, Heracl. Kal. *Led.* °*Lyc.* *Merc.* Mercurial. Mez. *Rhus.* °*Sec.* Tereb. Val.
Dorsal region, Ant. Ars. Bry. *Cinn.* **Lyc.* Magn. aust. Staph. Tart.
—, shoulders, Ars.
—, loins, Clem. Rhus.
—, cervia, Bry. Carb. an. Carb. veg. Caust. Cham. Clem. Nitr. °Petr. •Sec.
—, back, Alum. Baryt. Bry. °Carb. veg. Evon. Lach. Led. Merc. Mercurial. Natr. m. °Sep. Squill.
—, scapular region, Ant. Caust. Lach. Phos. ac.
—, arms, Alum. Berb. Bry. *Carb. an.* **Caust.* Lach. Led. Lyc. *Merc.* Phosph. Rhus. Sabin. Tart. Tax. Val. Zinc.
—, shoulder, Alum. Berb.
—, arm, °Caust. Rhus. Tart. Val.
—, upper arm, Led. Vip. torv.
—, elbow, *Merc.* Phosph. *Sabin.* Zinc.
—, forearm, Bry. *Carb. an.* *Caust.* Lach. Lyc. *Tax.* Zinc.

Hands, Alum. **Carb. veg.* Dig. *Hep.* Ipec. **Merc. Mur. ac. Nitr. ac.* Spig. *Sulph. Sulph. ac.*
—, wrist, Hep.
—, fingers, Caust. Corall. Galv. Graph. Mez.
Lower limbs, Hyos. Staph.
—, hips and nates, Borax. Natr. *Sulph.*
—, thigh, Alum. Calc. Cann. Caust. Merc.
—, knee, Anac. Ant. Bry. Carb. veg. Kal. *Led.* Merc. N. vom. Tereb.
—, legs, Agar. *Petr. Rhus.*
—, feet, Carb. an. *Graph. Led.* Rhus. Sulph. Tereb.
—, walking, Petr.

Eruptions, sanguineous.

In general, **Arn.* **Ars.* Aur. **Bell.* Berb. **Bry.* **Calc.* Canth. °Carb. an.? °Carb. veg.? Cham. Chin. °Clem.? Cocc. Con. Crotal. Dulc. Electr. Euphr. Ferr. °Hep. Hyos. °Kreas.? **Lach.* Laur. Led. °Lyc. °Merc. Natr. m. °Nitr. ac. N. mosch. *N. vom.* Oph. Par. Plumb. **Phosph.* Puls. **Rhus.* **Ruta.* **Sec.* °Sep. **Sil.* Stram. °Staph.? **Sulph.* **Sulph. ac.* °Tart. °Thuj.?
Blisters, vesicles, **Ars.* Aur. Bry. Canth. *Natr. m. Sec.* Sulph.
Pimples, *Ars.
Spots, **Arn.* Ars. Bell. Berb. °*Bry.* °*Calc.* Cham. Chin. °*Con.* Crotal. Dulc. Electr. Euphr. Ferr. °*Hep.* Lach. Laur. Led. Natr. Natr. m. **N. vom.* Oph. Par. Phell. **Phosph.* Plumb. °*Puls.* **Rhus.* Ruta. *Sec.* Sil. Stram. **Sulph.* **Sulph. ac.*
Tumours, Arn. Bry. Sec.

Head, °Ars.
Eyes, °*Calc.* °*N. vom.*
Nose, Sep.
Face, Stram.
Lips, °*Natr. m.*
Lower jaw, Par.
Back, Phell.
Arms, Berb. Sec.
Hands, *Berb.*
Lower limbs, Phosph.

Erysipelas.

In general, **Acon.* Amm. Amm. m. Anthrok. *Ant. Arn. Ars.* Baryt. **Bell. Borax.* **Bry.* Calc. **Camph.* Canth. **Carb. an.* Carb. veg. Caust. **Cham.* Chin. Chinin.? Clem. °*Crotal.* °*Dulc. Euphorb.* **Graph.* **Hep.* Hyos. *Jod.* Ipec. Kal. **Lach. Lyc.* Magn. c. Mang. **Merc.* Mur. ac. Natr. Natr. m. °*Nitr. ac.* Oph. Petr. **Phosph.* **Phos. ac.* Plumb. **Puls.* Ran. *Rhus.* Ruta. *Sabad. Samb.* Sassap. Sep. *Sil.* Spong. Stann. Staph. Stram. **Sulph.* Thuj. Vip. red. Zinc.
Boring, Euphorb.
Burning, Ars. Carb. veg. Petr. Phosph. Rhod. **Rhus.*
Creeping, Euphorb. **Rhus.*
Digging, Euphorb.
Gnawing, Euphorb.
Gangrenous, Acon. **Ars. Bell.* Camph. Chin. *Chinin.* Hyos. Lach. Mur. ac. Rhus. *Sabin.* Sec. Sil.
Hard, Sulph.

Inflamed, **Acon.* Ars. **Bell. Borax.* **Bry.* Camph. **Cham.* **Hep.* **Lach.* **Merc. Petr.* **Phosph.* **Puls.* **Rhus.* Sabad. **Sulph.* Zinc.
Itching, Euphorb. **Rhus.*
Peeling off, with, °Dulc. Puls. Rhus.
Stinging, Graph. Phosph. Puls. Rhus. Sulph.
Suppurating, Merc. Phosph.
Swollen, °*Acon.* Amm. °*Arn. Ars.* **Bell.* Bry. *Calc.* Canth. Carb. veg. Caust. *Chin.* Euphorb. Hell. °*Hep. Kal. Lyc.* Magn. c. **Merc.* Ruta. Samb. Sassap. Sep. Sil. Sulph. Thuj. *Zinc.*
Tensive, Rhus.
Vesicular, *Ars.* °*Bell.* Cist. *Euphorb.* °*Graph.* Hep. °*Lach.* Phosph. °*Puls.* Ran. *Ran. **Rhus.* Sep. Sulph.
Zone-shaped, °*Ars.* °*Graph.* °*Puls.* °*Rhus.*

Ears, Lach. Meph.
Nose, Canth. Plumb.
Face, **Bell.* Borax. Calc. Camph. Canth. °*Carb. an.* °Cham. Cist. Crotal. Euphorb. Gins. **Graph.* °Hep. **Lach.* Nitr. ac. °Puls. **Rhus.* Ruta. °Sep. Stram. °Sulph.
Abdomen, °*Graph.*
Mammæ and nipples, °Cham. **Phosph. Sulph.*
Dorsal region, Cist. °Graph. °Merc. °Rhus.
Arms, Petr. **Rhus.*
Hands, Graph. Rhod.
Lower limbs, legs, Borax. *Calc. Hep. Puls.* °*Sulph.*
—. tendo Achilles, Zinc.
Feet, °*Puls.* °*Rhus.*

Excoriating and Spreading, which is.

Blennorrhœas and expectoration, **Alum.* **Amm.* **Amm. m.* Anac. Ant. **Ars.* **Borax*, Bov. Calc. Cann. Canth. Carb. an. *Carb. veg. Cham.* Chin. *Con.* Euphorb. **Ferr.* Hep. *Ign. Jod.* Kal. Kal. hdr. *Kreas. Lach.* Lyc. Magn. arct. Magn. c. *Magn. m.* Mang. **Merc. Mez.* Mur. ac. **Natr. m. Nitr. ac.* °*N. vom.* **Phosph.* Phos. ac. Prun. **Puls. Ran.* °Ruta. **Sep.* **Sil. Spig. Squill.* **Sulph. Sulph. ac.* Thuj.

Blotches, Lach. °Sulph.

Blisters, vesicles, Amm. °*Ars.* Borax. Caust. °*Cham.* °*Clem.* °*Graph. Hep Kal. Magn. c.* Merc. °Natr. *Nitr. ac.* Oph. Petr. °*Sep.* **Sil.* Sulph.

Blood, Amm. Ars. Baryt. Bov. Canth. Carb. veg. Graph. Hep. *Kal. Nitr.* Rhus. Sassap. *Sil.* Sulph. Sulph. ac. Zinc.

Eruption, Alum. Amm. *Baryt. Borax. Calc.* Carb. veg. Caust. *Cham.* Chel. *Clem. Con.* Croc. *Graph.* Hell. *Hep.* Kal. Lach. Lyc. Magn. c. Mang. Merc. Mur. ac. *Natr. Nitr. ac.* N. vom. Oleand. Par. *Petr.* Phosph. Phos. ac. Plumb. *Rhus. Sep. Sil. Squill. Staph.* Sulph. Tarax. Viol. tr.

Erysipelas, Euphorb.

Herpes, °Alum. Caps. **Merc.* (Comp.: Scurfs spreading.)

Pus, Amm. Anac. **Ars.* Bell. Calc. *Carb. veg* **Caust.* Cham. Chel. Clem. Con. Cupr. Graph *Hep.* Ign. Jod. Kreas. Lach. *Lyc.* **Merc.* Mez Natr. Natr. m. *Nitr. ac.* N. vom. Phosph Plumb. Puls. *Ran.* Ran. sc. **Rhus.* Ruta

Sep. **Sil.* Spig. Squill. Staph. Sulph. Sulph. ac. Zinc.

Scurfs, crusts, Mang.

Ulcers, Amm. Anac. **Ars.* *Bell.* Borax. Calc. **Carb. veg.* *Caust.* °*Cham.* °*Chel.* °*Clem.* Con. Cupr. °*Graph.* *Hep.* Ign. Jod. *Kal.* Kreas. °*Lach.* °*Lyc.* Magn. c. **Merc.* *Mercurial.* Mez. °*Natr.* Natr. m. **Nitr. ac.* N. vom. Oph. **Petr.* Phosph. Plumb. *Puls.* **Ran.* **Ran. sc.* °*Rhus.* Ruta. °*Sep.* **Sil.* Spig. °*Squill.* Staph. °*Sulph.* *Sulph. ac.* Zinc.

Head, eruptions, ulcers, &c., °*Ars.* Caps. **Rhus.*

Ears, herpes, *Merc.*

Lips, Bell. *Mang.* Nitr. ac. Plat.

Buccal cavity, ulcers, *Merc.* Nitr. ac.

Sexual parts, ulcers, **Merc.*

Nipples, scurfs, °Lyc.

Hands, Ran. Rhus. Veratr.

Lower limbs, ulcers, Merc.

Feet, eruption, Sulph.

—, ulcers, °*Ars.* Caust. Con. °*Graph.* °*Natr.* Nitr. ac. °*Petr.* Selen. °*Sep.* *Sil.*

Excrescences.

n general, Acon. Agar. Agn. Alum. Amb. Amm. **Ant.* Arn. **Ars.* *Aur.* **Bell.* Bry. **Calc.* **Carb. an.* **Carb. veg.* **Caust.* Cic. **Clem.* *Cocc.* Colch. Dig. Euphr. **Graph.* *Hep.* *Jod.* Kal. Kreas. *Lach.* **Lyc.* Magn. aust. Men. Merc. Mez. Natr. *Natr. m.* **Nitr.*

ac. *N. vom.* Petr. *Phosph.* Phos. ac. *Plumb.* *Puls.* °Ran. Rhod. *Rhus.* Sabad. *Sabin.* Selen. Sep. **Sil.* Spong. Stann. **Staph.* **Sulph.* Sulph. ac. *Tart.* **Thuj.* Zinc.

Arthritic, s. ARTHRITIC.

Bloodvessels, of, s. BLOODVESSELS, SWELLING OF.

Callous, s. CALLOSITIES.

Chilblains, s. CHILBLAINS.

Comedones, Aur. Bry. Calc. Graph. °*Natr.* Natr. m. Nitr. ac. Plumb. Sabin. **Selen.* Sulph.

Corns, s. CORNS.

Disorganization of skin, °Ant.

Fleshy. **Staph.* **Thuj.*

Ganglia, s. GANGLIA.

Hangnails, s. NAILS.

Horny, **Ant.* °*Ran.* Sulph.

Humid, Nitr. ac.

Lupia, s. LUPIA.

Moles, °*Calc.* Carb. veg. Graph. Nitr. ac. Petr. Phos. ac. Sil. °*Sulph.* Sulph. ac.

Painful, Spig.

Polypi, s. POLYPI.

Proud flesh, s. ULCERS.

Red, **Thuj.*

Smooth, **Thuj.*

Spongy, s. SPONGY.

Sycosic, s. FIGWARTS.

Warty, s. WARTS.

Ears, spongy, Merc.

Buccal cavity, Merc. **Staph.* °*Thuj.* ?

Sexual parts, °Cinn. °Euphr. °*Lyc.* Magn. aust. °*Nitr. ac.* **Phos. ac.* *Sabin.* °Staph. °*Thuj.*

Sexual parts, corona glandis, Nitr. ac. Phos. ac. Staph. *Thuj.
—, os tincæ, °Thuj.
—, prepuce, *Nitr. ac. Sabin.
Feet, soles, **Ant.* (Puls.)
—, toes, **Ant.* Spig.

Exsudations, bloody.

In general, Arn. **Calc.* Cham. Clem. Cocc. *Crotal. Lach.* N. mosch. **N. vom. Oph.*
Eyes, °*Calc.* **N. vom.*

Eyebrows.

Burning, Asa. Dig. Dros. Merc. Spig.
Contracted skin, Bry. Hell.
Creeping, Croc. Ran.
Eruption, Clem. Cupr. Guaj. Kal. Par. Selen. Sil. Spong. Stann. Tarax.
Falling off of the lashes, *Agar.* Plumb. °*Selen.* (Bell. Caust. Hell. Kal. Par.)?
Figwarts, °*Thuj.*
Itching, Agar. Agn. Alum. Caust. Chin. Laur. Magn. arct. Par. Selen. Sil. Spig. Sulph. Viol. tr.
Swelling, *Kal.
Warts, **Caust.*

Eyes and Region of.

Bleeding, **Bell.* °Carb. veg. °Cham. Crotal. °Euphr. °N. vom. Ruta.

Bloated, *Ars.* Bry. Cham. Ferr. **Kal.* *N.* vom. Oleand. **Phosph.* Puls. Rhab. Ruta. **Sep.*

Bloody sweat, °Calc. **N. vom.*

Blotches, Sassap.

Blueness of whites, Veratr.

Burning, **Acon.* Aeth. Agar. Agn. Alum. Amm. *Amm. m.* Ang. *Arn.* **Ars.* *Asa.* **Asar.* Aur. Baryt. **Bell.* Berb. Bism. Bov. Bruc. **Bry.* Calad. **Calc.* Cann. Canth. Caps. Carb. an. **Carb. veg.* Cast. Caust. Cham. Chen. Chin. Cic. Cin. Clem. **Coloc.* Con. Corall. **Croc.* **Crotal.* Dig. *Dros.* Eug. **Euphr.* Ferr. Graph. Grat. Hell. Ign. Indig. *Kal.* **Lach.* Lact. *Laur.* Led. **Lyc.* Magn. art. Magn. arct. Magn. c. Magn. m. **Merc.* *Mur. ac.* *Natr.* Natr. m. Nicc. *Nitr.* Nitr. ac. N. mosch. **N. vom.* Ol. an. Par. Petr. Phell. *Phosph.* *Phos. ac.* Plat. Plumb. Puls. Ratanh. *Rhod.* °*Rhus.* Ruta. Sabad. Sassap. Seneg. *Sep.* Sil. Spig. **Spong.* Stann. Stront. Staph. Stram. **Sulph.* Sulph. ac. Tab. *Tarax.* Tart. Therid. Thuj. Tong. Val. Viol. od. Zinc.

Cataract, °Amm. Cann. °Dig. °Magn. c. Phosph. **Puls.* °Sil. *Sulph.*

Cicatrices from wounds, ulcers, °*Euphr.* °*Sil.*

Congestion of vessels, **Acon.* Aeth. **Amb.* Amm. °*Ars.* **Bell.* Bruc. Elect. Eugen. *Kal.* °Lach. Laur. Meph. **Merc.* Phosph. °Phos. ac. Spig. **Sulph.*

Congested vessels, **Acon.* Aeth. *Amb. Amm. °*Ars.* **Bell.* Bruc. Elect. Eugen. *Kal.* °Lach. Laur. Meph. **Merc.* °Phos. ac. Spig. **Sulph.*

Ecchymosis, °*Arn.* °*Bell.* °Calc. Cham. Crotal. **N. vom.* Plumb. Ruta. °Seneg.

Eruption, *Ars.* Calc. **Caust.* Con. °*Euphr.* Hell. ***Hep.*** Ign. **Kal.* *Merc.* Oleand. Par. Petr. Rhus. °*Selen.* Seneg. Sep. Sil. Spong. ****Staph.*** ****Sulph.*** Thuj.

Figwarts, Thuj.

Fungus hæmatodes, °Bell. ? °Calc. °Lyc. °Sep. °Sil.

Fungus medullaris, °Bell.

Herpes, °***Bry.*** Rhus. Sep.

Inflammation, ****Acon.*** Amb. Amm. ****Ant.*** °***Arn.*** **Ars.* Asar. Aur. ****Baryt.*** Bar. m. ****Bell.*** Borax. Bov. Bruc. ****Bry.*** ****Calc.*** Camph. °***Cann.*** Canth. Caps. Carb. veg. ****Caust.*** ****Cham.*** °***Chin.*** Cinn. ****Clem.*** °*Coloc.* Con. ***Cupr.*** Daph. ****Dig.*** ****Dulc.*** Eugen. Euphorb. Ferr. Galv. ****Graph.*** ****Hep.*** Hyos. °***Ign.*** Jod. ***Ipec.*** ***Kal.*** ****Lach.*** Led. ****Lyc.*** Magn. art. Magn. aust. Magn. c. Magn. m. ****Merc.*** Merc. corr. Mez. Mosch. **Natr.* ****Natr.*** *m.* Nitr. ac. **N. vom.* Ol. an. Op. °***Petr.*** ****Phosph.*** ****Phos. ac.*** Plumb. ****Puls.*** Ran. Ratanh. ****Rhus.*** Sabad. Sassap. ****Sep.*** ****Sil.*** °***Spig.*** Stann. Staph. ****Sulph.*** °***Sulph. ac.*** Tarax. Teucr. °***Thuj.*** °***Val.*** ***Veratr.*** Zinc.

Injuries, after, °***Arn.*** °Con. °***Hep.*** °***Puls.*** °Ruta. °*Sulph. ac.*

Itching, ***Agar.*** ***Alum.*** Amm. Ars. ***Asa.*** ***Baryt.*** Bell. Bov. ****Calc.*** Canth. Carb. an. Carb. veg. ***Caust.*** ***Chel.*** Con. Coloc. Cupr. ***Cycl.*** Ferr. ***Ign.*** Lach. Laur. Magn. art. Magn. arct. Magn. aust. Magn. c. ***Magn. m.*** ***Merc.*** Mosch. ***Mur. ac.*** ***Natr.*** ***Natr. m.*** Oleand. Petr. Phosph. Plat. ****Puls.*** Ran. Rhod. Sep. ****Sil.*** ***Spig.*** Squill. Stann. Stront. ****Sulph.*** Zinc.

Livid, whites, Plumb.

Pellicle, Cann. Chel. °*Euphr.* °Lach. Puls. °Ruta.
Petechiæ, °*Bell.* Calc. °*N. vom.* Ruta. °Seneg.
Pimples, Baryt. Chel. Guaj. Hep. Ign. Mosch. Par. Selen. ***Staph.*** Tarax. Thuj.
Purulent gum, Plumb.
Pustules, **Merc.* **Sep.*
Redness, ***Acon.*** Aeth. Agar. Alum. Amb. Amm. Amm. m. Ang. **Ant.* °*Arn.* **Ars.* °*Asar.* °Aur. Baryt. **Bell.* *Bism.* Borax. Bov. Bruc. ***Bry.*** **Calc.* Camph. Caps. Caust. **Cham.* Chel. ***Chin.*** Clem. Con. Crotal. Croton. *Cupr.* Dig. Electr. Eugen. °*Euphr.* Ferr. Galv. Gent. **Graph.* Grat. Hell. Hep. Hyos. °Ign. Jod. Ipec. *Kal.* Kal. chl. Kal. hdr. Kreas. °*Lach.* *Led.* Lyc. Magn. c. Magn. m. °*Meph.* **Merc.* Mosch. Mur. ac. Natr. m. Nicc. Nitr. *Nitr. ac.* °*N. vom.* Op. **Phosph.* Phos. ac. Plumb. ***Puls.*** Ran. sc. Rhus. Sassap. ***Sep.*** ***Sil.*** ***Spig.*** ***Spong.*** Staph. Stann. *Stram.* *Stront.* **Sulph.* Sulph. ac. Tab. Tart. Teucr. *Thuj.* Val. Veratr. Viol. od. Zinc.
Red spots, Phos. ac. *Puls.*
—, lids, Camph. Sil.
Red streaks, N. vom. Sassap.
Scurfs, Graph. **Merc.* Sep.
Cornea, vesicles, °*Euphr.*
—, inflammation, °*Euphr.*
—, specks, °Ars. °Aur.? °Calc. °*Cann.* °Cin. °Con.? °*Euphr.* °Gran.? °Hep. ***Nitr. ac.*** °Ruta. °*Seneg.* °Sep. °Sil. °Spig.
—, ulcers. °Ars. °Calc. °*Euphr.* °*Hep.* °Lach. °Merc. Natr. °*Sil.*
—, nets, Plumb.

Cornea, vesicles, obscuration, °Calc. **Cann.* °Chel. °Chin. °Euphorb. ? °*Euphr.* °*Magn. c.* *Nitr. ac. ****Puls.*** °*Sulph.*

Smarting, ****Agar.*** Agn. *Alum.* ***Amb.*** Amm. Ars. Aur. ****Bell.*** Bry. Calc. Camph. Canth. Carb. an. Carb. veg. Cast. Caust. *Chin. Clem.* Colch. **Con.* Croc. ***Dros.*** Eugen. Euphorb. Euphr. ***Graph.*** Hell. Kal. Kal. hdr. Kreas. Lact. Laur. Lyc. Magn. arct. Magn. c. Mang. **Merc.* Mez. Mosch. Mur. ac. Natr. Nicc. Nitr. ac. **N. vom.* Oleand. Ol. an. Par. Petr. Phosph. Phos. ac. Ratanh. ****Ran.*** Ran. sc. Rhab. Rhod. ****Rhus.*** Sabad. Sep. **Sil.* Stann. Staph. Stront. **Sulph. Sulph. ac.* Tart. Teucr. Thuj. *Val. Viol. tr. Zinc.

Spots on the eye, °Aur. °Bell. °Calc. °Cann. °Con. ? °*Euphr.* °*Hep.* °*Nitr. ac.* **N. vom.* Puls. °*Ruta.* °Seneg. °Sil. °*Sulph.*

Suppuration, Bell. Bry. **Caust.* °*Euphr.* Graph. Kal. °Kreas. °*Nitr. ac.* Plat.

Swelling, Ars. Baryt. ****Bry.*** Carb. veg. ****Guaj.*** Hep. Led. ****N. vom.*** Phosph. Plumb. ****Rhus.*** Ruta. Stram. ****Sulph.***

Tubercles, Aur. Bry. Calc. Ran. sc. Thuj.

Ulcers, °***Ars.*** °Calc. °Clem. °*Euphr.* °Hep. °Lach. °***Merc.*** Natr. Ruta. Sil. °*Sulph.*

Ulceration, Amb. Arn. Calc. Caps. Cham. °Clem. **Euphr.* Lyc. Phosph. *Sil.* Staph. **Sulph.*

Vesicles, Amm. m. Bell. Croton. °*Euphr.* Magn. arct. Seneg. **Sulph.*

Warts under the eyes, °*Sulph.*

Watery eye, Magn. c.

Yellowishness of sclerotica, **Acon.* °Amb. Ant. *Ars.* ****Bell.*** °Bry. Calend. Canth °*Cham.*

Chel. °*Chin.* °Cocc. °*Con. Crotal.* **Dig.* °Ferr. Ign. Jod. Magn. m. °*N. vom.* °Op. Phosph. Phos. ac. °*Plumb.* Puls. Rhus. Sep. °Sulph. Thuj. Veratr.
Yellow spots, Phos. ac.

Eyelids.

Bleeding, **Bell.*
Blotches, Aur. Bry. Calc. Ran. sc. Staph. Thuj.
Blueness, °Dig.
Burning, Alum. Amb. Ars. Asar. Bell. Berb. °*Bry.* **Calc.* Caps. *Caust.* Cin. Clem. Coloc. Con. Graph. Kal. Laur. Magn. arct. Magn. aust. Merc. Nitr. °*N. vom.* Oleand. Phell. Phosph. *Phos. ac.* Rhab. Ran. Ran. sc. Rhus. Sassap. *Seneg.* Sep. *Spig.* Spong. Stann. Sulph.
Ecchymosis, °Arn.
Herpes, °*Bry.* Rhus. Sep.
Itching, Agn. Alum. Amb. Amm. m. Ang. Ars. Baryt. **Bell.* **Bry.* **Calc.* Camph. Carb. an. Carb. veg. Caust. Chin. Cin. Cocc. *Croc. Cycl.* Dros. **Euphorb.* Euphr. Ferr. Graph. Jod. Kal. Kal. hdr. Kreas. Laur. Lyc. Magn. art. *Magn. arct. Magn. aust.* Magn. m. *Mez.* Mosch. Mur. ac. *Natr.* Natr. m. Nicc. **N. vom.* Oleand. Par. Petr. *Phosph.* Plat. Puls. *Rhus. Ruta.* Sep. **Sil.* Spong. Staph. **Sulph.* Sulph. ac. Veratr. Zinc.
Indurations, Bry. Ran. sc. °Spig. °Staph.
Inflammation, **Acön.* *Ant. *Arn.* **Ars.* Baryt. **Bell.* **Bry.* **Calc.* Carb. veg. **Caust.* **Cham.* Cinn. Cocc. °*Dig.* Euphorb. Euphr. Graph.

Hep. Hyos. °*Kreas.* Lach. Lyc. Magn. art. Magn. aust. Magn. c. **Merc.* **Natr.* **N. vom.* Phosph. *Phos. ac.* Puls. Rhus. Sassap. **Sep.* Spig. Spong. Staph. **Sulph.* Tarax. Thuj. Val. Veratr. Zinc.

Inflammation, eyelids, **Ars.* **Bry.* Caust. **Cham.* **Clem.* *Dig. **Euphr.* Kal. °Kreas. Lyc. **Merc.* Natr. Phosph. **Puls.* °*Spig.* **Staph.* **Sulph.* °Val.

Pimples, Alum. Canth. Hep. Lyc. Natr. m. Rhus. Selen. Seneg.

Redness, **Acon.* Amm. m. *Ant.* **Ars.* Baryt. **Bell.* Bism. Bry. **Calc.* °*Cann.* °*Cham.* Carb. veg. Caust. **Dig.* Ferr. Graph. Jod. Kal. hdr. Kreos. Lach. **Lyc.* Merc. Mosch. Mur. ac. Natr. m. Nicc. °*N. vom.* Par. Phosph. Phos. ac. Plumb. Puls. Rhod. Sabad. Sep. Spong. Stram. Sulph. Teucr.

Scales, °Bry. Sep.

Scurfs, Graph. Sep.

Smarting, Aur. Camph. Carb. veg. Caust. Clem. Ign. Nitr. Rhus. Spig.

Spots (red), Camph. Sil.

Styes, Alum. °*Amb.* Caust. **Con.* *Dig.* Ferr. **Graph.* Lyc. °*Merc.* Magn. aust. Men. Phos. ac. **Puls.* Rhus. Seneg. Sep. °Staph. Stann. **Sulph.*

Swelling, **Acon.* Agar. Alum. Ang. Arn. Ars. Asar. Aur. Baryt. **Bell.* **Bry.* **Calc.* Caust. °*Chamm.* Cocc. Colch. Cycl. °*Dig.* Euphorb. °*Euphr.* Ferr. °*Graph.* °*Guaj.* Hep. Hyos. °*Ign.* Jod. Kal. °*Kreas.* Lach. Lyc. Magn. aust. Magn. c. Mang. Men. **Merc.* Mosch. Mur ac. Natr. Natr. m. Nitr. ac. **N. vom.* Op.

Phosph. **Puls*. Rhod. **Rhus*. Ruta. Seneg. **Sep*. Sil. Spong. Squill. Stram. **Sulph*. Teucr. **Thuj*. Val.

Ulceration, °*Clem*. Colch. Croc. **Euphr*. Ign. Led. Lyc. Merc. Natr. Natr. m. N. vom. Phosph. Puls. Rhus. *Sil*. **Spig*. Staph. Stram. **Sulph*. Val.

Vesicles, Magn. arct. Rhus. Selen.

Warts, Nitr. ac.

FACE, SKIN, AND EXTERNAL PARTS OF.

Acne rosacea, °*Ars*. Calc. Calc. ph. Cann. ***Carb. an.*** Carb. veg. °Kreas. °Rhus. Ruta. Veratr.

Acne, like, *Bell. Carb. veg. Hep.°Lach.

Acne punctata, Dig. °Dros. °Nitr. ac. Sabin. °Selen. **Sulph*.

Blackish, Spig. Vip. torv.

Bleeds, that which, Lyc. Merc. Par.

Blisters, vesicles, Alum. Amm. Amm. m. Ant. Aur. Baryt. Bell. Bov. Bry. Canth. Carb. an. Caust. Cic. Clem. °*Euphorb*. Graph. Lach. Magn. c. Mang. Natr. Nitr. Nitr. ac. Ol. an. Petr. Phosph. **Rhus*. Sep. Sil. Stront. Sulph. Val. Zinc.

—, erysipelas, vesicular, **Rhus*.

Blisters, bloody, °Natr. m.

Blisters, watery, Bov. Coloc.

Bloatedness, **Acon*. Amm. °Arn. **Ars*. Aur. Baryt. Bell. **Bry*. **Cham*. **Chin*. Cin. Cocc. °Crotal. Dig. Dros. Dulc. °Ferr. **Hyos*. °Ipec. °Kal. Laur. Led. Lyc. Merc. Natr. **N. vom*. **Op*. **Phosph*. Plumb. °*Puls*. Rhus.

Samb. Sep. °Sil. °Spig. °*Spong.* Staph. °Sulph. °Tart. Teucr.

Bloatedness, around the eyes, **Ars.* **Bry.* *Cham. °*Ferr.* **N. vom.* Oleand. **Phosph.* °*Puls.* Rhab. Ruta. Sep.

—, glabella, Kal.

Blotches, tubercles, °*Alum.* Ant. °*Ars.* Baryt. Bry. Calc. Cann. Canth. Carb. veg. Cham. Chel. Cic. Con. Dig. Dulc. °*Graph.* Hell. Hep. Kal. Kal. hdr. Lach. *Led. Lyc.* Magn. arct. °*Magn. c.* Magn. m. *Merc.* Natr. Nitr. Nitr. ac. *N. vom.* Oleand. Op. *Puls.* Sep. Thuj. Viol. tr. Zinc.

Bone-pains, °Alum. °Aur. Asa. **Calc.* °Caps. Carb. veg. **Caust.* °Chel. *Chin. *Colch.* °Con. °Dros. **Hep.* **Mez.* **Natr. m.* **Nitr. ac.* N. mosch. **Phosph.* Ruta. Samb. *Spig.* **Staph.*

Boils, Alum. Amm. Arn. Baryt. Bell. °Bry. Calc. Carb. veg. Chin. Cin. Laur. Led. Mez. Mur. ac. Natr. Natr. m. Nitr. ac. Sil.

Broad margin, with a, Nitr. ac.

Brown, that which is, °Bry. °Dulc. Veratr.

Burning of the skin, Alum. Arg. Ars. Berb. Caps. Clem. Caust. Graph. Kal. Puls. Natr. Nitr. Sep. Stann. Viol. tr.

Burns, that which, *Amm.* Ant. **Ars.* Asa. Aur. Bell. Bry. Calc. Canth. Caust. Cic. Cin. Crotal. Dig. Euphr. Kal. Kal. chl. Kal. hdr. Led. Merc. Natr. m. Nitr. ac. Ratanh. Rhus. Samb. Sassap. Seneg. Senn. Teucr.

Burnt, as if, Clem. N. vom.

Caries, °Cist. °Sil.

Cancerous ulcers, °*Ars.*

Creeping, Acon. Alum. Amb. Anac. Ant. Arn. Bell. Calc. Cann. Colch. Euphorb. Evon. Ferr.

magn. Gran. Lact. Magn. m. Merc. N. vom. Ol. an. Pæon. Plat. Ran. Sabad. Sec. Thuj.

Callosities, Rhus v.

Comedones, Sabin. °Selen.

Confluent, Alum. *Cic.

Crusta lactea, °***Ars.*** °Baryt. ? °Bell. ? °Calc. ? °Carb. veg. ? °*Cic. ?* °Dulc. ? °Lyc. ? °***Merc.*** *?* °Natr. m. ? Phos.? °Phos. ac.? °***Rhus.*** °Sassap. ? °Sep. ? °***Sulph.*** °Viol. tr. ?

Drawing pain, with, Con. Magn. m. Staph.

Drunkards, as in, °Kreas. °Led. °Lach.

Dry, Amm. m. Baryt. Kal. hdr. Kreas. °Led.

Eruption in general, Agar. Agn. Alum. Amb. *Amm. Amm. m. Ant. Arg. Arn. Ars. ****Aur.*** ****Baryt.*** Bell. Borax. Bov. Bry. ****Calc.*** Calend. Cann. Canth. Caps. Carb. an. ****Carb.veg.*** Caust. Cham. Chel.**Cic.* Clem. Cocc.****Con.*** ****Crotal.*** Dig. ****Dulc.*** Electr. Euphorb. Ferr. magn. ****Graph.*** Hell. ****Hep.*** Hyos. °Ign. Kal. ****Kreas.*** Lach. Laur. Led. ****Lyc.*** Magn. arct. Magn. c. ***Magn. m.*** Magn. s. Mang. Merc. °Mur. ac. Natr. ****Natr. m.*** Nitr. ****Nitr. ac.*** N. vom. Oleand. Par. Petr. Phosph. ****Phos. ac.*** Puls. Rhus. Ruta. Sabad. Sabin. Sassap. Selen. ****Sep.*** Sil. Spong. Staph. Stront. ****Sulph.*** Sulph. ac. Tarax. Thuj. Veratr. Viol. tr. Zinc.

—, eyes, region of, Agn. ***Ars.*** Calc. Caust. Con. Hep. Ign. Kal. ****Merc.*** Natr. m. Oleand. Par. Petr. Rhus. Selen. Sep. ***Sil.*** Spong. ***Staph. Sulph.*** Thuj.

—, cheeks, region of, Agar. Agn. Alum. ***Amb.*** Amm. Anac. Agn. ***Ant.*** Arn. Asa. ****Baryt.*** ****Bell.*** Borax. ***Bov. Bry.*** ****Calc.*** ***Canth.*** Carb. veg. ***Caust. Cham.*** Chel. Cin. ***Con.*** Cycl. ***Dig.***

Dulc. Euphorb. Graph. Hep. Hyos. *Lach.* Laur. *Kreas.* **Led.* Magn. m. Merc. Mez. Natr. *Natr. m.* Nitr. Nitr. ac. N. vom. Oleand. Phosph. **Rhus.* Ruta. Sabad. Sabin. Sassap. Sep. Sil. Spong. *Staph.* Stront. Tarax. Thuj. Val. *Veratr.* Verbasc. Viol. tr.

Eruption in general, chin, region of, Agn. Alum. Amb. Amm. m. Anac. Ant. Bell. Borax. **Bov.* Calc. Canth. Caust. *Chel.* Cic. Clem. Con. Dig. Dulc. **Graph. Hep.* Hyos. Kal. °*Lach. Lyc.* Magn. art. Magn. aust. Magn. c. Merc. Mez. Natr. Natr. m. Nitr. ac. N. mosch. *N. vom.* Oleand. *Par.* Phosph. Phos. ac. Plat. Puls. **Rhus.* Sabin. Sassap. Sep. **Sil.* Spig. Spong. Squill. *Stront. Sulph. Tarax. Thuj. *Veratr.* Verbasc. Zinc.

—, lips, region of, Acon. Amm. m. Ant. Arn. **Ars.* Baryt. Bell. Bov. *Bry. **Calc.* Cann. Canth. Caps. Caust. Chin. Chinin. Coloc. Con. Dulc. Electr. °*Hell.* Hyos. Ign. Ipec. Kal. Kreas. Led. Magn. art. Magn. arct. Magn. m. Mang. Mur. ac. Natr. Nicc. N. vom. Par. °*Rhus.* Samb. Spig. Spong. Squill. Staph. Sulph. Tarax. Teucr. Veratr. °Zinc.

—, mouth, round the, Acon. Agar. Alum. Amm. Amm. m. Anac. Ant. Arn. Ars. Baryt. Bell. Borax. *Bov.* Bry. Calc. Cann. Canth. Caps. Carb. an. Carb. veg. Caust. Cham. Chin. Cic. Clem. Cocc. Con. Dig. Dulc. Graph. Hell. Hep. Hyos. Ign. **Ipec.* Kal. Laur. Led. Lyc. Magn. art. Magn. arct. *Magn. c.* Magn. m. Mang. Merc. Mez. Natr. **Natr. m.* Nitr. ac. N. vom. Par. Petr. Phosph. Phos. ac. Plat.

Rhod. ***Rhus.** Ruta. Sabad. Samb. Sep. *Sil.* Spig. Spong. Squill. *Staph.* Sulph. Tarax. Thuj. *Veratr.* Zinc.

Eruption, in general; mouth, corners of, Ant. ***Amm. m.** Arn. ***Bell.** ***Calc.** Carb. veg. Caust. Coloc. ***Graph.** Hell. Hep. ***Ign.** Kreas. Magn. arct. Mang. ***Merc.** Mez. Natr. Natr. m. °Nitr. ac. Petr. Phosph. Rhod. Sep. ***Sil.*** Veratr. Zinc.

—, nose, round the, Alum. Amm. ***Ant.*** ***Baryt.*** ***Bov.*** ***Caust.*** Dulc. Magn. arct. Magn. m. ***Natr.*** ***Rhus.*** ***Sep.*** ***Sil.*** *Sulph.* Zinc.

—, ears, round the, Ant. Magn. c. Mur. ac. Petr. Phosph. Sulph.

—, temples, on the, °***Alum.*** Amb. Anac. Ant. Arg. Arn. Baryt. Bell. Bry. Carb. veg. Caust. Cocc. Lach. Lyc. ***Mur. ac.*** Natr. m. Nitr. ac. Sabin. Spig. Sulph. Thuj.

—, forehead, on the, Agar. Amb. Amm. Amm. m. Ant. Arn. Baryt. ***Bov.*** Calc. Canth. Caps. Carb. veg. Cham. ***Clem.*** Cocc. Euphorb. ***Hell.*** Hep. Ipec. ***Led.** Magn. m. ***Natr. m.*** ***Par.*** Puls. Rhab. ***Rhod.*** Rhus. ***Sep.*** Sil. °***Staph.*** ***Sulph.** Sulph. ac.

Eruptions, bright-red, Bell. Carb. an. Carb. veg. Sassap. Teucr.

Eruption, fine, Caust. Nitr. ac. Phosph.

Eruptions, miliary, Alum. Natr. m. Phosph. Tab.

Erysipelatous, ***Bell.** Borax. Calc. Camph. Canth. °***Carb. an.*** °Cham. Cist. Crotal. Euphorb. Gins. ***Graph.** °Hep. ***Lach.** Nitr. ac. °Puls. ***Rhus.** Ruta. °Sep. Stram. °Sulph.

Excoriated, as if, °***Graph.***

Falling off of hair, Graph. Natr. m. Plumb.
—, whiskers, Agar. Amb. Calc. *Graph. Natr. Natr. m.* Nitr. ac. Plumb. Sil.
—, mustaches, Baryt. Kal. Plumb.
Fetid, °*Merc.*
Formication, Magn. m.
Freckles, °Alum. Amm. °Calc. °Graph. °Lyc. °Mur. ac. °Natr. °N. mosch. °Sulph.
Furfuraceous, °Aur. Lyc.
Glandular indurations, °Bry. (Comp.: LOWER JAW.)
Gnawing, Caps. Caust. °Con. Dig.
Green, that which is, Ars. Calc.
Hard, Anac. °Bry. Crotal. Magn. c. Puls. Veratr.
Hard and swollen, Amm. **Arn.* Ars. **Bell.* **Cham.*
Herpes, °Alum. *Amm.* Anac. Ars. °Baryt. °*Bov.* Bruc. Bry. Calc. Caps. °*Carb. veg.* Caust. °Chel. °Con. °Dulc. Graph. Kal. hdr. °Kreas. **Lach.* **Led.* °Lyc. Merc. Natr. **Natr. m.* Nicc. Nitr. ac. Petr. Phosph. °Phos. ac. **Rhus.* Sabad. °Sep. °Sil. °Sulph.
—, cheeks, Amb. Anac. °*Bov.* Bry. Caust. Merc.
—, chin, °*Bov.* Chel. Natr. m. N. vom. °Sil.
—, temples, °Alum.
—, forehead, *Caps. Caust.* °Chel. Colch. *Con. Dig. Dulc. Euphorb. Ferr. magn. Gins. Gran. Graph. Grat. Hep. Kal. Lach. Laur. *Lyc. Magn. c. Meph. Natr. *Natr. m. Natr. s. Nicc. *Nitr.* N. vom. Oleand. Ol. an. Op. Petr. Phell. *Phosph.* Phos. ac. Plumb. *Rhus.* Ruta. *Sabad. Sassap.* Sep. Sil. Spong. Squill.

Stann. Staph. *Stront.* Sulph. Tab. Thuj. *Veratr.* Viol. tr. Zinc.

Herpes, eyes, region of, Agn. Alum. **Con.* Caust. Lach. Oleand. Spong.

—, cheeks, Agar. *Agn.* Alum. Ant. Asa. **Bell.* Berb. Bov. Caust. Chel. **Con.* Cycl. Dig. Dulc. Graph. Hep. *Lach.* Laur. Magn. m. Natr. m. *Oleand. Rhus.* Sabad. Sil. *Spong. Staph.* Stront. Thuj.

—, whiskers, Agar. Amb. **Calc.* Nitr. Natr. m. Sil.

—, mouth, region of, Agar. Amm. m. Anac. Con. Hep. Ol. an.

—, forehead, Agar. Alum. Amb. Amm. m. Anac. Berb. Caps. Carb. an. Carb. veg. Caust. Canth. Cham. Chel. Croc. Laur. Led. Natr. m. N. vom. Oleand. Ol. an. Phell. Rhus. Samb. Sil. Spig. Squill. Veratr.

Herpes, mealy, Ars. Bruc. (Comp.: Furfuraceous.)

Hepatic spots, Laur.

Humid, that which is, °Alum. **Calc.* °Carb. veg. **Cic.* Coloc. Dulc. **Graph.* Kreas. °*Merc.* Natr. °Phos. ac. °*Rhus.* Sep. °*Sulph.*

Inflamed, that which is, Amm. m.

Insolation, as if from, Clem.

Itching, *Agar.* Agn. **Alum.* Amb. **Amm.* Anac. °Ant. Arg. Ars. Asa. Baryt. **Bell.* Berb. **Calc.* *Cann. Caps. Caust.* °Chel. Colch. *Con. Dig. Dulc. Euphorb. Ferr. magn. Gins. Gran. Graph. Grat. Hep. Kal. Lach. Laur. *Lyc. Magn. c. Meph. Natr. *Natr. m. Natr. s. Nicc. *Nitr.* N. vom. Oleand. Ol. an. Op. Petr. Phell. *Phosph.* Phos. ac. Plumb. *Rhus.* Ruta. *Sabad.*

Sassap. Sep. Sil. Spong. Squill. Stann. Staph. ***Stront.*** Sulph. Tab. Thuj. ***Veratr.*** Viol. tr. Zinc.

Itching, eyes, region of, Agn. Alum. ****Con.*** Caust. Lach. Oleand. Spong.

— cheek, Agar. ***Agn.*** Alum. Ant. Asa. ****Bell.*** Berb. Bov. Caust. Chel. ****Con.*** Cycl. Dig. Dulc. Graph. Hep. ***Lach.*** Laur. Magn. m. Natr. m. ***Oleand. Rhus.*** Sabad. Sil. ***Spong. Staph.*** Stront. Thuj.

— whiskers, Agar. Amb. **Calc.* Nitr. Natr. m. Sil.

—, mouth, region of, Agar. Amm. m. Anac. Con. Hep. Ol. an.

— forehead, Agar. Alum. Amb. Amm. m. Anac. Berb. Caps. Carb. an. Carb. veg. Caust. Canth. Cham. Chel. Croc. Laur. Led. Natr. m. N. vom. Oleand. Ol. an. Phell. Rhus. Samb. Sil. Spig. Squill. Veratr.

Lard, looking like, °Ars.

Livid, that which is, Gran.

Marbled, that which is, Phosph.

Mercurial, °Aur. °Nitr. ac.

Miliary, Amm. Kreas. Par. (Comp.: Rash.)

Mosquito-bite, like, *Ant.*

Œdematous, °Colch. Euphorb. Hell.

Ostitis, °Aur. °Staph.

Painful, Alum. Bell. Berb. Cham. Con. Eugen. Lach. Sabad. Stann. Val.

Painful, as if sore, Alum. Anac. Borax. Bry. Canth. Con. Dros. Magn. aust. Puls. Sil. Spig.

Pain, as if ulcerated, Acon. Caps. Chin. Lyc. Mang. Natr. Natr. m. Rhus. ***Staph.***

Peeling of, Amm. Canth. Phosph. °Puls. Rhus.

Petechiæ, Stram.

Pimples, Agar. Alum. Amb. Amm. m. **Ant.* Arn. Ars. Aur. *Baryt. ***Bell.*** Berb. Borax. ***Bov. Bry.*** *Cham.* **Calc.* Calc. ph. ***Canth. Carb. an.*** **Carb. veg.* *Caust.* *Cic. Clem. *Cocc.* Coloc. °Con. Dros. Dulc. Eugen. ***Graph.*** °Hep. ***Kal.*** Kal. chl. Kal. hdr. ****Kreas.*** Lach. Led. **Lyc.* Magn. c. Magn. m. Magn. s. Meph. **Merc.* Mosch. °Mur. ac. Natr. **Natr. m.* °*Nitr. ac.* Ol. an. Petr. °***Phosph.*** ****Phos. ac.*** Rhod. Rhus. Sabin. Sassap. **Sep. Sil.* Stann. ***Staph.*** ****Sulph.*** Tab. Tarax. Tart. Thuj. *Veratr.* Vinc. Zinc.

Pimples, close together, Sep.

Pimples and eruptions, clusters of, Sep. Sulph.

Pock-shaped, Ant. Arn. Hyos. Lach. Petr. Tart.

Pustules, Amm. Amm. m. Anac. **Ant.* Aur. **Bell.* Bov. Calc. ph. Carb. an. Caust. **Cic.* Clem. Cocc. Coloc. Crotal. Dros. Grat. Hyos. Kal. Kal. hdr. Magn. c. Magn. m. Magn. s. °*Merc.* Nitr. °*Nitr. ac.* Par. Phosph. ****Rhus.*** Sassap. Tarax. Veratr.

—, whiskers, °Ars.

Raised, that which is, Dulc. Oleand. Phosph. Sassap. Sulph. Teucr.

Rash, Sulph.

Red, that which is, Alum. Amm. Amb. Anac. Ant. Arn. °Ars. °Aur. ***Bell.*** Borax. Bry. Calc. ph. Carb. an. Caust. Cham. **Cic.* Crotal. Dig. Dros. °Euphr. Ferr. mur. °Ipec. Kal. Kal. hdr. °Kreas. Lach. Led. ***Merc. Nitr. ac.*** Par. Phosph. Phos. ac. *Puls. °Samb. ****Sep. Sulph.*** Tab. Thuj. Teucr. Veratr.

Red and swollen, **Arn.* **Bell.* Borax. °Bry. °Coloc. Crotal. Kal. *Lach. Natr. **N. vom.* Oleand. ***Rhus.** **Stram.* °Sulph.

With red areola, Tarax.

Rhagades, Sil.

Rough, Alum. Anac. Baryt. Bov. Merc. Nitr. ac. Phosph. °Rhus. Sassap. **Sep.* °*Sulph.*

Scaly, Amm. Anac. °Aur. °Led.

Scarlet-red, **Bell.*

Scrophulous, °Bov.

Scurfs, crusts, °Alum. Ant. **Ars.* **Baryt.* **Bell.* Bry. **Calc.* Carb. veg. **Cic.* °Coloc. °*Dulc.* **Graph.* Hep. Ign. *Lach. Lyc. °*Merc.* Mur. ac. Nitr. ac. Petr. Phosph. *Phos. ac.* Sassap. °*Sep.* Sil. Staph. Sulph. Thuj. Viol. tr. Zinc. (Comp. CRUSTA LACTEA.)

Semilateral, Arn. **Bell.* Bry. **Cham.* °Lach. **Magn. arct.* °Merc. **N. vom.* °*Puls.* **Sulph.*

Skin, adhesion of, Sabin.

—, shining as from grease, Plumb. Selen.

Skin, shining, Plumb. Selen.

Skin, thickening of the, Bell. °Sil. Viol. tr.

Smarts, that which, Bell. Bry. Calc. Coloc. Merc. Plat.

Sore, Cic.

Sore, as if excoriated, Bry. Natr. m. Sil.

Spots, blue, Ars. *Ferr.

Spots, eruption, Acon. Alum. Amb. Amm. Ars. Baryt. Bell. Berb. Bry. °*Calc.* Carb. an. Carb. veg. °Colch. Croc. Ferr. Ferr. m. Lyc. °*Merc.* °*Natr.* Nitr. ac. Par. Phosph. Samb. Sassap. **Sep.* Sulph. Tab. Vip. red. Zinc.

In spring, °Crotal.

Stinging, Ant. Asa. ***Bell.*** Bry. Calc. Calc. ph. Caust. Cham. Dros. Kal. Kal. hdr. Kreas. Lach. Led. Magn. arct. Natr. Nitr. ac. Plat. ***Rhus.*** Sulph. Teucr.

Syphilitic, °***Merc.***

Swelling, blue-red, Bell. °Bry. ****Cham.*** °Lach.

Swelling of bones, °Aur. °Sil. °Spig.

Swelling, inflammation, Borax. Sep.

Swelling, pale, Bov. °***Bry.*** Euphorb. Hell. N. vom. Rhus. Sep.

Swelling, Acon. Alum. Amb. Amm. Amm. m. **Arn.* **Ars.* Asa. **Aur.* **Baryt.* ****Bell.*** Borax. Bov. ****Bry.*** Calc. Cann. Canth. Carb. an. ***Carb. veg.*** Caust. Chel. Cic. °Colch. °Coloc. Con. Crotal. Dig. Dulc. Electr. ***Euphorb.*** Galv. Gran. ***Graph.*** Guaj. °Hell. ***Hep. Hyos.*** Kal. Kal. hdr. ****Lach.*** Laur. ****Lyc.*** Lupul. Magn. c. °Merc. Natr. Natr. m. Nicc. Nitr. ac. ****N. vom.*** Oleand. Oph. Op. Petr. ****Phosph.*** Plumb. ****Rhus.*** Rhus. v. Sabin. Sec. **Sep.* Sil. Spig. Spong. ***Stann.*** ****Stram.*** ****Sulph.*** Sulph. ac. Veratr. Vip. red. Vip. torv.

—, cheeks, **Arn.* ***Aur.*** Baryt. ****Bell.*** Bry. Canth. **Cham.* Chin. Ferr. °Lach. ****Magn. arct.*** °***Merc.*** °***N. vom.*** °***Puls.*** Spig. Spong. Staph. ****Sulph.***

Tearing and painful, Con.

Tensive, **Arn.* Baryt. Bov. Canth. Con. Crotal. Euphorb. Lyc. Magn. s. **Phosph.* Rhus. Staph. Vip.

Ulcers, °Ars. °Bry. °Con. Jod.Merc. Natr.Phosph.

Urticaria, Ant.

Warts, °***Caust.*** °Dulc. °Kal. Nitr. °Sep.

Wart-shaped, °Ars.

White, Amm. Anac. °Calc. Carb. veg. Clem. Coloc. Dros. Euphorb. Natr. Petr. ***Sulph.***

Yellow, that which is, Amb. Ant. **Cic.* °Colch. °Dulc. Euphorb. °Ferr. Hyos. Kreas. Lyc. Magn. m. °Merc. °*Natr.* **Sep.*

FEET AND PARTS OF FEET.

Arthritic, feet, *Amb.* Arn. °*Bry.* °*Chin. Graph.*

—, toes (gout), Amm. ? °*Arn.* °*Bry.* Con. Led. ? *Sabin.* °*Sulph.* Veratr.

Black, feet, Ant.

Black, blisters, °*Ars.* Natr. m.

—, pocks, *Sec.*

—, ulcers, °Ipec.

Bleeding, ulcers, **Ars.*

Blisters, vesicles, feet, °*Ars. Caust. Con. Graph. Lach. Phosph.* Selen. Sep. Tarax. Vip. torv. Zinc.

—, soles, Ars. Sulph.

—, heels, Calc. *Caust. Lach.* Lam. *Natr. Petr. Phosph.* Raph. *Sep.*

—, toes, *Graph. Lach.* Natr. Nitr. ac. *Phos. ac. Selen. Sulph.*

Blisters, phagedænic, feet, *Con. Selen.* °*Sulph. Zinc.*

—, heels, Caust. °*Natr.* °*Sep. Sil.*

—, toes. °*Ars.* °*Graph. Nitr. ac.* °*Petr.*

Blisters, watery, toes, *Phos. ac.*

Blotches, tumors, feet, Lyc.

—, toes, *Sulph. Zinc.*

Blueness, feet. Vip. torv.

Blue, spots, *Sulph.*

—, chilblains, Kal.

—, swelling, Ars.

Boils, feet, *Stram.*

—, heel, Calc.

Boils, sole, *Ratanh.*
Bone-pain, feet, Acon. Agar. *Alum.* Ars. *Asa. Aur.* Bell. Bism. *Carb. veg. Chin.* Cocc. *Cupr.* Lach. °*Merc.* Nitr. ac. Plat. *Ruta. Sabin.* Spig. Stann. ***Staph.*** Teucr. Veratr. Zinc. Zinc. ox.
—, heel-bone, Berb. Caps. Coloc. Crotal. Diad. Ign.
—, toes, Mez. Sep.
Bubbling, Berb. Chel. Lach.
Burning, feet, Ammoniac. Ang. Ant. Arn. *Berb. Bov.* **Calc.* Carb. an. Caust. Cham. Chin. Con. Croc. Crotal. Dulc. *Electr.* **Graph. Hep.* Heracl. *Ign.* Kal. Kreas. Laur. *Lyc. Magn. m.* Merc. *Mez. Natr.* **Natr. m.* Natr. s. *Nitr. ac. Ol. an.* Petr. *Puls.* Ratanh. *Rhab.* Rhus. Sabin. *Sec. Sep. Sil. Spig.* Squill. *Stann.* Staph. *Stram.* Stront. Sulph. *Tarax.* Thuj. Veratr. Zinc. Zing.
—, heels, Cycl. Graph. *Ign.* Magn. art. *Nitr.* Puls. Rhus. Sabin. Sep. Sulph. ac. Veratr. Zinc.
—, soles, Alum. **Amb.* Amm. **Anac.* Asar. Baryt. Bell. Berb. Bov. **Calc. Canth. Carb. veg.* Caust. Croc. Crotal. °*Cupr. Graph.* Hep. Kal. Kreas. Lach. Led. Lyc. *Magn. m.* Merc. Mur. ac. *Natr.* Natr. s. Nitr. N. vom. Petr. *Phos. ac.* Puls. *Sil. Sulph.* Tab. Tarax. Zinc.
—, toes, **Agar.* °*Alum.* Ammoniac. Amm. Ant. Asa. Atham. *Berb. Borax.* Calc. Carb. an. Caust. *Con.* Dulc. Hep. °*Kal.* Lach. Laur. *Lyc.* Magn. c. Meph. Merc. Mez. Mosch. Mur. ac. Natr. Nitr. ac. *N. vom.* Oleand. Paeon. Par. Phosph. Phos. ac. Plat. *Puls.* Ran. sc. Ratanh. Rhus. Ruta. Sabin. Sep. *Staph. Tarax.* Zinc.
Burning, spots, **Ars.* Lach.

Burning, swelling, Caust. Con. Kal. Merc. Nitr. ac. Petr. Phos. ac. **Puls.*

—, ulcers, Caust.

Callosities, heel, Lyc.

—, soles, °*Sil.*

Chilblains, feet and toes, *Agar. *Ant.* Hep. Kal. *Nitr. ac.* **N. vom.* *Phosph.* Rhus. °*Sulph.* °*Thuj.*

—, itching, redness and pain, as if from, **Agar.* *Alum.* *Amm.* Asar. Berb. Borax. Bry. Cann. Carb. an. Carb. veg. Caust. Chin. *Cocc.* *Colch.* *Kal.* *Lach.* Lyc. Magn. aust. *Nitr. ac.* *N. mosch.* **N. vom.* Petr. Phosph. **Puls.* Rhab. *Sabin.* *Staph.* *Zinc.*

Cold swelling, °*Asa.*

Contraction of tendons, s. Muscles.

Contraction of muscles, feet, **Caust.* Plumb. Vip. torv.

—, sensation, as of, Berb. *Carb. an.* Indig. *Sep.* *Spig.* Sulph.

—, tarsal joints, *Carb. an.* **Caust.* Plumb. *Sep.* *Spig.* Vip. torv.

—, soles, Berb. Indig. *Spig.* Sulph.

Cracked, blisters, Lach. Lam. Selen.

Creeping, feet, Alum. Amb. Amm. Ammoniac. Arn. Baryt. Bell. Berb. Carb. an. Croc. °*Dulc.* Euphorb. Magn. c. Mang. Mez. Mill. Phosph. Puls. *Rhod.* Rhus. Sassap. °*Sep.* Spong. *Stann.* Tax. Zinc. Zing.

—, soles, Arn. Berb. *Caust.* Clem. Con. Croc. Hep. *Kal.* Laur. Magn. m. Natr. m. Ol. an. Phosph. Plat. Puls. Raph. °*Sep.* Spig. Staph. Sulph. Thuj.

Creeping, heel, Amm. Caust. Ferr. magn. Graph. Natr. Phosph. Stront. Sulph.

—, toes, Alum. Amm. Asa. Berb. Cast. *Caust.* Chin. *Colch.* Euphr. *Hep.* Kal. *Lach.* Lact. Magn. m. Natr. Nicc. Nitr. ac. Plat. *Plumb.* Puls. Ran. sc. *Sec.* Spig. Staph. °*Sulph.* Veratr. Zinc.

—, feet, Arn. Phosph.

—, soles, Magn. m.

—, ankle-bone, Bell.

—, heel, Par.

—, toes, Ars. Spig.

Cutting, chilblains, Kal.

Dampness, feet, Mez. Selen.

Drawing, swelling, *Ferr.

As if ecchymosed, feet, Natr.

—, sole, *Led.* Puls.

—, heel, Aur.

Eruption, feet, Carb. an. *Graph.* *Led.* Rhus. Sulph. Tereb.

—, toes, Petr.

Erysipelas, feet, °*Puls.* °*Rhus.*

Excrescences, soles, **Ant.* (Puls.)

—, toes, **Ant.* Spig.

Formication, °*Dulc.* *Kal.* Phosph.

—, toe, *Sec.*

Ganglion, Ferr. magn.

Gangrene, Ant. Sec. Tart. Vip. torv.

Gnawing, feet, Agar. Anac. *Bell.* Berb. Bism. Cocc. Crotal. Dig. *Graph.* Led. Nicc. Plat. *Ran. sc.*

—, heel, *Graph.* *Ran. sc.*

—, soles, Plat. Tart.

—, toes, Berb. Cocc. Kal. *Ran. sc.* Sep.

Gnawing, eruption, Sulph.
Hard, eruption, Bov. *Lach.*
—, swelling, Chin.
Herpes, ankles, °*Natr. m.* °*Petr.*
—, toes, Alum.
Herpetic, soreness, °Graph.
Horny, excrescences, **Ant.*
—, soles, °*Graph.*
Humid, blisters, Lach. Phosph. Raph.
—, ulcers, °Petr.
—, sore, Selen.
Induration of muscles, feet, Vip. torv.
Induration, feet, Vip. torv.
—, soles, **Ars.*
Inflammation, ankles, *Mang.*
—, feet, °Rhus. Zinc.
—, dorsa of feet, Calc. **Puls.* Thuj.
—, toes, *Berb.* Carb. an. Caust. Lach. *Nitr. ac.* Phosph. *Phos. ac. Puls.* Sulph. Teucr. *Thuj.*
Inflamed, chilblains, *Kal. Lach.*
—, swelling, **Ars.* **Bry.* Calc. *Cann.* Caust. °*Chin.* Cocc. °*Led. Nitr. ac.* Petr. **Puls.* °*Rhus.* Sulph. *Thuj.* Zinc.
Itch, toes, °*Phos. ac.*
Itch-like, vesicles, feet, Lach. Squill.
Itching, feet, *Bell. Berb. Bov. Calc. Caust.* Cham. Cocc. Dulc. Electr. Gins. Grat. Hep. *Ign.* Kal. hdr. *Lach.* Laur. Led. Ran. sc. Selen. Stram. Veratr. Zinc.
—, dorsa of feet, Agar. Alum. Anac. Asa. *Bell.* Bism. Calc. *Caust.* Coloc. Dig. Hep. *Ign. Led.* Natr. m. Natr. s. Ran. sc. *Rhus.* Spig. Stann. Stram. *Tarax. Thuj.*
—, joints and ankles, Agar. Ant. Asa. Aur. Bo-

rax. Calc. *Cocc.* Dig. Grat. *Kal.* Lyc. Magn. m. Ol. an. *Oleand.* Petr. *Phos. ac.* Puls. *Rhus.* Selen. Sep. Stann. Staph.

Itching, heels, Calc. Caust. Cham. Ign. *Nicc.* Oleand. *Phosph. Phos. ac.* Puls. Ran. sc. Sabin. Sil. *Staph.* Veratr.

—, soles, *Alum. Amb.* Amm. Amm. m. Aur. Cham. Chin. Con. Cupr. Euphorb. Hep. Kreas. Mur. ac. *Natr.* Natr. s. *Oleand.* Ran. sc. Ratanh. Rhab. Sassap. Sep. Spig. Sulph. Tarax. Tart. Thuj. Zinc.

—, toes, **Agar. Alum. Amb.* Amm. Amm. m. Ant. Ars. Asa. *Berb.* Borax. *Carb. an.* Clem. *Cycl.* Dros. *Graph. Hep. Kal.* Lact. Magn. arct. Magn. aust. Magn. s. Mang. Merc. Mur. ac. Natr. Natr. m. *Natr. s.* Nitr. ac. **N. vom.* Paeon. Plat. *Puls.* Ran. sc. Rhab. Rhus. Sep. Spig. Spong. Stann. *Staph. Sulph.* Tarax. *Zinc.*

Itching, eruption, Calc. *Con.* Electr. Sep. *Sil.*

—, swelling, Caust. Cocc. Puls.

—, ulcers, °*Sil.*

—, scurfs, scald, Sil.

—, blister, phagedænic, Sil.

Marbled redness, *Caust.*

Numbness, feet, Acon. Amb. Ang. Ant. Ars. *Carb. veg. Con.* Electr. Graph. Hep. Lyc. Op. Par. Phos. ac. *Plat.* Rhus.

—, heels. Alum. Caust. Clem. *Ign.* N. vom. Sep. Stront.

—, soles, Bry. *Puls.* Sulph.

—, toes, Arn. Chel. Crot. Cycl. Lach. °*Plumb.* Puls.

Pain, as if contused, toe, Berb. Daph. Mez. Ruta.

Pain, as if burnt, Amm. Zinc.

Pain, as if bruised, feet, Hell. Ol. an. Tart.
—, heel, Caps. Magn. m.
—, toe, Ruta.
Pain, as if dislocated, feet, Agn. *Anac.* Ang. Ant. Ars. *Baryt. Berb.* **Bry.* Camph. Chel. Cupr. Gran. Laur. *Led. Magn. art.* Magn. aust. *Merc.* Mur. ac. Natr. m. Natr. s. *Phosph.* Phos. ac. Plat. Puls. Ran. Rhus. *Sulph.* Veratr. Zinc.
—, heel, *Merc.*
—, toe, Zinc.
Pain, as from a splinter, heel, Mang. Natr. Nitr. ac. Petr. Phos. ac.
Pain, as if sore, feet and joints, Ars. Berb. Chin. Evon. **Hep.* Mur. ac. Natr. Phos. ac. *Plat.* Spig.
—, heel, Borax. Cast. Cycl. Euphorb. *Ign.* Laur. Magn. arct. N. vom. Phos. ac. Sep.
—, toes, Agar. °*Ars.* Berb. Camph. Clem. Cycl. *Lyc. Magn. art.* Magn. aust. Mur. ac. *Natr.* Natr. m. Plat. *Ran.* Sep. Zinc.
Pain, as if sprained, feet and joints, Ang. Arg. Arn. Ars. Bell. **Bry.* Calc. *Caust.* Chin. Cocc. Croton. *Cycl.* Dig. Dros. Hell. *Ign. Lyc.* Magn. art. Magn. aust. *Men.* Mosch. °*Natr.* Nitr. Nitr. ac. N. vom. Plumb. *Prun. Rhab. Rhus.* Ruta. Sil. Sulph. *Val. Zinc.*
—, heel, Cycl. Euphorb. Laur. Nitr.
—, toe, °*Amm.* Arn. Aur. Carb. an. Kal. Mosch. Petr. Ratanh. Sil.
Painful, eruption, Lyc. Phosph. Spig. °*Sulph.*
—, swelling, °*Bry.* Con. °*Daph.* Ferr. *Led.* °*Merc.* Phosph. Phos. ac. Rhus. Sabad. *Sulph.*
Paleness, heel, Sep.
—, toes, Sec.

Rhagades, toes, Carb. an. Eugen. **Lach.*
Rheumatic, feet, **Hep.* Ruta. Stram. Zinc.
—, toes, Cinn.
Scurf, *Sil.*
Shining, swelling, Alum. **Ars. Sabin.* °*Sulph.* Thuj.
Smarting, feet, Berb. Grat. Merc.
—, heel, Lam. Sep.
—, toe, Berb.
Smarting, ulcer, Lam.
Softening, soles, *Sulph.*
Sore, pimples, Bov.
—, swelling, Natr.
—, ulcer, Lam.
—, callosities, Lyc.
Soreness, soles, N. vom. Sil.
—, toes, *Carb. an.* Coff. **Graph.*
Spreading, ulcers, °*Ars.* Caust. Con. °*Graph.* °*Natr.* Nitr. ac. °*Petr.* Selen. °*Sep.* Sil.
Spots, feet, Ant. **Ars.* Led. Sec. Squill. *Sulph. Thuj.*
—, soles, *Rhus.*
—, toes, Lach. *Natr.*
Stinging, eruption, Calc. Zinc.
—, spots, Lach.
—, chilblains, *Kal.*
—, swelling, °*Carb. veg.* Lyc. Merc. *Phosph.* **Puls.*
Suppurating, tumor, *Lach.* Sassap.
—, blisters, *Con. Graph. Natr. Selen.*
—, chilblains, °*Lach.*
—, scurf, *Sil.*
—, ulcers, **Ars.*
Suppuration, heel, Borax.

Suppuration, toes, Lach.
Swelling, feet, °*Amb.* **Amm.* Arn. **Ars.* °*Asa.* Bar. m. *Bov.* **Bry.* *Calc.* *Carb. an.* Carb. veg. *Caust.* Cham. **Chin.* Chinin. Cocc. Colch. Con. Crotal. °*Dig.* Electr. **Ferr.* **Graph.* Hyos. Indig. Jod. **Kal.* Kreas. **Lach.* **Led.* Lyc. **Natr.* °*Natr. m.* Nitr. ac. N. vom. Op. **Petr.* **Phosph.* °*Phos. ac.* Plumb. **Puls.* **Rhus.* Sabad. °*Samb.* Sassap. Sec. **Sep.* **Sil.* **Stann.* °*Stront.* **Sulph.* *Veratr.* Vip. torv. *Zinc.*
—, dorsa of feet, *Calc.* Carb. an. Lyc. *Merc.* *N. vom.* **Puls.* Staph. Thuj.
—, joints, *Ferr.* *Merc.*
—, ankles, Amb. Ars. °*Asa.* Berb. Calc. **Hep.* Kal. *Led.* Lyc. *Mang.* Puls. Sil. *Stann.* Sulph. Zinc.
—, bones, °*Merc.* *Staph.*
—, heels, *Con.* *Merc.* *Raph.*
—, soles, *Cham.* *Kal.* Kreas. °*Lyc.* Natr. Petr.
—, toes, Amm. Ammoniac. Carb. an. °*Carb. veg.* °*Daph.* Gins. **Graph.* *Merc.* *Mur. ac.* *Natr.* *Nitr. ac.* Oph. *Phos. ac.* Plat. *Sabin.* **Sulph.* *Thuj.* Zinc.
Swelling, sensation as of, Plat. Sassap.
—, soles. Bry. °*Calc.*
—, toes, Mur. ac.
Swelling, watery, (Œdematous), °*Ferr.* Hep. *Jod.* Kreas. °*Led.* °*Puls.* *Rhod.* °*Samb.*
—, dropsical, *Sec.*
Tearing, swelling, Natr.
Tensive, swelling, Cann. Chin. **Puls.*
Titillation, feet, Ign. Rhod.
—, heel, Laur. Mur. ac. Ol. an. Ratanh. Rhod.

Titillation, soles, Alum. Euphorb. Graph. Hep. Mang. Ratanh. Ruta. **Sil.*

—, toes, Agar. Amb. Ars. Caust. Euphr. Kal. Sep.

Thickening, soles, **Ars.*

Tubercles, Carb. an.

Ulcers, feet, *Con.* °*Ipec.* *Phosph.* Puls. Selen. °*Sulph.* *Zinc.*

—, heels, **Ars.* Caust. Lam. °*Natr.* °*Sep.* *Sil.*

—, soles, **Ars.* **Sep.* Sulph.

—, toes, °*Ars.* Carb. veg. **Graph.* *Nitr. ac.* °*Petr.* Plat.

Ulcerated, blisters, **Sulph.* Zinc.

Ulcerated, pain as if, feet, Amm. m. **Bry.* Caust. Hep. Indig. Lyc. **Natr. m.* Nitr.

—, soles, Amb. *Baryt.* Calc. *Canth.* *Graph.* °*Ign.* Kreas. Laur. Lyc. Magn. s. Nitr. °*Phosph.* Prun. *Puls.* *Spig.* Sulph. Zinc.

—, heel, Amm. Amm. m. Berb. Carb. an. *Caust.* Euphorb. Graph. Kal. hdr. Laur. Natr. s. Zinc.

—, toes, Amm. Carb. an. Carb. veg. Caust. Con. Kal. hdr. *Natr.* Phos. ac. *Sil.* Val. Zinc.

—, swelling, Cann. Caust.

Varices, Sulph.

White, eruption, *Cycl.* *Graph.* *Lach.* Sulph.

—, swelling, Kreas.

Fetid, which is.

Pus, Amm. **Ars.* °*Asa.* Aur. Bar. m. Bell. Bov. Bry. *Calc.* Caust. **Carb. veg.* Chel. *Chin.* Chinin. Cic. Con. Cycl. *Graph.* **Hep.* Kreas. **Lach.* *Lyc.* Mang. Mez. Mur. ac. Natr. Nitr. ac. N. mosch. N. vom. Phosph. *Phos. ac.*

Plumb. Puls. Rhus. Ruta. Sabin. Sec. *Sep.* **Sil.* Staph. **Sulph.* Sulph. ac. Thuj. Vip. red.
Herpes, Oleand.
Ulcers, °*Amm.* **Ars.* °*Asa.* Bar. m. Calc. °*Carb. veg.* Caust. Chin. °*Con.* Graph. °*Hep.* Lach. °*Lyc.* Mang. *Merc.* Mur. ac. Phosph. Plumb. °*Rhus.* °*Sec.* °*Sep.* **Sil.* **Staph.* Vip. red. (Comp.: Putrid, and Pus, fetid.)
Scurfs, crusts, Graph. Lyc. *Merc.* Plumb. Staph. **Sulph.*

Head, *Graph. °Lyc. Nitr. ac.
Ears, °Aur. °Bov. °Carb. veg. Caust. °Cist. °Graph. °Hep. Hyos. Merc. Zinc.
—, behind the ears, herpes, °Oleand.
Face, °*Merc.*
Lips, ulcers, Merc.
Sexual parts, ulcers, Hep. Nitr. ac.
Arms, pocks, °*Ars.*

FIERY-RED.

Eruption, **Acon.* Bell. Stram. °*Sulph.*
Spots, Ferr. magn.

FIGWARTS.

In general, °Calc.? °Euphr. °*Lyc.* °Magn. aust. **Nitr. ac.* °N. vom. **Phos. ac.* °Sabin.? °Sassap. °Staph. °Sulph. **Thuj.*
Bleeding, Magn. aust. *Thuj.*
Burning, Thuj.
Dry, after mercurial-treatment, °*Sassap.* °*Sulph.*

Horny, °*Thuj.*
Humid, Thuj.
Itching, Euphr. Thuj.
Painful, Sabin.
Painful, as if sore, Sabin. Thuj.
Pedunculated, °*Lyc.*
Stinging, Euphr. Thuj.
Suppurating, * *Thuj.*
Titillating, Thuj.

Eyes, Thuj.
Eyebrows, °*Thuj.*
Nose, °Nitr. ac.
Anus, * *Thuj.*
Sexual parts, °Cinn. °Euphr. Magn. aust. °*Nitr. ac.* °Phos. ac. °Sassap. Sabin. °Staph.? °Thuj.

Fine, that which is.

Eruption, Agar. Alum. *Ars.* Bell. Bry. * *Carb. veg.* Caust. Clem. Cocc. Con. Dulc. Graph. Hep. Jod. Ipec. Kreas. Led. Merc. Mez. Natr. m. Nitr. ac. N. vom. Par. Phosph. Phos. ac. Puls. Rhus. Sassap. Sulph. Val. Zinc.
Pimples, Kal.

Face, eruption, Caust. Nitr. ac. Phosph.
Lips, eruptions, Lyc.
Sexual parts, eruptions, Kal. Merc.
Hands, eruption, * *Carb. veg.*
Lower limbs, eruption, Alum.

Fistulous.

Blisters, vesicles, Aur. **Calc.* Petr.
Ulcers, °*Ant.* Ars. °*Asa. Aur.* °*Bell.* Bry. **Calc.* °*Carb. veg.* °*Caust.* Chel. Clem. °*Con. Hep.* Kreas. *Lach.* Led. °*Lyc.* Merc. Natr. Natr. m. °*Nitr. ac.* Petr. °Phosph. Phos. ac. °*Puls.* Rhus. °*Ruta.* Sabin. Selen. *Sep.* °*Sil.* Stann. Staph. Stram. °*Sulph.* Thuj.

Canthi, ulcers, °Bry. ? °*Calc.* °Natr. °Petr. ? °Phosph. ? °Puls. ? °Sil. ? °Stann. ?
Gums, ulcers, Canth. °*Caust.* Lyc. °Natr. m. Sulph.
—, pain, as if ulcerated, Aur. **Calc.* Petr.
Anus, ulcers, °*Caust.* Petr. °Thuj.
Mammæ and nipples, °Phosph. °Sil.
Lower limbs, ulcer, °*Ruta.*

Flaccidity.

Of the skin, in general, Agar. Ang. Borax. **Calc.* Caps. Cham. **Chin.* Clem. **Cocc.* Con. Croc. Crotal. Cupr. Dig. Euphorb. Ferr. Graph. Hell. Hyos. **Jod.* Ipec. Lach. °*Lyc.* Magn. c. Merc. Natr. Oph. Puls. Rhab. Sabad. **Sec.* Seneg. Sil. Spong. Sulph. Sulph. ac. Veratr. Vip. red. Vip. torv. Zinc.
Glands, Ars. Cham. Chin. °*Con.* **Jod.* Kal. °*Nitr. ac.* N. mosch. Phos. ac. Sec. Sil. Veratr.

Flea-bite, like.

Spots, Acon. Bell. Dulc. Graph. Mez. Sec. Stram. Tart.

Thoracic region, spots, Mez.
Dorsal region, itching, Alum. Laur. Squill.

Flat, that which is.

Eruption, *Amm.* Ang. *Ant.* *Ars.* *Asa.* *Bell.* Carb. an. Euphorb. *Lach.* *Lyc.* Merc. *Natr.* Nitr. ac. Petr. Phosph. *Phos. ac.* Puls. Ran. *Selen.* *Sep.* *Sil.* Staph. Sulph. Tart. Thuj.
Pimples, Ant.
Ulcers, Amm. Ang. *Ant.* °*Ars.* °*Asa.* °*Bell.* Carb. an. Carb. veg. *Chin.* Corall. **Lach.* °*Lyc.* **Merc.* Natr. **Nitr. ac.* *Petr.* Phosph. °*Phos. ac.* °*Puls.* Ran. °*Selen.* °*Sep.* °*Sil.* Staph. Sulph. Tart. **Thuj.*
Warts, Dulc. Lach.

Sexual parts, ulcers, Corall. **Nitr. ac.* **Thuj.*
Lower limbs, ulcers, Staph.
—, pimples, Ant.

Flesh, as if loose.

Arms, *Dros.* Ign. *Staph.* *Thuj.*
—, shoulder, joint, Staph.
—, upper arm, Thuj.
Hands, Ol. an.
Lower limbs, Sulph.
—, nates and hips, Zinc.
—, thighs, Electr. Led. Mosch. Natr.
—, legs, Canth. Stann. Sulph.
Bones, **Bry.* Canth. *Dros.* Electr. **Ign.* Kreas. Led. Mosch. Natr. *Nitr. ac.* *N. vom.* Ol. an. **Rhus.* *Stann.* *Staph.* *Sulph.* *Thuj.* Zinc.

Formication.

In general, Agn. Alum. Amm. Arg. Aur. Baryt. Borax. Bov. Calc. Cann. Caps. Carb. veg. Caust. Laur. Led. *Lyc.* Magn. aust. Magn. c. Magn. m. Mang. Mur. ac. ***Natr.*** Nitr. ac. N. vom. *Oleand.* Phosph. ***Phos. ac. Plat.*** Ran. Ran. sc. ***Rhod.*** Rhus. ***Sabad. Sec.*** Sil. Spig. Spong. Staph. Sulph. Zinc. Compare: Creeping.

Face, Magn. m.

Buccal cavity, gums, Sec.

Thorax, Magn. m.

Dorsal region, neck, Electr. Sec.

—, back, Evon. Graph. *Natr.* Sassap.

Hands, Alum. Sec.

Lower limbs, Alum. ***Ol. an. Rhod.*** Tab. Zinc.

Feet, °***Dulc. Par.*** Phosph.

—, toe, ***Sec.***

Freckles.

In general, °***Amm.*** °***Ant.*** Bry. ****Calc.*** Carb. veg. *Con.* ***Dros.*** °***Dulc.*** °***Graph.*** Hyos. Jod. ***Kal.*** Lach. Laur. **Lyc. Merc.* Mez. Natr. Nitr. ac. ***N. mosch. Petr.*** ****Phosph.*** Plumb. °***Puls.*** °***Sep. Sil.*** Stann. ****Sulph.*** Tart. Thuj.

Nose, Phosph. °*Sulph.*

Face, °Alum. Amm. °Calc. °Graph. °Lyc. °Mur. ac. °Natr. °N. mosch. °Sulph.

Chest, Nitr. ac.

Lower limbs, Phosph.

Fungus articularis.

In general, **Ant. Ars.?* Clem.? Con.? Kreas.? °*Jod. Lach.?* Petr.? Phosph.? Rhus.? Sabin.? °*Sil. Staph.? Sulph.?*
Knee, °*Ant.* °*Jod.* °*Sulph.*

Funguses.

In general, **Ant.* Ars.? *Bell.* °*Calc. Carb. an.? Carb. veg.?* Clem.? Con.? **Jod.* Kreas.? *Lach.?* °*Lyc.* Merc.? *Nitr. ac.?* N. vom.? Petr.? °*Phosph.* Rhus.? Sabin.? °*Sep.* °*Sil.* Staph.? Sulph.? Tart.? Thuj.?
Fungus hæmatodes, Ars.? °*Bell.* Calc.? *Carb. an.?* Carb. veg.? Clem.? Kreas.? Lach.? °*Lyc.* Merc.? Nitr. ac.? N. vom.? °*Phosph.* Rhus.? °*Sep.* °*Sil.?* Staph.? *Sulph.?* Thuj.
Fungus articularis, **Ant. Ars.?* Clem.? *Con.?* Kreas.? °*Jod. Lach.?* Petr.? Phosph.? Rhus? Sabin.? °*Sil. Staph.?* Sulph.?
Fungus medullaris, °*Bell.* Carb. an. °*Phosph.* Sil.? Sulph.? Thuj.?

Ears, Merc.
Lips, Ipec.
Lower limbs, knees, °*Ant.* °*Jod.* °*Sulph.*

Fungus hæmatodes.

In general, Ars.? °*Bell.* Calc.? *Carb. an.?* Carb. veg.? Clem.? Kreas.? Lach.? °*Lyc.* Merc.? Nitr. ac.? N. vom.? °*Phosph.* Rhus.? °*Sep.* °*Sil.?* Staph.? Sulph.? Thuj.

Eyes, °Bell. ? °Calc. °Lyc. °Sep. °Sil.

Fungus medullaris.

Eyes, °*Bell.* Carb. an.? °*Phosph.* Sil. ? Sulph. ? Thuj. ?

Furfuraceous, that which is.

Eruption, Agar.
Pustules, Merc.
Herpes, *Ars. °Bry. Bruc. °Dulc. °Kreas. °Lyc. *Merc.* °Phosph. °Sulph.

Eyelids, °Bry. Sep.
Nose, herpes, *Ars.
Face, °Aur. Lyc.
—, herpes, Ars. Bruc.
Nipples, covering, Petr.
Arms, eruption, Agar.
Herpes, °Phosph.
Hands, eruptions, Alum.

Ganglia.

In general, °Amm. Plumb. °*Phosph.* Phos. ac. °*Sil.* °*Zinc.*

Hands, ***Amm.*** Magn. m. ***Phos. ac. Plumb.*** Prun. Rhod. *Sil.*
—, dorsa of hands, Zinc.
Feet, Ferr. magn.

Gangrene.

In general, **Acon.* **Ars.* Asa. **Bell.* Camph. Caps. Carb. veg. **Chin.* °Chinin. ? Con. *Crotal.* Electr. *Euphorb.* Hell. Hyos. **Lach.* Merc. Mur. ac. Oph. Phosph. Plumb. Ran. Rhus. *Sabin.* **Sec.* **Sil.* *Squill.* Sulph. Sulph. ac. Tart. *Vip. red.* *Vip. torv.*
—, humid gangrene, Chin. Hell. Phosph. Vip. red.
—, hot, °Acon. Ars. Bell. Mur. ac. Sabin. Sec.
—, cold, *Ars.* *Asa.* Bell. Con. *Euphorb.* *Lach.* Merc. *Plumb.* Ran. *Sec.* *Sil.* *Squill.* Sulph. Sulph. ac. Tart.

Nose, Sec.
Buccal cavity, **Ars.* Chinin. Lach.
Sexual part, *Ars.* *Canth.* Laur. Plumb. °Sec.
—, scrotum, Plumb.
—, penis, Canth. Laur. Plumb.
—, uterus, °Sec.
Arms, *Ran.* Sec.
Lower limbs, *Sec.*
—, tibiæ, *Sec.*
Feet, Ant. Sec. Tart. Vip. torv.
Bones, Ars. Asa. Euphorb. ? Phosph. ? Plumb. *Sabin.* *Sec.* °*Sil.*

Gangrenous, that which is.

Anthrax, carbuncle, **Ars.* °Bell. Caps. Electr. *Hyos.* Lach. Rhus. *Sec.* °*Sil.* Tart. Vip. torv.
Blisters, vesicles, Acon. Ars. Bell. *Canth.* Carb. veg. Hyos. Lach. Mur. ac. *Ran.* Sabin. *Sec.*

Spots, Crotal. ***Cycl.*** Hyos.
Swelling, Ars. Euphorb. Vip. torv.
Ulcers, Acon. °***Ars.*** °*Asa.* Bell. °***Chin.*** Con. Mur. ac. Rhus. °***Sabin.*** °Sec. Squill. Vip. red.
Erysipelas, Acon. **Ars.* ***Bell.*** Camph. Chin. ***Chinin.*** Hyos. Lach. Mur. ac. Rhus. ***Sabin.*** Sec. Sil.
Scarlatina, °Amm. °Ars. °Lach.

Arms, boils, °*Lach. Sec.*
Hands, pocks, Sec.
—, ulcers, fingers, °*Lach. Sec.*
Lower limbs, vesicles, Hyos.
—, spots, *Cycl. **Hyos.***
—, ulcers, °*Lach.*

Glands, affections of.

In general, Acon. Agn. Alum. Amb. *Amm. Amm. m. Ant. Arg. Arn. *Ars. °Asa. °Aur. *Baryt. Bar. m. *Bell. Berb. Borax. Bov. *Bry. Calad. *Calc. Calend. Camph. Canth. Caps. **Carb. an.* **Carb. veg.* Caust. *Cham. Chin. Cic. Cinn. °*Cist.* Clem. Cocc. Coloc. **Con.* Corall. Croc. Cupr. Cycl. Dig. ****Dulc.*** °Electr. Euphorb. Ferr. °Gran. ? ****Graph.*** °Hell. ****Hep.*** Hyos. ****Ign.*** ****Jod.*** **Kal.* °Kreas. ****Lach.*** Led. **Lyc.* Magn. c. Magn. m. Mang. ****Merc.*** Mez. Mur. ac. Natr. °***Natr. m.*** ****Nitr. ac.*** °N. vom. Oph. *Petr. ****Phosph.*** Phos. ac. Plumb. Prun. Puls. Raph. Ran. Ran. sc. Rhod. °***Rhus.*** Ruta. Sabad. Sabin. Samb. Sassap. ****Sep.*** **Sil.* Spig. ****Spong.*** Squill. Stann. ****Staph.*** Stram. Stront.

Sulph. Sulph. ac. Tart. Teucr. °*Thuj.* Veratr. Viol. od. Zinc.

Aching-pressing, Alum. Arg. ***Ars.*** ***Aur.*** ***Bell.*** *Calc.* Carb. veg. *Caust.* Chin. Cin. Cocc. Con. Cycl. ***Ign.*** Kal. ***Lyc.*** Magn. arct. Magn. m. Mang. Men. ***Merc.*** Natr. m. Nitr. ac. Par. Phos. ac. Puls. Rhab. ***Rhus.*** Sabin. ***Spong.*** Stann. Staph. Stram. ***Sulph.*** Veratr. ***Zinc.***

Air, passing through, as if, Spong.

Beating, Amm. m. Arn. Asa. Bell. Bov. Bry. Calc. Caust. Cham. Clem. Kal. Lach. Lyc. Magn. art. Merc. Natr. Nitr. ac. Phosph. Rhod. Sabad. Sep. Sil. Sulph. Thuj.

Blueness, Arn. Ars. Aur. Carb. an. Carb. veg. Con. Hep. Lach. Mang. Merc. Puls. Sil. Sulph. ac.

Boring, Bell. Lyc. Puls. Sabin.

After bruising, °Con. Jod.

Burning, Ars. Bell. Cann. Carb. veg. Cocc. Hep. Laur. Merc. Phosph. °Puls. Rhab. Sil. Tereb.

Cancerous ulcer, s. CANCER.

In children, °***Ars.*** °Baryt. °Bell. °Cham. °*Calc.* *Hep. °Sil. °***Sulph.***

Choking, Amm. ***Chin.*** Ign. Magn. arct. N. vom. Plumb. ***Puls.*** ***Spong.***

Cold swellings, s. Painless.

During contact, Cocc.

Contraction, ***Acon.*** Alum. Arn. ***Bell.*** ***Borax.*** ***Chin.*** Cocc. Con. ***Ign.*** Jod. Lyc. ***Mang.*** ***Nitr. ac.*** N. vom. Phosph. ***Plumb.*** ***Puls.*** ***Rhus.*** Sep. ***Sulph.*** Sulph. ac.

After contusion, fall, hurt, °Con. °Jod. °Petr. °Phosph.

Crampy feeling, Amm. m. Anac. Ang. Bell.

Bov. Calc. Carb. veg. Caust. Chin. Jod. Kal. Lyc. Magn. arct. Magn. aust. Natr. Phos. ac. Plat. Sabad. Sep. Sil.

Creeping, Bell. Calc. Laur. Sep. Spong. Sulph.

—, as if of some things alive, Ign. Merc. Rhod. Spong. Sulph.

Cutting, Arg. Bell. Calc. Con. Graph. Ign. Lyc. Natr. Phos. ac. Sep. Sil. Staph. Sulph.

Darting, jerking pain, Arn. ***Asa.*** Aur. ***Bell.*** Bry. ***Calc. Caps. Caust.*** Chin. ***Clem.*** Graph. Lyc. Men. Merc. Natr. ***Natr. m.*** Nitr. ac. ***N. vom.*** Petr. ***Puls. Rhus.*** Sep. Sil. ***Sulph.***

Digging, Acon. Amm. m. ***Arn.*** Asa. ***Bell.*** Bov. Bry. Calc. ***Dulc.*** Kal. Natr. ***Phosph.*** Plat. ***Rhod. Rhus.*** Ruta. Sep. ***Spig.*** Stann.

Drawing, pulling, Alum. Ign. ****Merc.*** ****Puls. Sil. Zinc.***

Dwindling, withering, Ars. Cham. Chin. °***Con.*** ****Jod.*** Kal. °***Nitr. ac.*** N. mosch. Phos. ac. Sec. Sil. Veratr.

With emaciation, °Arn. ? °***Ars.*** °Baryt. ? °Bell. ? °***Calc.*** °***Cham.*** °Chin. ? °***Cin.*** °Ferr. ? °Jod. ? °N. mosch. °***N. vom.*** °***Sulph.***

Gnawing, Baryt. Cham. Mez. °Phos. ac. Plat. Ran. sc. Spong. Staph.

Hardness, induration, °***Agn.*** Amb. Amm. Ant. Arn. Ars. Aur. ****Baryt.*** Bar. m. ****Bell.*** Bov. °Bry. ****Calc.*** Camph. Cann. Canth. Caps. ****Carb. an.*** ****Carb. veg.*** Caust. ****Cham.*** Chin. ****Clem.*** Cocc. Coloc. °***Con.*** Cupr. Cycl. Dig. ****Dulc.*** Ferr. ****Graph.*** Hep. Hyos. Ign. ****Jod.*** Kal. ****Lyc. Magn. m.*** Mang. Merc. Natr. Nitr. ac. N. vom. ****Petr.*** Phosph. Plumb. Puls. Raph.

Rhod. ***Rhus.** Sep. **Sil.* Spig. **Spong.* °Squill. ? ***Staph.** *Sulph.* Thuj. Veratr.

Heat, °***Acon.*** Amm. Ant. ***Arn.*** Asa. ****Bell.*** ****Bry.*** Calc. Canth. Carb. an. ***Carb.*** *veg.* Chin. Clem. Cocc. Euphorb. Hep. Kal. Led. Merc. N. vom. Petr. Phosph. Puls. Rhus. Sassap. Sil. Sulph.

Heaviness, sensation of, Bell. Chin. Cupr. Magn. arct. Merc. N. vom. Phosph. Puls. Rhus. Sil. Stann. Staph. Sulph.

Herpes, with eruption, °Dulc. °Graph.

Inflammation, °Acon. °*Arn.* Ars. Aur. ****Baryt.*** **Bell.* Berb. °***Bry.*** Calc. Camph. Canth. ***Carb. an.*** °*Carb. veg.* Cham. *Con.* Dulc. °Gran. ? ****Graph.*** Hep. Kal. Lach. Laur. Lyc. Magn. aust. Magn. m. **Merc.* **Nitr. ac.* N. vom. Petr. ****Phosph.*** Phos. ac. Plumb. Puls. Rhus. Samb. Sassap. **Sil.* Spig. Squill. Staph. **Sulph.* Sulph. ac. Thuj. Veratr. Zinc.

Itching, Amm. Anac. Ant. Canth. Carb. an. Carb. veg. Caust. Cocc. Con. Kal. Magn. c. Merc. Phosph. Ran. sc. Rhab. Rhus. Sabin. Sep. Sil. Spong.

After abuse of Mercury, °*Aur.* °*Carb. veg.* °*Nitr. ac.* °*Thuj.*

Pain, as if contused, Arg. Arn. Ars. Carb. an. Caust. Chin. Cic. Con. Cupr. Jod. Kal. Magn. arct. Natr. m. Phosph. Plat. Puls. Rhod. Rhus. Ruta. Sep. Staph. Sulph. Sulph. ac.

Pains in the evening, Con.

Pain, as if ulcerated, Amm. Amm. m. Aur. Bell. Bry. Calc. Canth. Caust. Cham. Chin. Cic. Cocc. Graph. Hep. Ign. Kal. Merc. Mur. ac. Natr. Natr. m. Nitr. ac. Petr. Phosph. Puls. Rhus. Ruta. Sil. Staph. Sulph. ac. Teucr. Zinc.

Painfulness, **Acon.* Alum. Amb. Amm. Ant. Arn. Ars. Aur. **Baryt.* **Bell.* Berb. Borax. Bry. **Calc.* Calend. **Cann.* Canth. **Carb. an.* Carb. veg. Caust. Cham. Chin. Cic. Clem. Cocc. *Coloc.* Con. Corall. Dulc. **Graph.* Hell. Hep. Ign. **Jod.* Kal. **Lyc.* Magn. arct. Magn. c. Magn. m. **Merc.* Murex. Natr. m. Nitr. ac. N. vom. Petr. **Phosph.* °Phos. ac. Puls. Rhab. Rhus. Selen. °Sep. **Sil.* *Spig.* *Spong.* Squill. Stann. Staph. Stram. **Sulph.* Sulph. ac. Tart. Thuj. Veratr.

Painlessness, (when swollen or suppurating), Ars. Asa. **Calc.* *Cocc.* *Con.* Cycl. *Dulc.* Ign. Lach. Nitr. ac. *Phosph. ac.* Plumb. Rhod. *Sep.* Sil. Spig. Staph. Sulph.

Pinching, Bry. Calc. Magn. arct. Men. Mur. ac. Prun. Rhod. Rhus. Sabad. Stann. Sulph. Veratr.

Pulling, s. Drawing.

Redness, s. Inflamed.

Sensitiveness, Arn. Aur. Baryt. Bell. Cham. Chin. Cocc. Con. Cupr. Graph. Hep. Ign. Kal. Laur. Lyc. Magn. c. Natr. Nitr. ac. N. vom. Petr. Phosph. Phos. ac. Puls. Sep. Sil. Spig. Squill. Sulph. ac.

Sore, as if excoriated, Con. °*Sulph.*

Sore pain, Alum. Ant. Arn. Bry. Calc. Caust. Cic. Clem. *Con.* *Graph.* *Hep.* *Ign.* Kal. Merc. Mez. Natr. m. *N. vom.* Phosph. Plat. Puls. Rhus. *Sep.* Staph. Sulph. Sulph. ac. Teucr. *Zinc.*

Stiffness, Arg.

Stinging, Acon. Agn. Alum. *Amm. m.* Ang. Arg. Arn. *Asa.* Baryt. *Bell.* Berb. Borax. *Bry.* *Calc.*

Carb. an. Caust. Chin. *Cocc. Con.* Cupr. Cycl. Euphr. *Electr.* Graph. Grat. Hell. Hep. *Ign.* Jod. Kal. Lach. Lyc. Magn. art. Magn. arct. **Merc.* Mez. Murex. Mur. ac. Natr. *Natr. m.* Nitr. ac. N. vom. Ol. an. Phell. *Phosph.* Phos. ac. Plumb. *Puls.* Raph. *Ran. sc.* Rhab. Rhus. Sabad. Sang. **Sep.* Sil. Spig. *Spong.* Stann. Staph. *Sulph.* Sulph. ac. Thuj. Veratr. Zinc.

Suppuration, °*Aur.* Bar. m. **Bell.* **Calc.* *Canth.* °*Cist.* Coloc. *Dulc.* **Hep.* Hyos. Ign. Kreas. *Lach. Lyc.* **Merc.* **Nitr. ac.* Petr. °*Phosph.* Sassap. *Sep.* **Sil.* Squill. **Sulph.*

Swelling, Acon. Agn. Alum. Amb. **Amm.* Amm. m. Ant. Arg. *Arn.* **Ars.* °Asa. °Aur. **Baryt.* Bar. m. **Bell.* Borax. Bov. **Bry.* Calad. **Calc.* Camph. Cann. Canth. Caps. **Carb. an.* **Carb. veg.* Caust. **Cham.* Chin. Cic. Cinn. °*Cist.* Clem. Cocc. Coloc. **Con.* Corall. Croc. Cupr. Cycl. Dig. **Dulc.* °Electr. Euphorb. *Ferr.* **Graph.* °Hell. **Hep.* Hyos. Ign. **Jod.* *Kal.* °Kreas. °*Lach.* Led. **Lyc.* Magn. c. Magn. m. Mang. **Merc.* *Merc. corr.* Mez. Mur. ac. *Natr.* Natr. m. **Nitr. ac.* °N. vom. Oph. **Petr.* **Phosph.* Phos. ac. Plumb. *Puls.* Raph. Ran. Ran. sc. Rhod. **Rhus.* Ruta. Sabad. Sabin. Samb. Sassap. **Sep.* **Sil.* *Spig.* **Spong.* *Squill.* Stann. **Staph.* Stram. Stront. **Sulph.* Sulph. ac. Tart. Tereb. Teucr. °*Thuj.* Veratr. Viol. od. Zinc.

Swollen, sensation as if, Ant. *Aur. Bell. Bry.* Carb. veg. Chin. Con. Dulc. *Hep. Ign.* Lach. Magn. art. Magn. arct. *Merc.* Natr. m. *Nitr.*

Nitr. ac. N. mosch. N. vom. *Puls Rhus.* Sabin. Spig. *Spong.* Staph. Sulph. Zinc.

Swollen cords, Calc. Dulc. Hep. Jod. Lyc. Rhus.

Tearing, *Amb.* Amm. *Arn.* Baryt. Bell. Bov. *Bry. Calc.* Cann. Caps. *Carb. an. Carb. veg.* Caust. *Cham. Chin.* Cocc. Con. Cycl. *Dulc.* Ferr. Graph. Grat. *Kal. Lyc.* **Merc.* Mez. Natr. Nitr. ac. N. vom. Ol. an. Phell. Phosph. **Puls. Rhod. Rhus.* Selen. Seneg. Sep. *Sil. Sulph.* Thuj. *Zinc.*

Tension, Alum. Amb. Amm. Ang. Arg. Arn. Aur. Baryt. Bell. Bov. Bry. Calc. Carb. an. Caust. Clem. Coloc. Con. Dulc. Graph. Kal. Lyc. Magn. art. Magn. arct. Merc. Mur. ac. N. vom. Phosph. **Puls.* Rhus. Sabad. Sabin. Sep. Sil. Spong. Staph. Stront. Sulph. Thuj.

Tickling, Kal. Plat.

Titillation, Acon. Arn. Canth. Cann. Con. Magn. aust. Merc. Natr. Phos. ac. Plat. Puls. Rhod. Rhus. Sabin. Sep. Spong. Sulph. Zinc.

Tubercles, °Bry. Calc. **Carb. an.* *Cham. Clem. Dulc. °Graph. Ign. Lyc. °Nitr. ac. °Phosph. Puls. Rhus.

Twitching, Ang. Bell. Calc. Kal. Mez. Natr. Sil.

Ulcers, °*Bell.* °Clem. °Con. °*Hep.* °*Lach.* °*Merc.* °*Phosph.* °*Sil.* °*Sulph.*

Lachrymal glands, °Bry. °*Calc.* °Natr. °Petr. °Phosph. °*Puls.* °Sil. °Stann. ?

Parotid glands, Amm. Arg. Arn. Aur. Baryt. Bell. Bry. Calc. Caps. Carb. an. °*Carb. veg.* Caust. Cham. Chin. Cocc. Con. Dig. Dulc. Euphorb. Graph. Hep. Hyos. Ign. **Kal.* Lyc. Magn. c. Mang. **Merc.* Mez. Natr. Nitr. ac. N. vom. Petr. Phosph. Phos. ac. Puls. Rhus. Sabad. Sep. Sil. Staph. Sulph. Thuj.

Face, tubercles, °Bry.

Lips, ulcers, Ign.

—, induration, Con. Sulph. Zinc.

Lower jaw, *Amm. Amm. m. Arg. Arn. **Ars.* Aur. **Baryt.* °*Bell.* **Calc.* *Chin.* Cic. Clem. Cocc. *Corall.* Croton. °Dulc. *Graph.* Ign. Jod. Kal. °Kreas. Lact. Led. °*Lyc.* Magn. art. Magn. arct. Magn. aust. Magn. c. °*Merc.* Mez. Natr. **Natr. m.* *Nitr. ac.* *Petr. Phosph. Phos. ac. Puls. Raph. *Rhus.* Sep. **Sil.* Spong. Squill. Stann. **Staph.* **Sulph. ac.* Veratr. Zinc.

Inguinal glands, °Ars. °*Aur.* *Calc.* °*Carb. veg.* Clem. **Dulc.* *Graph.* Lyc. **Merc.* Natr. **Nitr. ac.* Phosph. Stann. Stram. **Staph.* **Sulph.* °Thuj. Tereb.

Axilla, Amm. Amm. m. Ars. Asar. Baryt. **Bell.* Calc. Calend. °*Carb. an.* Clem. Coloc. Cupr. *Hep.* Jod. *Kal.* *Lyc.* *Natr. m.* **Nitr. ac.* *Phosph.* Phos. ac. Prun. *Rhus.* *Sep.* **Sil.* °Staph. **Sulph.* Sulph. ac.

Neck, Alum. °*Amm.* *Arn.* Bar. m. **Bell.* **Calc.* Caps. **Carb. an.* Carb. veg. *Caust.* Cinn. °*Cist.* Cupr. °Electr. *Ferr.* *Graph.* Hell. Ign. *Kal.* °Kreas. °*Lach.* **Lyc.* *Magn. m.* **Merc.* *Natr.* Natr. m. **Nitr. ac.* °Phosph. Puls. Selen. **Sil.* *Spig.* *Spong.* °Staph.? **Sulph.* Tart. Viol. tr.

Nape of neck, Baryt. Calc. •Hell. °Jod. °Mur. ac. °Petr. °Phosph. **Sil.* °Staph. ? **Sulph.*
—, tubercles, °Ign. *Nitr. ac.* Phosph.
(Comp. MAMMÆ, TESTICLES, GOÏTRE, TONSILS, &C.)

GNAWING, GNAWING-ITCHING.

Of the skin, in general, *Agar.* **Agn.* *Alum.* Amb. Anac. *Ant.* Arg. Ars. °*Baryt.* Bell. Berb. *Bism.* Bry. *Canth.* *Caps.* Caust. Cham. Clem. Cocc. Con. °*Cycl.* °*Dig.* °*Dros.* Euphorb. Evon. Graph. Guaj. Hell. Hep. Hyos. *Kal.* °*Led.* **Lyc.* Magn. art. Magn. aust. *Men.* Merc. Mez. Natr. N. vom. **Oleand.* *Par.* Phell. *Phosph.* *Phos. ac.* **Plat.* *Puls.* °*Ran. sc.* Rhod. *Rhus.* °*Ruta.* Sep. Spig. °*Spong.* Squill. Stann. **Staph.* Sulph. Tarax. Thuj. * *Veratr.* Vinc.

Scalp, Agn. Alum. Ars. *Baryt.* *Berb.* Bry. Caps. Cham. *Dros.* N. vom. Oleand. Rhus. Ruta. Sep. Staph. Thuj. Veratr.
Ears, Arg. Dros. Indig. Kal. hdr. Mur. ac. Plat. Sulph.
Anus, Agn. Ars. Ferr. Phosph. Phos. ac. Stann. Tarax.
—, perineum, Agn. Ars. Tarax.
Sexual parts, °Kal. °Lyc. N. vom. Plat.
—, testicles, °Phos. ac.
—, scrotum, Plat.
—, labia, °Kal. °Lyc.
Thoracic region, Bell. Berb. Phos. ac.
Dorsal region, Agar. Alum. Anac. Berb. Dig. Guaj. Spig.

Dorsal region, axilla, Mez.
—, neck, Magn. m.
—, hips, Amm.
—, small of back, Amm. Canth. Magn. m. Nicc. Phosph. Stront. Sulph.
—, loins, Phos. ac.
—, back, Bell. Hell. Magn. aust. Magn. m.
—, scapulæ, Alum. Natr.
—, os sacrum, Alum. Kal.
Arms, Ars. Hell. Lam. Led. °*Lyc.* Phell. Phosph. Plat. Ruta. **Sulph.*
—, shoulder, Berb.
—, axilla, Agn.
—, elbow, Berb. Dulc. Phosph. Puls.
—, upper arm, Led.
—, forearm, Rhus.
Hands, Baryt. Berb. Gran. Lam. Merc. Platin.
—, wrists, Berb. Plat. Veratr.
—, fingers, Berb. Oleand., Phos. ac.
—, thumb, Oleand.
Lower limbs, Alum. Bell. °*Lyc.* **Sulph.*
—, nates and hips, Amm. m. Berb. Euphorb. Evon. Kal. hdr. Led. Staph. Sulph.
—, thighs, Agar. Anac. Ars. Berb. Canth. Chel. Dig. Euphorb. Kal. hdr. Led. N. vom. Par. Phosph. Ran. sc. Spig. Stront. Tarax.
—, knees, Berb. Ran. sc. Zinc.
—, legs, Aur. Berb. Euphorb. Natr. Natr. m. Phos. ac. Tarax.
—, tibiæ, Bism. Coff. Lam. Laur.
Feet, Agar. Anac. *Bell.* Berb. Bism. Cocc. Crotal. Dig. *Graph.* Led. Nicc. Plat. *Ran. sc.*
—, heels, *Graph. Ran. sc.*
—, soles, Plat. Tart.

Feet, toes, Berb. Cocc. Kal. *Ran. sc.* Sep.
Bones, periosteum, *Amm. m.* Arg. Bell. Canth. *Con. Dros.* Graph. Lyc. *Mang. Phosph. Phos. ac.* Puls. °*Ruta.* Samb. Staph. Stront.
Nails, Alum.
Glands, Baryt. Cham. Mez. °Phos. ac. Plat. Ran. sc. Spong. Staph.

GNAWING-PAINFUL.

Ulcers, Agn. *Baryt.* Bell. Calc. *Cham.* Cycl. **Dros.* Hyos. *Kal.* Led. *Lyc.* Mang. *Merc.* Mez. Natr. *Phosph.* Phos. ac. °*Plat.* °*Puls.* °*Ran. sc.* Rhus. Ruta. **Staph. Sulph.* Thuj.
Tumors, Rhus.
Nails, on the, Alum.

Face, Caps. Caust. °Con. Dig.
Mouth, Kal. *Merc.* Puls.
Hands, eruption, Ant.

GOÏTRE.

Dorsal region, °Amm. °*Calc.* Con. **Jod.* Kal. hdr. °*Lyc. Natr.* Natr. m. Plat. °*Spong.*
—, itching, Natr.
—, as if alive within, Spong.
—, constrictive, Jod.
—, hard, Spong.
—, indurated, **Jod. Spong.*
—, jerking, Lyc.
—, painful, Jod. Plat.
—, pressing, from within outward, Spong.
—, sensitive, Kal. hdr.

Dorsal region, soft, Kal. hdr.
—, tensive, Jod.
—, tickling, Plat.
—, throbbing, Jod. Lyc.

GRAPE-SHAPED.

Eruption, Agar. **Calc. Rhus.* Staph. Veratr.
Blisters, *Rhus.*

Arms, eruption, Calc.
Hands, eruption, Rhus.

GRAY.

In general, gray colour of, °*Carb.veg.* Kreas. Lach. Laur. Sec.
—, livid, sallow, **Ars.* Bism. *Borax. Bry. Canth.* °*Carb. veg.* **Chin.* Cic. °*Croc.* Euphorb. Ferr. *Ign.* °*Ipec.* °*Kreas. Lach.* Laur. *Lyc.* Magn. c. **Merc.* Mosch. Natr. m. Nitr. ac. *N. vom.* Op. Phosph. Plumb. °*Samb.* Sec. *Sep. Sil.* Zinc.

GRAY, THAT WHICH IS.

Blennorrhœa, expectoration, *Amb.* Anac. *Arg.* Ars. Carb. an. Caust. Chin. Cop. Kreas. Lach. Magn. m. Merc. Sep. *Sil.* Thuj.
Tumors, Nitr. ac.
Pus, *Amb.* Ars. Carb. an. **Caust.* Chin. Lyc. Merc. Sep. *Sil.* Thuj.
Spots, Nitr. ac.
Ulcers, (Comp.: Pus, gray.)

Scurfs, crusts, Ars. Merc.

Hands, spots, Nitr. ac.
Lower limbs, crusty ulcer, Ars.

Gray-yellow.

Herpes, °*Sulph.*

Greasiness.

Of the skin, Agar. Aur. °*Bry.* Calc. Chin. Magn. c. °*Merc.* °*Natr. m.* Plumb. Selen. Stram.

Nose, shining like oil, Calc.
Face, shining, Plumb. Selen.
Lips, Amm. m.

Green.

Colour of skin, Ars. °*Carb. veg.* Veratr.
Crusts, scurfs, **Calc.*
Spots, Ars. °*Con.* Crotal. Vip. torv.
Ulcers, (Comp.: Pus, greenish) Staph.

Face, Ars. Calc.

Hæmorrhage.

In general, **Acon.* Agar. Alum. Amb. Amm. Amm. m. Anac. **Ant.* Arg. **Arn.* **Ars.* Asar. Baryt. **Bell.* Bism. Borax. Bov. **Bry.* **Calc.*

*Cann. **Canth.* Caps. Carb. an. **Carb. veg.* Caust. **Cham.* **Chin.* Cin. Clem. Cocc. Coff. Colch. Coloc. Con. **Croc.* *Crotal.* *Cupr.* **Diad.* Dig. Dros. Dulc. Euphr. **Ferr.* Graph. Hep. *Hyos.* Ign. Jod. **Ipec.* Kal. Kreas. Lach. *Led.* *Lyc.* Magn. art. Magn. arct. Magn. aust. Magn. c. Magn. m. **Merc.* *Mercurial.* Mez. Mosch. Mur. ac. Natr. Natr. m. Nitr. **Nitr. ac.* N. mosch. **N. vom.* Oph. Op. Par. Petr. **Phosph.* Phos. ac. **Plat.* Plumb. **Puls.* Rhod. *Rhus.* Ruta. Sabad. **Sabin.* Sassap. Sec. Selen. **Sep.* *Sil.* Stann. Staph. *Stram.* **Sulph.* Sulph. ac. Tarax. Tart. Thuj. Val. Veratr. Vip. torv. Zinc.

Eyes, **Bell.* °Carb. veg. °Cham. Crotal. °Euphr. °N. vom. Ruta.

Eyelids, **Bell.*

Ears, Bry. Caust. Cic. Galv. °*Graph.* *Merc.* Oph. Petr. Phosph. °*Rhus.* Sep.

Nose, **Acon.* Agar. Amb. **Amm.* *Anac. Ant. Arg. **Arn.* *Ars.* *Baryt.* *Bell. Berb. Borax. **Bry.* **Calc.* **Cann.* Canth. Caps. *Carb. an.* **Carb. veg.* *Caust.* **Cham.* **Chin.* Chinin. Coff. Colch. Con. Corall. **Croc.* Crotal. Cupr. ac. Diad. Dig. **Dros.* Dulc. Electr. °Euphr. Ferr. Galv. *Graph.* Hep. Hyos. *Ign. *Jod.* Ipec. *Kal.* Kal. chl. *Kal. hdr.* Kreas. Lach. Led. *Lyc.* Magn. art. Magn. arct. *Magn. c.* Magn. m. Magn. s. Meph. **Merc.* Merc. d. Mosch. Mur. ac. Natr. *Natr. m.* Natr. s. **Nitr. ac.* N. vom. Oph. Par. *Petr.* **Phosph.* Phos. ac. **Puls.* Ratanh. Rhod. **Rhus.* **Ruta.* Sassap. Sec. **Sep.* **Sil.* Spong.

Stann. **Sulph.* Sulph. ac. Tarax. Thuj. Veratr. Zinc.

Lips and mouth, region of, Ars. °Bry. Carb. an. Gins. **Ign.* Kal. Phos. ac. Plat.

Mouth, Agar. *Alum.* Amm. Anac. Ant. °*Arn.* °Ars. Arum. Baryt. **Bell.* Borax. Bov. **Calc. Canth.* °*Carb. an.* **Carb. veg.* Caust. *Chin.* °Chinin. **Cist.* Con. Crotal. Croton. Euphr. Ferr. magn. °Gran. ? Graph. °*Jod.* Kal. Kal. chl. Lach. °*Led.* Lyc. *Magn. m.* **Merc. Merc. d.* Natr. *Natr. m.* Nitr. *Nitr. ac.* N. mosch. N. vom. Oph. *Phosph. Phos. ac.* Ran. sc. Ruta. Sec. *Sep.* °*Sil.* Staph. **Sulph.* Sulph. ac. *Tereb. *Tong.* **Zinc.*

—, Buccal cavity, hæmoptysis. °*Arn.* **Bell.* Canth. Chin. °Chinin. Lach. °Led. Merc. N. vom. Oph. Sec.

—, gums, Agar. *Alum.* Amm. Anac. Ant. °*Ars.* Arum. Baryt. Bell. Borax. Bov. **Calc.* °*Carb. an.* **Carb. veg.* Caust. *Cist.* Con. Crotal. Croton. Euphr. Ferr. magn. °Gran. ? Graph. °*Jod.* Kal. Kal. chl. Lach. Lyc. *Magn. m.* **Merc. Merc. d.* Natr. *Natr. m.* Nitr. °Nitr. ac. N. mosch. *Phosph. Phos. ac.* Ran. sc. Ruta. *Sep.* °Sil. Staph. **Sulph.* Sulph. ac. °Tereb. Tong. **Zinc.*

Anus, Alum. **Amm.* **Amm. m.* °*Anac.* Ant. Ars. Asar. Baryt. Borax. Calc. Caps. *Carb. an.* **Carb. veg.* Cast. **Caust.* Chinin. Coloc. **Con.* Croc. Crotal. *Cupr. Ferr.* Graph. Hep. Ign. *Kal.* °*Lach.* Lam. Led. Lyc. Magn. arct. Magn. m. **Merc.* Mercurial. **Merc. corr.* Mur. ac. Natr. m. Nitr. Nitr. ac. **N. vom.* Oph. **Petr.* **Phosph.* Plat. Prun. *Puls.*

Raph. Ratanh. Sabad. Sabin. °*Sassap.* Selen. **Sep.* Sil. Stram. **Sulph.* Tart. Thuj. Val. Vip. torv. Zinc.

Sexual parts, (metrorrhagia), **Acon.* Amm. **Bell.* Bry. *Calc. **Cham.* **Chin.* °Chinin. ? Cin. °Cinnam. ? Cocc. °Coff. ? **Croc.* °Diad. ? **Ferr.* °Hyos. °Ign. ? **Ipec.* Jod. °Kreas. °Led. ? Magn. arct. °Magn. aust. *Merc.* °Natr. Natr. m. N. vom. °*Plat.* °*Puls.* °Rhus. °Ruta. ? Sabin. **Sec.* Squill. *Stram.* °Sulph. ? °Sulph. ac.

—, urethra, Amm. °Arn. *Ars. °Calc. **Canth.* °Caps. ? °Caust. °Chin. ? °*Con.* °Cop. ? Crotal. °Euphorb. ? **Ipec.* **Lyc.* **Merc.* Mez. °Mill. Murex. °N. vom. Op. *Phosph.* °*Puls.* *Sec.* Tereb. Uv. Zinc.

Nipples, Sep. °Sulph.

Nails, Crotal.

Hair, diseases of the.

Cold, Sab.

Contractive sensation, **Chin.*

Desiccated, Alum. **Kal.*

Dry, Alum. **Kal.*

Dry, as flax, °Phos. ac.

Hair, stands on end, Amm. Arn. Baryt. Cann. Canth. Cin. Cocc. Croc. Dulc. Laur. Lyc. Magn. c. Merc. Mez. Mur. ac. N. vom. Puls. Ran. Sil. Spig. Spong. Veratr. Zinc.

Entangled, Borax.

Fetid, Natr. m.

As if glued together, Borax. Natr. m.

Growing, Electr. Lyc.

19*

Greasy, Bry.
Turning gray, °Lyc. °Phos. ac. Sulph.
As if moving, Carb. veg.
Painful, Agar. Amm. **Amb.* **Ars.* **Bell.* Calc. Caps. *Carb. veg.* °*Chin.* Cinn. *Ferr.* Hep. *Ign. Mez. Natr. m. Natr. s. Nitr. ac. **N. vom.* Par. Spig. Spong. Sulph. Thuj. * *Veratr.*
Plica polonica, Borax. °Natr. m. ?
Sensation as if pulled at, **Acon.* Alum. Arn. Baryt. Bell. Bry. Canth. Kal. Kreas. °*Laur.* Lyc. Magn. m. Mur. ac. Nitr. Phosph. Phos. ac. Rhus.
Sensation, as if torn out, °Chin. Indig. °Lyc. Selen. Sulph.
Wilted, °Phos. ac.

HAIR, FALLING OFF OF.

Eyebrows, Agar. *Bell.* Caust. Hell. **Kal.* Par. Plumb. Selen.
Whiskers, Agar. Amb. °*Calc.* °*Graph.* Natr. **Natr. m.* Nitr. ac. Plumb. Sil.
Baldness, °*Baryt.* °*Lyc.*
Occiput, Calc. °*Carb. veg.* Hep. °*Petr.* Sep. Sil. Staph. Sulph.
Head, in general, Alum. *Amb. °Amm. °Ant. Ars. Aur. °*Baryt.* Bell. Bov. **Calc.* Canth. **Carb. an.* **Carb. veg.* Caust. Chel. Colch. *Con. Cycl. Dulc. *Ferr.* Ferr. magn. **Graph.* Hell. **Hep.* Ign. Jod. **Kal.* *Kreas. °Lach. **Lyc.* *Magn. c.* **Merc.* Natr. **Natr. m.* **Nitr. ac.* Op. Par. Petr. *Phosph.* *Phos. ac.* Plumb. Puls. Rhus. *Sassap. Sec. Selen. **Sep.* **Sil.* Staph. **Sulph. ac.* Tab. Zinc.

Headache, after frequent attacks of, °Hep.
Body, on the whole, Ars. *Calc. Carb. veg. Graph.* Hell. Kal. Lach. *Natr. m.* Op. Oph. Phosph. *Sabin. Sec.* Sulph.
Diseases, after severe, °*Carb. veg.* °Chin. Ferr. °*Hep.* °*Phosph.*
Chagrin, grief, after, °Ign. °Lyc. °Phos. ac. °Sulph. ac.
Moustaches, Baryt. *Kal.* Plumb.
Abuse of mercury, after, °Hep.
Nostrils, Calc. *Caust. Graph.* Sil.
Sexual parts, Bell. Hell. Natr. *Natr. m.* Nitr. ac. *Rhus.* Selen.
Temples, Calc. *Kal.* Lyc. Merc. *Natr. m.* Par. Sabin.
Vertex, **Baryt.* Calc. Carb. an. °*Graph. Hep.* Lyc. *Nitr. ac.* Plumb. Selen. °*Sep.* Sil. Zinc.
Pregnancy, during, °Lach, Merc.
Sides of the head, Bov. °*Graph.* Kal. Phos. ac. Staph. Zinc.
Bald spots, Hep. Phosph.
—, as if from scaldhead, Nitr.
Sinciput, °Ars. *Bell. Hep.* °*Merc.* °*Natr. m.* °*Phosph.* Sil.
In lying-in females, °*Calc.* °Natr. m. °*Sulph.*

Hairy parts, on.

Eruption, Kal. Lyc. *Merc. Natr. m.* Nitr. ac. Phos. ac. *Rhus.*

Hairy Scalp and Scalp in general.

Abscesses, °*Calc.* Lyc.

Acne, eruption, Bov.
Biting in the skin, Agn. Bry. Coloc. Dros. Grat. Jod. Magn. arct. Merc. Mez. Ran. Rhod. Thuj. Zinc.
Blisters, bloody, °Ars.
Bloatedness, Acon. Berb. Rhus. Ruta. Staph. Sulph.
Boils, Baryt. Bell. Calc. Kal. *Led. Magn. m. Mur. ac. Nitr. ac. Rhus.
Bone-pains, Ang. *Ant.* *Arg.* **Aur.* Baryt. *Bell.* Bry. *Calc.* Canth. Carb. veg. Caust. Cham. **Chin.* Cocc. Cupr. Graph. Guaj. **Hep.* Ign. Ipec. *Lyc.* Mang. **Merc.* *Mez.* Natr. m. Nitr. **Nitr. ac.* N. vom. *Phosph.* *Phos. ac.* Puls. Rhod. Rhus. **Ruta.* Sabad. Sabin. Samb. *Sep.* *Sil.* Spig. Staph. Sulph. Veratr. Viol. tr. Zinc.
Bony tumors, **Aur.* °Daph. °*Merc.*
Burning of the skin. Ars. Baryt. **Bry.* **Calc.* *Caps.* Clem. Coloc. Cupr. Dros. Grat. Indig. Lach. Laur. Lyc. *Merc.* Mur. ac. Natr. m. Oleand. *Ol. an.* Par. Phell. Phosph. Phos. ac. Plat. Ran. Ruta. Sep. Spig. Spong. Staph. Sulph. Thuj. Veratr. Viol. tr. Zinc.
Burning of the eruption, Ars. Baryt. Nitr. ac.
As if burnt, Lach.
Contact, being painful, Amb. Arg. Ars. Aur. Baryt. *Bell.* *Bry.* *Calc.* *Carb. veg.* **Chin.* Cinn. Ferr. Hell. Graph. Hep. Ign. Lyc. Magn. **Merc.* Mez. *Mosch.* Natr. c. Natr. m. Nitr. Nitr. ac. **N. vom.* *Par.* *Petr.* Phosph. Phos. ac. Rhod. Rhus. Sabin. Sassap. *Spig. **Staph.* **Sulph.*
Contraction of skin, *Carb. veg.* **Chin.* Lyc. Natr. m. Par. Plat. Rhus. Stann.

Crawling, Alum. Ant. Baryt. Ran. Rhus. Sil. Spig. Thuj.
Creeping, Alum. Cann. Chin. Kal. Kal. chl. Ran. Sil. Staph. Thuj.
Cutting in the skin, Clem.
Drawing-up of the skin, Carb. an.
Early in bed, Carb. veg.
Ears, behind the, Alum. Amb. Amm. Amm. m. Anac. Ant. Ang. Arg. Arn. Aur. **Baryt.* Bell. Bry. **Calc.* Cann. **Canth.* Carb. an. Carb. veg. **Caust.* Chel. Chin. Cic. Cin. Cocc. **Con.* Dros. **Graph.* Hell. *Hep.* Kal. Lach. *Lyc.* Men. Merc. Mez. *Mur. ac.* Nitr. Nitr. ac. **Oleand.* **Petr.* Phosph. Phos. ac. Puls. Rhus. Ruta. Sabad. Sabin. Sassap. Selen. *Sep.* **Sil.* Spong. Stann. **Staph.* *Sulph.* Tarax. Thuj. Verb. Viol. tr. Zinc.
Ecchymosed, as if, Arn. **Ars.* Asa. Baryt. Calc. *Ferr.*
Eruption, in general, *°Baryt.* Bar. m. **Calc.* *°Carb. an.* Cic. *°Clem.* **Lyc.* **Merc.* **Oleand.* *Petr. *Rhus.* *Ruta.* Spig. *Staph.
Eruptions, dry, *°Baryt.* *°Calc.* Merc. °Mez.
Eruptions, fetid, *Graph. °Lyc. Nitr. ac.
Eruptions, hard, Ant. Carb. an. Natr. m.
Eruptions, humid, *°Baryt.* **Calc.* °Clem. **Graph.* °Hell. *°Hep.* **Merc.* **Nitr. ac.* *°Oleand.*
Eruptions, itching, **Alum.* Baryt. Bov. Graph. **Merc.* °Mez. °Nitr. ac. Oleand. Phosph. Sep. Sil. Staph.
Eruptions, painful, °Clem. °Daph. *Graph. Hell. Kal. Magn. c. Merc. N. vom. Par.
Eruptions, suppurating, **Ars.* Cic. Nitr. ac. (Comp. Ulcers.)

Eruptions, ulcers, &c., spreading. °*Ars.* Caps. **Rhus.*

Forehead, Alum. Amb. Ant. Aur. Baryt. Bell. Bov. Calc. Carb. an. Carb. veg. Caust. °Clem. Con. Cupr. Dros. Gran. Graph. Hep. Jod. Kal. Laur. Led. Lyc. Men. Merc. Mur. ac. Natr. m. Nitr. ac. Par. Phosp. Phos. ac. Rhus. Sep. Sil. Spig. Staph. Viol. od.

Glandular swellings, °Ars. °*Baryt.* **Calc.* Lyc.

Gnawing on skin, Agn. Alum. Ars. *Baryt. Berb.* Bry. Caps. Cham. *Dros.* N. vom. Oleand. Rhus. Ruta. Sep. Staph. Thuj. Veratr.

Hair, s. Falling off, Diseases of.

— borders of, Calc. Natr. m. Sep.

Herpes, Baryt. Cupr. Kal. Petr. Rhus.

Itching, Agar. Agn. Alum. **Amm.* **Amm. m.* Anac. °Ant. Arg. Arn. *Ars.* Asar. *Baryt. Berb. Bov.* **Calc.* Calc. ph. Caps. Carb. an. *Caust. Cham.* Chin. Coff. Con. *Crotal.* Cycl. Dros. **Graph.* Grat. *Kal.* Lach. *Laur. Lyc.* Magn. arct. Magn. c. Magn. m. Mang. Meph. **Merc.* Mez. Mur. ac. *Natr. m.* Nitr. °Nitr. ac. *Oleand. Ol. an.* Par. Petr. Phell. **Phosph.* Phos. ac. Puls. Ran. sc. Ratanh. *Rhod. *Rhus.* Ruta. Sabad. **Sassap.* **Seneg.* **Sep.* **Sil.* Spig. Staph. Stront. Sulph. Sulph. ac. *Thuj. Veratr.

Itching, like nettlerash, Ant. Calc.

Itching, as of vermin, Bov. Caps. Laur. Merc. *Mez. Oleand.* Rhod. Ruta. Sabad. Staph.

Lupia, °Calc. °Lyc. ? (Comp. Abscesses.)

Liable to take cold, Baryt. Borax. Calc. °Carb. veg. **Kal.* Led. Lyc. Natr. Natr. m. Phos.

At night, Bry. Chin. Hep. Led. Lyc. Oleand. Par. Rhus. Staph. Thuj.

Occiput, principally, *Amb.* Amm. Amm. m. *Ars.* **Baryt.* Bell. Berb. *Borax.* Bry. *Calc. Carb. an. Carb. veg.* Caust. Chel. Chin. °*Clem.* Cupr. Cycl. °*Daph.* Euphorb. Graph. *Hep.* Jod. Lach. Laur. *Lyc.* Merc. Mez. Natr. Natr. m. Nitr. ac. Oleand. *Petr.* Puls. Rhus. Ruta. *Sep. Sil.* Spig. *Staph. Sulph. Thuj.* Viol. od. Zinc.

Pain, as if contused, bruised, Arn. Dig. Par.

Open air, walking in the, Calc.

Pain, as if sore, *Amb. Anac. Ars. Bry. Calc. *Dros.* Gran. Graph. **Hep.* Jod. Magn. c. **Merc.* **Mez.* Natr. c. Natr. m. N. vom. *Ol. an.* Par. Petr. Phosph. Phos. ac. Ran. Ruta. Staph. Stront. Zinc.

Pain as if ulcerated, Agar. Arg. *Ars. Colch. Graph. Kal. hdr. *Kreas.* **Merc.* Mur. ac. Nitr. ac. *Petr.* Phosph. Rhod. Rhus. Ruta. Sil. Spig. Stann. Sulph. ac. Tarax. Zinc.

Painfulness, Agar. Alum. Amb. Amm. Ant. **Ars. Baryt. Bell. Bry. Calc. Carb. veg.* **Chin.* Cinn. *Ferr.* Ign. *Lact.* Lyc. Magn. c. **Merc.* Mez. *Mosch.* Natr. c. Natr. m. Nitr. Nitr. ac. **N. vom.* Par. *Petr.* Phosph. Phos. ac. Rhod. Rhus. Sabin. Sassap. *Spig. Staph. Sulph.*

Peeling off, Lach.

Pimples, Agar. Alum. Anac. Ant. Amb. Arg. **Ars.* Baryt. Bar. m. Berb. Bov. Calc. °Clem. *Con.* Cycl. Hell. **Hep.* Kal. **Led.* Lyc. Magn. art. Magn. arct. Mur. ac. Natr. °*Natr. m.* Nitr. N. vom. Oleand. Par. Petr. Puls. Rhus. Sil. Tarax. Zinc.

Pityriasis, Magn. art. °*Oleand.?* °*Sabad.?* °*Sulph.?*

Pocks, Bov.

Pustules, Arn. **Ars.* Bov. Gran. Kal. Mur. ac. N. vom. Puls. Rhus. Sil.

Rash, Natr. m. Spong. Tart.

Red eruptions, pimples and spots, Agar. Amb. Anac. Ant. Ars. Bov. Kal. *Mosch.* Natr. c. N. vom.

With red areola, Anac.

Rhagades, Ruta.

Scales, **Alum.* Calc. Crotal. Graph. Kal. Lach. °Mez. **Oleand.* °Rhus. Staph.

Scaly scaldhead, °*Oleand.*

Scurfs, crusts, °Alum. **Ars.* °Baryt. **Calc.* °*Carb. an.* °Chel. Electr. Ferr. magn. **Graph.* °Hell. °Kal. Magn. c. **Merc.* Mur. ac. **Natr. m.* Nitr. ac. **Oleand.* Par. Petr. Phosph. **Rhus.* Ruta. Sil. Sulph.

Sensitive skin, Alum. Amb. Ars. **Baryt. Bell.* Borax. Bov. *Bry. Calc.* Carb. an. *Carb. veg.* **Chin.* Chinin. *Ferr.* Grat. Ign. *Lach.* Lyc. Magn. c. Magn. m. Mang. Natr. c. Natr. s. Nitr. *Nitr. ac. **N. vom.* Par. *Petr.* Phosph. Phos. ac. Rhus. Sassap. Selen. *Sep. Sil.* Spig. Spong. Squill. *Sulph.* *Zinc.

Sides of the head, Baryt. Caust. Laur.

Skin, adhesion of, Arn. Berb. Magn. art. Par.

Skin, rough, Natr. m. Ruta.

Scratch, desire to, Alum. Amm. Baryt. *Bov.* Lyc. Mur. ac. Natr. m. Oleand. Par.

—, relieved by, *Grat.* Mez. Ol. an.

—, until blood is drawn, Alum. Bov. Carb. an. Magn. c. Mur. ac.

Scratching, causes pain, Alum. Anac. Ars. *Calc. Caps. Kal. Lach. Laur. *Oleand. Par.
—, causes the symptom to shift, Cycl. Mez.
—, aggravates, Caps.
—, does not remove the symptom, Bov. Calc.
Smarting eruptions and ulcers, Agn. Bry. Coloc. Dros. Jod. Magn. art. Ran. sc.
Soft, that which is, °Calc. °Daph.
Soreness, Bov. °*Calc.*
Spots, °*Ars.* Mosch. Kal. Zinc.
Spots, like scalds, Nitr.
Spots, brownish, °Ars.
Spreads, that which, Ars. **Merc.*
Stinging in the skin, Agn. Ant. Arn. Asa. *Asar. Berb.* Caust. Chin. Cupr. Cycl. Mez. Petr. Phos. ac. Sulph. Thuj.
Swelling, **Ars. Bell.* Cham. Crotal. Cupr. °Daph. Dig. Merc. Op. Petr. Phosph. Puls. *Rhus.* Ruta. Sep. Stram. Sulph.
Temporal region, Anac. °*Alum.* Asar. Ant. Ars. Bell. Bov. Carb. veg. Caust. Guaj. Merc. Mur. ac. Ran. sc. Ratanh. Sassap. Spig. Thuj.
Tightness, of the skin, Asar. Baryt. Berb. Carb. an. Caust. Lam. Par. Ruta. Sabad. Stront. Spig. Staph.
Titillation, Acon. Alum. Amm. Arn. Ars. Baryt. Calc. Carb. veg. Chel. Croton. Lach. Laur. Led. Nitr. ac. *N. vom.* Plat. Ran. Rhod. Rhus. Sabad. Spig. Veratr.
Tumors, blotches, tubercles, Anac. Baryt. **Calc.* Carb. an. °*Daph.* Hell. Kal. *Lyc.* Natr. m. N. vom. Puls. Phosph. Phos. ac. Ruta. Sil.
Ulcers, **Ars.* Nitr. ac. Ruta.
On the vertex, Agar. Asa. Arn. *Aur. Baryt.* Bo-

rax. Bov. Bry. Calc. *Carb. an.* Carb. veg. Caust. *Cupr.* Electr. Graph. Hep. Lyc. Men. Mez. Nitr. ac. Par. Phosph. Plumb. Ran. sc. Ruta. Selen. Sep. Sil. Spig. Spong. Staph. Sulph. Veratr. Zinc.

Vesicles, Bov. °Clem. Ol. an.

When getting warm in bed, Bov.

Watery swellings, °Daph.

In wet weather, Magn. c.

White, Ant.

Yellowish-white, Calc.

Yellow spots, Kal.

Hands and Fingers.

Arthritic (swelling), °*Calc.* °*Carb. an.* Carb. veg. Caust. °*Cocc.* Gent. Graph. Hep. **Lyc.* Magn. art. Mur. ac. Petr. Sep. Teucr. Veratr.

—, nodosities, wrists, °*Calc.*

—, fingerjoints, °*Agn.* °*Calc.* °*Clem.* °*Graph.* °*Lyc.* Staph. ?

Black, swelling, Lach. Vip. torv.

Bleeding, rhagades, **Alum.* *Merc.* **Petr.*

Blisters, vesicles, hands. Ant. Bov. *Bruc.* Canth. Caust. °*Clem.* *Cocc.* Daph. °*Hep.* *Kal.* *Kal. chl.* *Kal. hdr.* *Lach.* Magn. c. *Merc.* *Mez.* *Natr. m.* Phosph. *Rhus.* *Selen.* *Sep.* *Sil.* *Squill.* *Sulph.*

Blisters, vesicles, wrists, *Amm. m.* Merc. *Rhus.*

—, fingers, Bell. °*Clem.* Cupr. *Cycl.* Electr. *Graph.* Grat. Hell. °*Hep.* *Kal.* Lach. Laur. Magn. c. Mang. *Natr.* *Natr. m.* Nitr. s. *Nitr. ac.* Phosph. *Phos. ac.* *Plumb.* *Ran.* *Rhus.* *Sassap.* *Sep.*

Blisters, finger-joints, Cyc. Hell. Hep.
—, thumbs, *Hep. Lach. Natr.* Natr. s. *Phos. ac. Sep.*
Blotches, tubercles, hand, Ars. Carb. an. *Kal. chl. Merc. Rhus.* Rhus. v. Sep. *Spig.* Stram.
—, wrist-joints, Amm. m.
—, fingers, Berb. Caust. Cocc. *Con. Lach. Led.* Lyc. Natr. Rhus. Veratr. Zinc.
—, finger-joints, *Zinc.*
Blisters, phagedænic, hand, °Clem. Magn. c.
—, fingers, °*Clem. Graph.* Hep. *Kal. Magn. c.* Nitr. ac. *Sil.* Sulph.
—, wrist-joints, Hep.
—, thumb, *Hep.* Nitr. ac.
Blisters, transparent, Mang. Ran.
Blueness, hands, Acon. Amm. Cocc. Lach. **N. vom.* Spong. Zinc.
Blue, eruption, *Ran.*
—, swelling, Lach.
Bones, affections of, hand, Aeth. Agar. Anac. Anis. Arg. Asa. Atham. *Aur.* Bell. *Berb. Bism.* Carb. an. **Carb. veg.* Caust. *Chel. Chin. Euphr.* Ign. Jod. Kal. Lach. Lact. Laur. Led. Magn. c. Magn. m. *Mang. Merc.* Mez. Natr. Natr. s. Nitr. Ol. an. Par. *Phosph.* Phos. ac. Ran. sc. Rhod. *Sabin.* Samb. Sassap. *Spig. Stann.* Staph. Sulph. Sulph. ac. Tax. *Teucr.* Zinc.
—, fingers, Crotal. Daph.
Brittle, Graph. *Natr. Natr. m.* Petr.
Brown, eruptions, Natr. m.
—, spots, Natr. m. °Petr.
—, scald, Amm. m.
—, swelling, Lach.

Burning, hands, Anac. Anis. Arg. Asar. Baryt. Berb. Bry. Calc. *Canth.* Carb. an. Cham. Cop. Dulc. Graph. Galv. *Hep.* Kal. °*Lach.* *Laur.* Lyc. Magn. c. Merc. Natr. Natr. m. *Natr. s.* Nicc. N. mosch. *N. vom.* Ol. an. *Petr.* **Phosph.* Phos. ac. Plat. Ran. Rhod. Rhus. Sassap. *Sec.* Spig. Spong. Stann. *Stront.* Sulph. Tab. Tax. Zinc.

—, wrist-joints, Arg. Asar. Berb. Mez. Phosph. Plat. Plumb. *Stront.* Thuj. Zinc.

—, finger, **Agar.* Asa. *Berb.* Borax. Calc. Carb. veg. *Caust.* Coloc. Con. Croc. Dig. Euphorb. Gran. Graph. *Kal.* °*Lach.* Laur. Lyc. Magn. art. Magn. arct. Magn. m. Mang. Merc. Mez. Mill. Mosch. *Natr.* Natr. s. Nicc. Nitr. ac. N. vom. *Oleand.* Ol. an. Petr. Ran. Ran. sc. *Rhod.* Sassap. Sabad. Sabin. Sil. Spig. Staph. *Sulph.* Sulph. ac. Tarax. *Teucr.* Therid. Veratr. Vip. torv. *Zinc.*

—, finger-joints, Berb. Carb. veg. Caust. Sabin. Spig.

—, thumb, Gran. Graph. Lach. Laur. Magn. art. Merc. N. vom. Oleand. Ol. an. Sassap. Staph.

Burning eruptions, itching, &c., **Agar.* Amm. m. Berb. Carb. an. Cic. Gran. Graph. Jod. *Laur.* Lyc. Magn. arct. Magn. m. Merc. Natr. m. Natr. s. Nitr. ac. N. vom. Oleand. Plumb. Rhus. Sassap. Sil. Spig. *Stront.* Sulph.

—, phagedænic blisters, Graph. Sil.

—, swelling, Oleand. Vip. torv.

—, ulcers, °*Ars.* Ran.

—, erysipelas, Rhod.

Bubbling, hand, Berb. Rhus.
—, fingers, Berb. Par. Spig. Teucr.
Callosities, hand, °*Graph.*
Carbuncle, finger, °*Lach. Sec.*
Chilblains, hand, Nitr. ac. *Stann. Zinc.*
—, fingers, Carb. an. *Lyc.* °*Petr.* °*Puls.* ***Sulph.*** Sulph. ac.
—, itching and redness, as if from, **Agar. Berb.* Borax. *Lyc.* Magn. arct. **N. vom.* Spig. **Sulph.*
Cobweb, sensation as of, hand, Borax.
Confluent eruptions, Cic.
Contraction of tendons, s. Muscles.
Copper-coloured, spots. °*Nitr. ac.*
Cracked, callosities, Graph.
Crawling, finger, Lach.
Creeping, hand, Arn.
Drawing-painful, swelling, Chin.
Dryness, hand, *Anac. Baryt.* Bism. Ferr. magn. *Hep.* Lach. **Lyc. Natr. Natr. m.* Phosph. *Phos. ac. Sabad. Sulph.* Tax. *Thuj.*
—, finger, Anac. *Sil.* Tart.
Eczema, hand, Mez. Phosph.
—, finger, *Sil.*
Eruptions, close together, Rhus.
Eruptions, dry, Bov. Lyc. Veratr.
Eruptions, fine, **Carb. veg.*
Eruption, gnawing, Ant.
Eruption, hands, Alum. **Carb. veg.* Dig. *Hep.* Ipec. **Merc. Mur. ac. Nitr. ac.* Spig. *Sulph. Sulph. ac.*
—, wrists, Hep.
—, fingers, Caust. Corall. Galv. Graph. Mez.

Eruptions, raised, Bruc. Kal. Lach. Rhus v. *Sulph. ac.*
Erysipelas, hand, Graph. Rhod.
Flesh as if loose, Ol. an.
Formication, Alum. Sec.
Furfuraceous, eruptions, *Alum.*
Ganglia, hand, *Amm.* Magn. m. *Phos. ac. Plumb.* Prun. Rhod. *Sil.*
Gangrenous blisters, hand, Sec.
Gnawing, hand, Baryt. Berb. Gran. Laur. Merc. Plat.
—, wrist-joint, Berb. Plat. Veratr.
—, fingers, Berb. Oleand. Phos. ac.
—, thumb, Oleand.
Granular, eruptions, °*Carb. veg.* Graph. Hep.
Grape-shaped, eruption, *Rhus.*
Gray, spots, Nitr. ac.
Hardness, skin of hand, Sulph.
—, finger, Tart.
Hard, eruption, Amm. m. Bov. Led. Phos. ac. Rhus. Spig.
—, callosities, *Rhus v.*
Hepatic spots, hand and finger, Ferr. magn.
Herpes, hand, **Dulc.* °*Ipec.* Kreas. Merc. Natr. Sassap. Sep. Staph. Veratr. °*Zinc.*
—, fingers, Amm. Caust. °*Graph. Merc.* °*Nitr. ac.*
Herpetic, eruption, °Graph. Ipec. Nitr. ac.
—, scald, *Ran.*
Horny, scald, *Ran.*
—, callosities, °*Graph.*
Humid, eruption, Bell. Electr. Hell. Kal. Mang. Merc. Ran. Rhus.
Impressions, deep, from instruments, Bov. Merc.
Indurations, hand, Borax.

Induration, muscles of fingers, ***Caust.***
Inflammation, hand, Bry. Cupr. Natr. m.
—, fingers, *Ran. Sil.*
—, finger-joints, ****Lyc.***
—, thumb, Natr. Sassap.
Inflamed, eruptions, Agar. Bell.
—, swelling, °***Bry.*** °*Cocc.* Gran. Hep. ****Lyc. Magn. s.*** N. vom. Rhus.
—, callosities, ***Phosph.***
Itching, hand, Agar. Alum. Amb. Amm. m. Anac. Arg. Aur. Baryt. ***Berb.*** Borax. Calc. *Carb. an.* ***Carb. veg.*** *Caust.* Cin. *Colch.* Dig. Euphorb. Galv. ***Grat. Gran.*** Graph. ***Hep.*** Ipec. Kal. Kal. hdr. ***Kreas.*** Lach. Lam. Lupul. *Lyc.* Magn. c. Magn. s. Mang. ***Merc.*** Mur. ac. Natr. Natr. m. *Nitr. ac.* Ol. an. Petr. ***Phell. Phosph.*** Phos. ac. Plat. Ran. ***Rhus.*** Rhus v. Ruta. ***Sassap.*** Sep. *Sil.* *Spig.* Staph. *Stann.* Stram. ***Sulph.***
—, wrist-joint, Agar. Amm. m. Arg. Berb. Kal. Led. Plat. Plumb. Selen. Veratr.
—, fingers, ****Agar.*** Alum. Amb. Amm. m. *Anac.* Ant. Ars. ***Berb.*** Borax. Calc. Carb. an. Carb. veg. Caust. ***Cocc. Con. Cycl.*** Euphorb. Grat. ***Lach.*** Lact. Laur. ***Lyc.*** Magn. arct. Magn. c. Mang. *Merc.* ***Natr. m.*** Natr. s. N. vom. Oleand. Ol. an. Petr. Phos. ac. Plat. ***Plumb.*** Prun. ***Ran.*** Ran. sc. ***Rhod.*** *Spig.* Sulph. Therid. Veratr. Verb. ***Zinc.***
—, finger-joints, Alum. Arn. Camph. Caust. Crotal. Ign. Natr. m. N. vom. Petr.
—, thumb, Ant. Carb. veg. Cocc. Grat. Natr. Oleand. Ol. an. Plumb. Spong. Staph.

Itching, eruptions, ***Agar.*** Amb. Amm. m. Ant. Baryt. Berb. Canth. Carb. an. **Carb. veg.* Caust. Dros. Electr. ***Hep.*** Jod. Ipec. Kal. Kal. chl. Laur. Led. ***Lyc. Magn. c.*** Mur. ac. Natr. m. ***Nitr. ac. Rhus. Rhus v.*** Sabad. Sassap. Selen. ***Sulph.*** Tarax. Zinc.
—, herpes, Amb. Caust.
—, blisters, phagedænic, Graph. Sil.
—, swelling, Canth. Lach. Sulph.
—, ulcers, Dros. Ran.
Itch-like, eruption, hand, Ant. ***Lach. Rhus. Selen.*** Squill. °*Sulph.*
—, finger, °Lach. °*Sulph.*
Livid, swelling, Gran.
Marbled, spots, Natr. m.
—, swelling, Gran.
Miliary, eruption, ***Agar.***
Nettle-rash, like, eruption, hand, *Berb.* Euphorb. °*Hep.* Natr. *Natr. m.* Natr. s. *Sulph.*
—, finger, °*Hep.*
Numbness, hand, Acon. Ars. Bov. Bry. Cann. Carb. an. *Carb. veg.* Cocc. Graph. Lach. Lam. °*Lyc.* Nitr. Puls. °*Ruta.* Sep. Sil. Zinc.
—, wrist-joints, Bov. Plumb.
—, fingers, Anac. Ang. Calc. Cann. Caust. Cic. Cin. Coff. Colch. Con. Crotal. Cupr. Dig. *Electr. Euphr.* Ferr. Kal. Kreas. *Lach.* Lyc. Magn. m. Mur. ac. Nicc. *Ol. an. *Phosph.* Phos. ac. Plat. Rhod. Rhus. *Sec. Sep. Sil.* Spong. Staph. Stront. *Sulph.* Tart. Thuj. Verbasc. Zinc.
—, finger-joints, Anac.
—, thumb, Cin. Kal. Plat. *Stront.* Verbasc. Zinc.

Œdematous, s. Watery.
Pain, as if bruised, hand, Bov. Calc. Graph. Jod.
—, fingers, Cin. Cupr. Ruta.
—, thumb, Cin.
Pain as if contused, hand, Dros. Spig.
—, finger, Caust. Prun. *Ruta.* Verb.
—, thumb, Plat.
Pain as if ecchymosed, finger, Par.
Boils, hand, °*Calc. Lyc.*
—, finger-joints, Calc.
—, thumb, *Nitr.*
Pain as if luxated, hands and wrists, **Amm.* Amm. m. **Arn.* Berb. Bry. **Calc. Carb. veg. Caust.* Hep. *Lach. Laur.* Lyc. Petr. *Puls. Rhod.* Sabin. Sil. *Stann. Verb.*
—, fingers and joints, Ang. Berb. Camph. Cham. Cupr. *Kreas. Phosph.*
—, thumb, Camph. *Kreas. Magn. art. Phosph.* Prun.
Pain as if sore, smarting, hand, Berb. Calc. Carb. veg. **Hep.* Lam. Nicc. °*Nitr. ac.* **Rhus.*
—, finger, Amb. Berb. °*Graph. Kal.* Petr. Sulph. ac.
—, thumb, Magn. art. Mez. Spong.
Pain as from splinter, finger, **Arn.* Bell. Carb. veg. Colch. °*Hep.* °Lach. **Nitr. ac.* Petr. Puls. Ran. *Sil.* Sulph.
Pain as if sprained, hand and wrist, Alum. **Amm.* Anac. *Arn.* Baryt. Bov. *Bry.* **Calc. Carb. an. Caust.* Cin. Cist. Con. Ferr. magn. Graph. *Ign.* Lach. Mez. N. vom. Phosph. Prun. *Rod. Rhus.* °*Ruta.* Sassap. Seneg. Sil. *Stann. Sulph.* Thuj. Zinc.

Pain as if sprained, fingers and joints, Acon. Alum. °*Graph.* *Ign.* *Laur.* Lyc. Magn. c. *Natr. m.* *Nitr.* N. mosch. *Phosph.* Rhod. Stann. *Sulph.*

—, thumb, Con. °*Graph.* *Laur.* *Magn. art.* Natr. m. Nitr. Petr. *Phosph.* Prun. *Sulph.* Veratr.

Pain, as if ulcerated, hand, Plat. Sil. Sulph. ac. Teucr.

—, wrist-joint, Bov.

—, finger, Berb. Bry. Carb. veg. Caust. Graph. Kal. Par. Plat. Sassap. *Sil.*

—, finger-joints, Kal.

Painful as if sore, that which is, Baryt.

Painful, Amb. Ars. Borax. Calc. Led. Magn. arct. Mang. Sec. Sulph. ac. Zinc.

—, rhagades, *Graph.* Mang. *Merc.* **Sulph.* Zinc.

—, ulcers, Lyc.

—, swelling, Chin. Hep. Merc. Nitr. ac. N. vom. Phosph. Sec.

Painless, swelling, Euphr. Lyc.

Panaritia, s. NAILS, ulcers.

Paleness, fingers, Cic. *Kreas.* Lach. Par. Sec.

Pale, swelling, **Bry.* *N. vom.* Sec.

Pale-red, eruption, *Ars.* *Rhus.*

Peeling off, hands, Alum. Amm. Amm. m. Baryt. Eugen. Ferr. *Merc.* Natr. m. *Sep.*

—, finger, Baryt. Sabad. Sulph.

Peels off, that which, eruptions, Ferr. Jod.

Pemphigus, hand, °*Sep.*

Petechiæ, *Berb.*

Phagedænic, Ran. Rhus. Veratr.

Pimples, hands, Agar. Amm. m. Ant. Bov.

Canth. *Kreas. Lyc.* Mur. ac. Par. *Rhus. Selen. Tarax. Zinc.*

Pimples, wrists, Baryt. Bry. *Rhus.*

—, finger, Anac. Ant. Arn. Ars. Berb. Canth. Cycl. *Kal. Lyc.* Magn. c. Mur. ac. *Phos. ac. Spig.* Squill. Tab. Tarax. *Therid. Zinc.*

—, finger-joints, Cycl.

—, thumbs, Ant. *Kal. Lyc. Therid.*

Pocks, finger, *Lach.*

Prickling, hand, Lach. *Plat.* Seneg. Sil.

—, finger, Ferr. magn. Natr. m. *Ol. an.* Sil. *Sulph.*

—, thumb, Ol, an.

Pustules, hand, Cic. Natr. m. Rhus. °*Sep.* Sil.

—, finger, Anac. Baryt. Borax. *Sassap.* Spig. Zinc.

Rash, hand, Bruc. Bry. Cupr. Dig. *Led.*

Rash-like pimples, **Carb. veg.*

With red areola, eruption, Anac. Borax. Bov. Canth. Cycl. Natr.

Redness, hands, Baryt. Carb. an. *Dulc.* Hep. Indig. *Natr. s.* N. vom. Ran. Sabad. Staph. Sulph.

—, wrist-joints, Magn. c. Merc. acet.

—, fingers, **Agar.* Berb. Borax. Gent. Laur. *Lyc.* Magn. c. Mur. ac. **N. vom.* Ran. Rhod. Therid. *Thuj.*

—, finger-joints, Gent. **Lyc.* Spong. *Sulph.*

—, thumb, Lach.

Red, eruptions, Bell. Berb. Bov. Bruc. Canth. Carb. an. Cic. Cycl. Lyc. *Merc. Ran.* Spig. Spong. **Sulph.* Sulph. ac. Veratr.

—, spots, Alum. Berb. Dros. Elect. Kal. Magn.

m. Mang. Natr. Natr. m. *Phos. ac. Plumb. Sabad.* °*Sulph. Tart.* Zinc.
Red, scald, Amm. m.
—, swelling, **Bell.* Electr. Hep. **Lyc. Magn. c. Mur. ac.* Ran. Sulph. *Therid.*
—, Callosities, Lach. Phosph.
Rhagades, hands, **Alum.* Graph. Kal. Kreas. **Lach.* °*Magn. c. Merc. Natr. Natr. m.* °*Nitr. ac.* °*Petr.* Sil. **Sulph.* **Zinc.*
—, fingers, Baryt. Kal. Mang. Merc. **Petr.* Phosph. Zinc.
—, joints, Phosph. **Sulph.*
Rheumatic, hand, Ang. Borax. Lach. Zing.
—, wrist-joints, Amb. *Gran.* Grat. *Lach.* Ruta. Zinc.
—, fingers, Ammoniac. Colch. °*Lach.*
Roughness, hands, **Alum.* Baryt. *Hep. Kal.* Laur. °*Nitr. ac.* Petr. Phosph. Phos. ac.
—, fingers, Laur. °*Petr.*
Scaly, Hep. Laur.
Scarlet-coloured, swelling, **Bell.*
Scurfs, hand, Sassap. °Sep.
—, fingers, Anac.
Scurfy, eruption, Hell. Mur. ac. *Sassap.*
Shining, swelling, *Ran.*
Shortening of muscles, fingers, **Caust. Sulph.*
Smarting, hands, Berb. Natr. m. Zinc.
—, fingers, Berb. Mez.
Smarting, eruption, Mang.
Spots, hands, Acon. Bell. Berb. Corall. *Dros.* Electr. Ferr. magn. *Jod. Kal. Natr. Natr. m.* °*Nitr. ac. Sabad. Sep.* Squill. Stann. *Tart.* Vip. torv. Zinc.
—, wrist-joint, *Kal. Merc.* °*Petr.*

Spots, finger, *Con.* Corall. Ferr. magn. Lyc. Mang. *Natr. m. Phos. ac. Plumb.* Sabad. Squill. Tart.
—, thumb, Lyc.
As if from stings of insects, Spong.
Stings, that which, in general, Arn. Berb. Calc. Canth. Dros. Lyc. Magn. c. Oleand. Puls. Rhus. Sulph.
—, phagedænic blister, Magn. c.
—, swelling, Oleand.
—, ulcers, Mang. Ran.
Suppuration, hand, Eugen.
—, finger, Borax. **Mang.* N. vom.
—, thumb, N. vom.
Suppurating, eruptions, Spig.
—, phagedænic blister, Graph.
—, ulcer, Mang.
Swelling, hands, Acon. Amm. m. Ars. Bar. m. **Bell.* °*Bry.* °*Calc. Caust.* °*Cham.* Chin. Clem. °*Cocc.* Cupr. *Dig. Electr. Ferr.* Galv. *Hep. Hyos.* °*Lach.* Laur. *Lyc. Merc. Mez. Natr. Natr. m.* Nitr. Nitr. ac. N. vom. Phosph. °*Rhod. Rhus.* Sec. Sep. Spong. **Stann.* Sulph. Vip. red.
—, wrist-joints, Aur. m. *Carb. veg.* Crotal. °*Euphr.* °*Lach.* Magn. c. Merc. Merc. acet. Phosph. Sec. Sep.
—, fingers, Alum. Ammoniac. Amm. Ant. Ars. Berb. Borax. Bry. Calc. Canth. Chin. *Hep.* Jod. °*Lach. Led.* Magn. c. °*Mang.* Mur. ac. *Nitr. ac.* Oleand. *Phosph.* Ran. Ran. sc. Rhus. *Sulph.* Thuj. Vinc. Vip. torv.
—, finger-joints, Amb. Berb. Canth. *Carb. veg.*

Euphr. Graph. *Hep.* **Lyc.* *Nitr. ac.* Spong. *Sulph.*
Swelling, thumb, Gran. Led. N. vom. *Phosph.*
Tearing, swelling, **Lyc.*
Throbbing, phagedænic blisters, Sil.
Tickling, hands, Arg. Ars. Cin. Grat. Lach. Mang. Merc. Mur. ac. Plat. Ruta. *Staph.*
—, fingers, Anac. Ars. Calc. Cocc. Grat. Hell. Merc. Ran. sc. Ratanh. Sep. Verbasc.
—, thumbs, Merc. Ratanh.
Tickling, eruptions, Agar. Canth.
Titillating, hand, Anis. Arn. Ars. *Baryt.* Berb. Bry. Caust. Hyos. Lach. Lam. Mez. Ol. an. Op. Par. Phosph. Phos. ac. Plat. °*Ruta.* Sec. Seneg. Spig. *Sulph.* *Veratr.*
—, wrist-joint, Calc.
—, fingers, *Acon.* Agar. *Alum.* *Amm. m.* Baryt. °*Calc.* *Cann.* Cin. Croc. Hep. Kal. Kreas. Lach. Lact. Laur. *Magn. arct.* *Magn. aust.* Magn. m. *Magn. s.* Mur. ac. °*Natr. m.* *Natr. s.* Nitr. ac. *Ol. an.* Op. Pæon. *Ran.* *Rhod.* Rhus. *Sec.* *Sep.* °*Sil.* Staph. *Sulph.* Tab. *Teucr.* Thuj. Veratr. Verb.
—, finger-joints, Sulph.
—, thumb, Amb. Cin. Magn. art. *Natr.* *Ol. an.* Plat. Plumb. Sabad. *Teucr.* Zinc.
Titillating, eruption, Sil.
—, swelling, Caust. Lach.
Tumours, hands, Ars.
—, fingers, Ant.
Ulcers, hand, Dros. °*Sil.*
—, fingers, Alum. Ars. Carb. veg. Kreas. *Lyc.* Mang. Plat. *Ran.* *Sep.*
—, finger-joints, Sep.

Ulcerated, eruptions, Phosph. Ran.
Ulcerated, rhagades, *Merc.*
—, warts, Petr.
Violet-red, swelling, Lach.
Warts, hand, Anac. Berb. °*Calc. Dulc.* Ferr. magn. *Lach. Lyc.* Natr. m. °*Nitr. spir.* Phosph. °*Rhus.* **Sep.* **Thuj.*
—, fingers, Berb. Ferr. magn. Lach. °*Rhus.* °*Sulph.* Thuj.
—, thumbs, *Lach.*
Wart-shaped, pimples, Lyc.
—, indurations, Borax.
Watery vesicles, hand, Bell. *Cocc.* Magn. art. *Rhus v. Sassap.*
—, fingers, Cupr. Magn. c. Natr. s. *Plumb. Puls. Rhus v.*
White, that which is, in general, Bov. Cycl. Magn. c. Natr. Nitr. ac. Phos. ac.
—, spots, Electr. Nitr. ac.
—, streaks, Magn. c.
Wrinkles, fingers, Amb. Cupr. Phos. ac. Sulph.
Yellow colour, hands, Ign. Spig.
—, fingers, Chel. Phos. ac.
Yellow eruption, Ran. Sil. Spig.
—, spots, Sabad.

Hangnails.

In general, **Calc.* Lyc. Merc. Natr. m. **Rhus.* Sabin. Stann. **Sulph.*

Hard, indurated.

Blisters, vesicles, Lach. Phos. ac. Sil.
Bloodvessels, swelling of, °*Sep.*

Blotches, tubercles. Amm. Amm. m. Ant. Bov. **Bry.* Con. *Lach. Magn. c. Magn. s.* Natr. m. Phosph. Rhus. Val.

Eruption, Ant. Aur. Mez. Ran. Rhus. Spig. Val.

Erysipelas, Sulph.

Pimples, *Bov.* Sabin. Veratr.

Pustules, Anac. Crotal.

Spots, Vip. torv.

Swelling, Acon. Agn. Alum. Amm. Amm. m. *Ant.* **Arn.* **Ars.* *Asa.* Aur. **Bell.* Bov. **Bry.* **Calc.* Canth. **Carb. an.* *Caust.* **Cham.* *Chin.* Cin. *Con.* Dig. *Dulc.* **Graph.* Hell. Hep. *Kal.* Lach. **Led.* **Lyc.* Magn. c. *Merc.* Mez. N. vom. Oph. Par. **Phosph.* Phos. ac. Plumb. **Puls.* **Rhus.* *Sabin.* *Samb.* Sep. **Sil.* Spig. Spong. Squill. °*Staph.* *Stront.* **Sulph.* *Thuj.*

Ulcers, Arn. °*Ars.* °*Asa.* Bell. Bry. *Calc.* Carb. an. *Carb. veg.* *Caust.* Cham. Cic. Cin. Clem. Graph. Hep. °*Lach.* **Lyc.* °*Merc.* Mez. Natr. N. vom. Petr. Phosph. Phos. ac. °*Puls.* Ran. Sep. **Sil.* Staph. **Sulph.* Thuj.

Warts, Ant. Borax. Dulc. Ran. Sil. °*Sulph.*

Head, eruptions, Ant. Carb. an. Natr. m.

Face, eruptions, Anac. °Bry. Crotal. Magn. c. Puls. Veratr.

—, swelling, Amm. m. **Arn.* Ars. **Bell.*. **Cham.*

Buccal cavity, swelling, Ign. Merc. Par.

Sexual parts, eruptions, Bov. Kreas.

—, swelling. Carb. veg, Merc.

Chest, pimples, Bov.
Dorsal region, blotches, Ant. Phosph. Zinc.
—, swelling, Amm. m. *Calc.* °*Carb. an.* *Kal.* °Lyc. °Sil. Spig. °Spong.
Arms, eruptions, Mez. Sep. Sil.
—, swelling, Led.
Hands, eruptions, Amm. m. Bov. Led. Phos. ac. Rhus. Spig.
—, callosities, *Rhus v.*
Lower limbs, eruption, Aur.
—, swelling, Aur. Bov. *Chin.* Graph. °*Led.* Magn. c. Mez. Rhus.
Feet, eruption, Bov. *Lach.*
—, swelling, Chin.

Hardness, of Skin.

In general, Amm. **Ant.* *Ars.* Bov. Chin. Cic. Clem. °*Dulc.* °*Graph.* Kal. *Lach.* Led. *Lyc.* Par. Phosph. *Ran.* **Rhus.* **Sep.* °*Sil.* Sulph. *Thuj.* Veratr.
Peeling off, with, Amm. Ant. Borax. °*Dulc.* *Graph.* *Lach.* Ran. *Rhus.* °*Sep.* *Sil.* Sulph.
Horny, **Ant.* *Graph.* *Ran.* Sulph.
Parchment-like, **Ars.* *Chin.* Dulc. Kal. Led. °*Lyc.* Phosph. °*Sil.* Squill.
Callous skin, Amm. **Ant.* Borax. **Graph.* Lach. *Ran.* **Rhus.* **Sep.* °*Sil.* Sulph.
Thick skin, Amm. *Ant. Ars. Borax. Cic. Clem. °*Dulc.* *Graph.* *Lach.* Par. *Ran.* **Rhus.* **Sep.* °*Sil.* Sulph. *Thuj.* Veratr.

Nose, Alum. Canth. Rhus. Thuj. Zinc.
Chin, Staph.

Arms, upper arm, Magn. c.
—, forearm, Carb. an.
Hands, skin, Sulph.
—, fingers, Tart.
Lower limbs, knee, Led.
—, legs, Graph.
—, tibia, Rhus.
—, calves, Ars.

Hepatic.

Spots, °*Ant.* Caust. Con. Ferr. Hyos. °*Laur.* **Lyc.* Natr. Nitr. ac. Petr. Phosph. Sep. **Sulph.* (Comp.: Brown, Yellow, &c.)

Face, Laur.
Lips, °Sulph.
Thoracic region, °*Lyc. Sulph.*
Dorsal region, back, Sulph.
—, shoulders, Ant.
Arms, Ant.
Hands and fingers, Ferr. magn.

Hernia.

In general, °*Acon.* Alum. Amm. Asar. °*Aur. Cocc.* °*Coloc.* Con. Lach. °Laur.? ᵈLyc. °*Magn. arct.* °Magn. c. Natr. m. Nitr. ac. **N. vom.* °Op. °Petr. °Phosph. °Spig. °Staph. °*Sulph.*? Zinc.
—, incarcerated, °*Acon.* Alum. °Cocc.? °*N. vom.* °Op. Phosph. °*Sulph.*

HERPES.

In general, **Alum.* **Amb.* *Amm. Anac. *Ars. °Aur. Baryt. Bar. m. Borax. °*Bov.* °Bry. **Calc.* Caps. *Carb. veg. *Caust. °Chel. °*Clem.* °*Con.* Cupr. **Dulc.* **Graph.* Grat. °Hep. Hell. Hyos. Ipec. °Jod.? **Kal.* °Kreas. Lach. **Led.* **Lyc.* Magn. arct. Magn. c. Magn. m. Magn. s. Mang. *Merc. Merc. corr. Mosch. °*Natr.* Natr. m. Nitr. °*Nitr. ac.* N. vom. °Oleand. **Petr.* °Phosph. °Phos. ac. Plumb. *Ran. bulb.* **Rhus.* Sassap. **Sep.* °Sil. Sol. m. °Spig. Stann. *Staph.* **Sulph.* Tax. °Thuj. °Veratr. °Zinc.
Bleeding, °Dulc. °Lyc.
Brown, °Dulc.
Burning, °Amb. °Amm. Anac. **Ars.* °Bov. °Bry. Calad. Calc. °Carb. veg. **Con.* Led. Magn. arct. **Merc.* Mosch. Rhus. °Sep. *Staph.* °Sulph.
During change of moon, °Clem.
Chronic, °Clem. °Con. °Lach. °Sulph.
Circinnatus, Clem. Magn. c. °*Natr.* Natr. m. °*Sep.*
Cracked, Graph. °Lyc. Magn. arct.
Dry, Amm. m. °Clem. °Dulc. Kal. hdr. °Kreas. **Led.* Merc. Nicc. °Phosph. °Phos. ac. °Sulph. Tax. °Veratr. (Comp.: Dry scurfs, and, DRY, THAT WHICH IS.)
Dysentery, alternating with, °*Rhus.*
Fetid, Oleand. (Comp.: SCURFS, and, FETID, THAT WHICH IS.)
Furfuraceous, *Ars. °Bry. Bruc. °Dulc. °Kreas.

°Lyc. ***Merc.*** °*Phosph.* °Sulph. (Comp.: FURFURACEOUS, THAT WHICH IS.)

Gonorrhœal, Zinc.

Grayish-yellow, °Sulph.

Humid, Amm. m. Baryt. °Bov. **Calc.* °Carb. veg. **Caust.* °Clem. °*Con.* **Dulc.* **Graph.* Hell. **Kreas.* Led. **Lyc.* **Merc.* Natr. Natr. m. Oleand. **Phos. ac.* °Sep. *Sil.* **Sulph.* (Comp.: HUMIID SCURF, and, HUMID, THAT WHICH IS.)

Impetiginous, °Merc.

Inflamed, Graph. (Comp.: INFLAMED, THAT WHICH IS.)

Itching, Alum. Amb. °Amm. °Ars. °*Bov.* °Bry. *Caps.* **Caust.* Clem. °Con. Cupr. **Graph.* Ipec. Kal. hdr. **Led.* **Lyc.* Magn. s. Mang. **Merc.* Nicc. **Nitr. ac.* *Petr. Plumb. **Rhus.* °Sep. Staph. °*Sulph.* Tax.

Itch-like, Grat.

Mercurial, °Aur. °Mosch.? °Nitr. ac.

Painful, °Dulc. (Comp.: PAINFUL, THAT WHICH IS.)

Pale-red, Clem. °Dulc.

With peeling off of the skin, °Dulc. Magn. *Merc.* Sep.

Pustules, °Kreas.

Raised, Merc. (Comp.: RAISED, THAT WHICH IS.)

Red pimples, °Bov.

Red, °Amm. °Ars. °Clem. °Dulc. Kreas. °*Lach.* Magn. Magn. s. Oleand. °Sulph. Tax.

With red areola, °Dulc.

Rough, °*Bov.* Oleand.

Round, °Dulc. Hell. Phosph.

Scaly, Anac. °Ars. °*Clem.* Cupr. °***Dulc.*** Kreas. °Led. °*Lyc.* Magn. c. °***Merc.*** Sulph. Teucr. (Comp.: Scaly scurfs under SCALY, THAT WHICH IS.)
Scrofulous, °Aur.
Scurfy, °Bov. ****Calc.*** *Clem.* °***Con.*** Graph. °Lach. °Lyc. °Sep. °***Sulph.***
Without sensation, °Lyc.
Small, °Dulc. °Lach. Magn. Magn. s.
Smarting, biting, Alum.
Smooth, Magn.
Spreading, °Alum. Caps. ****Merc.*** (Comp.: SPREADS, THAT WHICH.)
Stinging, Anac.
Suppressed, °Alum. ? Amb. °*Calc.* °***Lach.*** °***Lyc.*** °Natr. ? °Sep. ? °***Sulph.***
Suppurating, Clem. °Dulc. °Lyc. °Merc. Natr. (Comp.: SUPPURATES, THAT WHICH.)
Syphilitic, °Nitr. ac. °Thuj.
Tearing, Magn. arct.
Ulcerated, Zinc.
Vesicular, °***Sulph.***
With watery vesicles, °Sulph.
White, whitish, Anac. °Zinc. (Comp.: White scurfs, under WHITE, THAT WHICH IS.)
Wrinkled, Lyc.
Yellow-scaly, Cupr.
Yellow, Cupr. °***Dulc.*** Hell, °***Lyc.*** °***Sulph.*** (Comp.: YELLOW, THAT WHICH IS.)
Head, Baryt. Cupr. Kal. Petr. Rhus.
Eyes, °***Bry.*** Rhus. Sep.
Eyelids, °***Bry.*** Rhus. Sep.
Canthi, Tax.

Ears, Amm. m. Caust. ***Graph.*** Creas. Magn. m. °***Oleand.*** °***Sep.*** Teucr.
—, behind the ears, Amm. m. °Graph. °***Oleand.*** °***Sep.***
—, lobules, Caust. °*Sep.* Teucr.
—, in front of ears, °Oleand.
Nose, Nitr. ac. Spig.
Face, °Alum. *Amm.* Anac. Ars. °Baryt. °***Bov.*** Bruc. Bry. Calc. Caps. °*Carb. veg.* Caust. °Chel. °Con. °Dulc. Graph. Kal. hdr. °Kreas. ****Lach.*** ****Led.*** °Lyc. Merc. Natr. **Natr. m.* Nicc. Nitr. ac. Petr. Phosph. °Phos. ac. ****Rhus.*** Sabad. °Sep. °Sil. °Sulph.
—, cheeks, Amb. Anac. °***Bov.*** Bry. Caust. Merc.
—, chin, °***Bov.*** Chel. Natr. m. N. vom. °Sil.
—, temples, °Alum.
—, forehead, Caps.
Lips and mouth, region of, Anac. Ars. Caust. Magn. c. Natr. Par. Phosph. °Rhus. Sassap. Sep.
—, corners of mouth, Carb. veg. Phosph. Sep.
Chin, Bov. Chel. Natr. m. N. vom. °*Sil.*
Buccal cavity, bluish, °Zinc.
Anus, Ipec. Natr. m. Petr.
—, perineum, Petr.
Sexual parts, Croton. °***Dulc.*** Natr. m. °***Petr.*** ***Sassap.***
—, scrotum, Croton. Natr. m.
—, between scrotum and thigh, °Petr.
—, labia. °Dulc.
—, prepuce, Sassap.
Chest, Magn. °***Petr.*** Staph.
Mammæ and nipples, °Caust. °Dulc.

Dorsal region, axilla, °Carb. an. °Lyc. °Sep.
—, neck, Lach.
—, nape of neck, Caust. °Lyc. °Petr. °Sep. *Sulph.*
Arms, *Con. Cupr.* °*Dulc.* Grat. *Hell.* Kreas. Lach. Magn. s. *Mang.* **Merc.* °*Phosph. Sep.*
—, arm, °*Dulc. Hell.* Lach. Merc. Natr. m. °*Phosph.*
—, elbow, *Cupr.* Kreas. *Sep.*
—, upper arm, Grat. Magn. s.
—, forearm, *Con.* Magn. s. *Mang.* **Merc.*
Hands, **Dulc.* °*Ipec.* Kreas. Merc. Natr. Sassap. Sep. Staph. Veratr. **Zinc.*
—, fingers, Amb. Caust. °*Graph. Merc.* °*Nitr. ac.*
Lower limbs, °*Clem.* Kal. Lach. Merc. *Staph.*
—, nates and hips, Borax. Caust. Nicc.
—, thighs, °*Graph.* **Merc.* Mur. ac. *Nitr. ac.*
—, knee, °*Ars.* °*Carb. veg.* °*Dulc.* °*Graph.* Kreas. Merc. **Natr. m.* °*Petr.* Phosph.
—, legs, Ars. Calc. °*Graph. Kal.* °*Lach.* Lyc.
Feet, ankles, °*Natr. m.* °*Petr.*
—, toes, Alum.

HERPETIC.

Eruption, Amm. *Anac.* Ipec. **Rhus.* Sep.
Blisters, vesicles, Nitr. ac.
Spots, Crotal. Graph. *Hyos.* Lyc. **Merc.* Mur. ac. Natr. m. Phosph. Sabad. Sassap. **Sep.* Sil. Zinc.
Ulcers, °*Zinc.*
Scurfs, °Bov. **Calc. Ran.* °*Sep.* Sulph.

Dorsal Region, spots, Hyos. Sep.
Arms, eruption, *Natr. m. Sep.*
Hands, eruption, °Graph. Ipec. Nitr. ac.
—, Scurfs, *Ran.*
Lower limbs, spots, Graph. Mur. ac. Sassap.
Feet, soreness, °Graph.
Glands, eruption, °Dulc. °Graph.

Horny.

Eruption, **Ant. Ran.*
Excrescences, **Ant.* °*Ran.* Sulph.
Figwarts, °*Thuj.*
Scurfs, *Graph. Ran.*
Hard skin, **Ant. Graph. Ran.* Sulph.
Corns, **Ant.* Graph. Ran. Sulph.
Callosities, **Ant.* °Graph.
Warts, Ant. Borax. Graph.? Ran. °*Sulph.* °*Thuj.*

Hands, scurf, *Ran.*
—, callosities, °*Graph.*
Feet, excrescences, **Ant.*
—, soles, °*Graph.*

Humour, Secreting a.

Blisters, vesicles, Electr. *Hell.* Hep. Lach. Mang. *Merc.* Phosph. Ran. Ran. sc. Raph. *Rhus.* Sulph. Vip. torv.
Blisters, phagedænic, Kal.
Bloodvessels, swelling of, Alum. Amm. Bary. Caust. Natr. m. Sep. Sulph. Sulph. ac.
Blotches, Nitr. Selen.

Eruption, Alum. Ars. Baryt. Bell. *Bov.* Bry. **Calc.* Carb. an. **Carb. veg.* Caust. **Cic.* **Clem.* Con. Daph. **Graph.* °Grat. ? Hell. Hep. Heracl. **Kal.* Kreas. Lach. Led. **Lyc.* **Merc.* *Mez.* *Natr.* Natr. m. Nitr. ac. Oleand. Petr. Phosph. Phos. ac. **Rhus.* Ruta. Sabin. *Selen.* **Sep.* Sil. Squill. **Staph.* **Sulph.* Sulph. ac. Tarax. Thuj. Viol. tr.

Excrescences, Nitr. ac.

Figwarts, Thuj.

Herpes, Amm. m. Baryt. °Bov. **Calc.* °Carb. veg. **Caust.* °Clem. °*Con.* **Dulc.* **Graph.* Hell. **Kreas.* Led. **Lyc.* **Merc.* Natr. Natr. m. Oleand. **Phos. ac.* °Sep. *Sil.* **Sulph.*

Itch, Calc. ? °*Carb. veg.* °*Caust.* Clem. ? Dulc. ? °*Kreas.* *Graph.* °*Lyc.* ? °*Sep.* Staph. ? °*Sulph.*

Pimples, **Calc.* Graph. Kal. Natr. s. Ol. an. Puls. Sil. Sulph. Thuj. Zinc.

Pustules, Bell.

Rhagades, Aloë.

Spots, Ant. Ars. Carb. veg. *Hell.* Kal. Lach. Selen. **Sil.* °*Sulph.* Tarax.

Swelling, Sulph.

Scurfs, crusts, °*Alum.** *Ars.* *Baryt.* **Calc.* Chinin. **Cic.* °*Clem.* **Graph.* **Hell.* °*Hep.* **Lyc.* **Merc.* °*Mez.* °*Oleand.* Plumb. Ran. °*Rhus.* °*Ruta.* Sep. °*Sil.* **Staph.* **Sulph.*

Warts, Ars. Bov. °*Calc.* °*Caust.* °*Hep.* Sil. °*Thuj.*

Head, eruptions, °*Baryt.* **Calc.* °Clem. **Graph.* °Hell. °*Hep.* **Merc.* **Nitr. ac.* °*Oleand.*

Ears, eruption, Bov. Calc. Lyc. Mez.

Ears, herpes, Amm. m. Kreas. Merc. Oleand.
Nose, Graph.
Face, °Alum. **Calc.* °Carb. veg. **Cic.* Coloc. Dulc. **Graph.* Kreas. °*Merc.* Natr. °Phos. ac. °*Rhus.* Sep. °*Sulph.*
Lips, Kal. Squill. Zinc.
Anus, varices, Alum. Amm. Baryt. Caust. Natr. m. Sep. Sulph. Sulph. ac.
Dorsal region, eruption, Clem.
—, herpes, Caust. °Sep.
—, spots, Lach.
—, swelling, Sulph.
Arms, herpes, °*Con.* Hell.
—, scurfs, °*Alum.*
Hands, eruption, Bell. Electr. Hell. Kal. Mang. Merc. Ran. Rhus.
Lower limbs, eruption, Merc. Puls. Selen.
—, spots, °*Sulph.*
Feet, blisters, Lach. Phosph. Raph.
—, ulcers, °Petr.
—, wound, Selen.

Impressions.

Deep, from instruments, Bov. Merc. Veratr.
On the hands, Bov. Merc.

Indented, which is.

Ulcers, Hep. Lach. **Merc.* °*Phos. ac.* Sil. Staph. Sulph. Thuj.
Warts, Calc. Euphr. Lyc. Nitr. ac. °*Phos. ac.* °*Rhus.* Sabin. Staph. °*Thuj.*

Indurations.

In general, °*Agn.* Alum. Amb. °*Arn.* *Ars.* Asa.

Aur. **Baryt.* Bar. m. **Bell.* °Bov. °*Bry.* **Calc.* Camph. Cann. Caps. **Carb. an.* **Carb. veg.* Caust. **Cham.* Chel. **Chin.* Cin. **Clem.* Cocc. **Con.* Cupr. Cycl. °*Dulc.* Ferr. **Graph.* Hep. Hyos. Ign. **Jod.* Kal. **Lach.* °*Led.* **Lyc.* Magn. c. Magn. m. Merc. Mez. Natr. N. vom. Oph. Op. °*Petr.* **Phosph.* Plumb. **Puls.* Ran. ? *Rhod.* **Rhus.* Sec. Selen. **Sep.* **Sil.* Spig. °*Spong.* Squill. *Staph. Stram. **Sulph.* Thuj. Val. Veratr.

Scirrhous, °Bell. Carb. an. ? Carb. veg. ? °*Clem.* Cic. ? °*Con.* Jod. ? Lach. ? °*Petr.* Phosph. ? Ran. ? °*Rhus.* °Sep. °*Sil.* °Spong. ? °Sulph.

Eyelids, Bry. Ran. sc. °Spig. °Staph.

Face, skin, Bell. °Sil. Viol. tr.

Lips, °Bell. Cycl. °Sil.

Lower jaw, Staph.

Sexual parts, testes, °Agn. °Aur. °*Clem.* Cop. N. vom. °Spong. ? Sulph.

—, scrotum, Clem. Rhus.

—, neck of womb, Chin. Jod. °Sep.

—, prostate gland, Cop. °Jod.

—, labia, Merc.

—, prepuce, °Lach.

Mammæ and nipples, °Bell. °Bry. **Cham.* *Clem.* °*Con.* °Merc. °Ol. jec. ? °Sil. °Sulph.

—, nipples, °Bry.

Arms, upper muscles, Petr.

—, forearm, cellular tissue, °*Sil.*

Hands, Borax.

—, fingers, muscles of, **Caust.*

Feet, Vip. torv.

—, soles, **Ars.*

Glands, °*Agn.* *A*mb. Amm. Ant. Arn. Ars. Aur. **Baryt.* Bar. m. **Bell.* Bov. °Bry. **Calc.* Camph. Cann. Canth. Caps. **Carb. an.* **Carb. veg.* Caust. **Cham.* Chin. **Clem.* Cocc. Coloc. °*Con.* Cupr. Cycl. Dig. **Dulc.* Ferr. **Graph.* Hep. Hyos. Ign. **Jod.* Kal. **Lyc.* *Magn. m.* Mang. Merc. Natr. Nitr. ac. N. vom. **Petr.* Phosph. Plumb. Puls. Raph. Rhod. **Rhus.* Sep. **Sil.* Spig. **Spong.* °Squill.? **Staph.* *Sulph.* Thuj. Veratr.

Indurations of Muscles.

In general, Alum.? Baryt.? Bry.? °*Carb. an.* Carb. veg. °*Caust.* Con.? Dulc. Hep. °*Jod.* °*Kal.* Lach. °*Lyc.* Natr.? N. vom.? °*Puls.* Rhod.? Rhus.? Sassap.? Sep.? Sil.? Spong.? °*Sulph.* Thuj.? Vip. torv.?

Arms, upper arm, Petr.
—, forearm, cellular tissue, °*Sil.*
Hands, fingers, **Caust.*
Lower limbs, Ars. Graph. Vip. torv.
Feet, Vip. torv.

Inflamed, that which is.

Bloodvessels, swelling of, **Arn.* **Ars.* Calc. °*Cham.* Kal. Kreas. Lyc. N. vom. °*Puls.* °*Sil.* °*Spig.* **Sulph.* Thuj. Zinc.
Blotches, tubercles, Amm. m. Rhus.
Chilblains, °Ars. Bell. Cham. Hep. Lyc. °*Nitr. ac.* Phosph. °*Puls.* Rhus. Staph. °*Sulph.*

Corns, Borax. ? Calc. ? Hep. ? °*Lyc.* °*Puls.* °*Rhus.* **Sep.* °*Sil.* Staph. ? **Sulph.*
Eruption, Ars. Calc.
Erysipelas, **Acon.* Ars. **Bell.* *Borax.* **Bry.* Camph. **Cham.* **Hep.* **Lach.* **Merc.* *Petr.* **Phosph.* **Puls.* **Rhus.* Sabad. **Sulph.* Zinc.
Herpes, Graph.
Nails, Con. Hell. Kal. Lyc. Natr. m. Phos. ac. Teucr.
Pimples, Agar. Berb. Petr.
Pustules, Rhus. Stram.
Scurfs, crusts, Lyc.
Spots, Ars. Bell.
Swelling, °*Acon.* Agn. Amm. *Ant.* **Arn.* **Ars.* °*Asa.* *Aur.* **Bell.* **Borax.* **Bry.* Calc. *Cann.* Canth. *Carb. veg.* *Caust.* **Chin.* **Cocc.* *Colch.* Con. Crotal. Gran. **Hep.* Hyos. **Jod.* Kal. **Lach.* °*Led.* **Lyc.* *Magn. c.* °*Mang.* **Merc.* Mez. Mur. ac. Natr. *Natr. m.* Nitr. *Nitr. ac.* **N. vom.* Oph. Petr. **Phosph.* Phos. ac. Plumb. **Puls.* **Rhus.* Sassap. Seneg. **Sep.* **Sil.* Stram. **Sulph.* *Thuj.* Veratr. *Zinc.*
Tumors, °Hep. °Mang. **Merc.* °*Phosph.* °*Sil.*
Ulcers, **Acon.* Agn. Ant. Arn. **Ars.* Asa. Baryt. °*Bell.* Borax. Bov. °*Bry.* *Calc.* Caust. **Cham.* Cin. Cocc. *Colch.* Con. Croc. Cupr. Dig. Galv, **Hep.* Hyos. Ign. Kreas. Led. **Lyc.* Magn. arct. Mang. **Merc.* *Mez.* *Natr.* *Nitr. ac.* N. vom. Petr. **Phosph.* Plumb. °*Puls.* Ran. °*Rhus.* °*Ruta.* Sassap. Sep. °*Sil.* Staph. *Sulph.* Thuj. Veratr. *Zinc.*
Vesicles, *Amm. m.* Baryt. Bell. Nitr.
Warts, Amm. Bov. Calc. **Caust.* Hep. Lyc. **Natr.* *Nitr. ac.* Rhus. Sep. **Sil.* Staph. °*Sulph.*

Ears, scurfs, Lyc.
Face, eruption, Amm. m.
—, swelling, Borax. Sep.
Mouth, eruptions, Baryt. Spig.
—, swelling, °*Acon.* **Bell.* Berb. Borax. Carb. veg. **Hep.* °Ign. Jod. °*Lach.* °*Merc.* Natr. m. Natr. s. °*N. vom.* Nitr. *Nitr. ac.* Sil.
Anus, eruptions, Calc.
Sexual parts, swelling, °Arn. *Merc.* Phos. ac. °*Puls.*
Dorsal region, swelling, °Merc. Sil. °Sulph.
—, blotches, Amm. m.
Arms, swelling, *Bry.* °*Lyc.* Sep.
—, erysipelas, *Petr.*
Hands, eruptions, Agar. Bell.
—, swelling, °*Bry.* **Cocc.* Gran. Hep. **Lyc.* *Magn. c.* N. vom. Rhus.
—, callosities, *Phosph.*
Lower limbs, pimples, Petr.
—, swelling, Borax. Calc. **Chin.* Crotal. °*Jod.* °*Led.* *Natr.* **Puls.* Sabad. °*Sil.* °*Sulph.* *Zinc.*
—, ulcers, Ars. Graph. N. vom.
Feet, chilblains, *Kal. Lach.*
—, swelling, **Ars.* **Bry.* Calc. *Cann.* Caust. °*Chin.* Cocc. **Led.* *Nitr. ac.* Petr. **Puls.* °*Rhus.* Sulph. *Thuj.* Zinc.

Inflammations.

In general, **Acon.* Agn. Alum. Amm. Ant. °*Arn.* **Ars.* °*Asa.* °Aur. Baryt. **Bell.* *Borax.* Bov. **Bry.* **Calc.* Camph. Cann. Canth. Carb. an. Caust. **Cham.* **Chin.* Chinin. Cin. Cocc. Colch. Con. Croc. Crotal. Croton. Cupr. Cupr.

ac. Euphorb. Ferr. Galv. Gran. **Graph.* **Hep.* Hyos. **Lach.* Lact. Lyc. **Magn. arct.* °*Mang.* **Merc.* *Merc. d.* Mez. Natr. *Natr. m.* °*Nitr. ac.* Oph. **Petr.* **Phosph.* Plumb. *Puls.* Ran. **Rhus.* °Ruta. Sep. **Sil.* °*Staph.* Stram. **Sulph.* Veratr. Zinc.

Arthritic, °Acon. °*Arn.* °Bell. °*Bry.* °Carb. an. °*Chin.* °Chinin. ? °Clem. °*Cocc.* °*Colch.* °Cycl. ? °Graph. °Hep. °*Kreas.* °*Lach.* °Led. ? °Lyc. °*Merc.* °Nitr. °N. vom. °*Puls.* °Rhod. °*Rhus.* °Sassap. °Sep. °*Sulph.*

Erysipelatous, s. ERYSIPELAS.

Rheumatic, °*Acon.* °*Arn.* °*Bell.* °Berb. Bry. °Calc. ph. °*Cham.*

Eyes, **Acon.* Amb. Amm. **Ant.* °*Arn.* **Ars.* Asar. Aur. **Baryt.* Bar. m. **Bell.* Borax. Bov. Bruc. **Bry.* **Calc.* Camph. °*Cann.* Canth. Caps. Carb. veg. **Caust.* **Cham.* °*Chin.* Cinn. **Clem.* °*Coloc.* Con. *Cupr.* Daph. **Dig.* **Dulc.* Eugen. **Euphorb.* **Euphr.* Ferr. Galv. **Graph.* **Hep.* Hyos. °*Ign.* Jod. *Ipec.* *Kal.* *Lach.* Led. **Lyc.* Magn. art. Magn. aust. Magn. c. Magn. m. **Merc.* Merc. corr. Mez. Mosch. **Natr.* *Natr. m. Nitr. ac. **N. vom.* Ol. an. Op. °*Petr.* **Phosph.* **Phos. ac.* Plumb. **Puls.* Ran. Ratanh. **Rhus.* Sabad. Sassap. **Sep.* **Sil.* °*Spig.* Stann. *Staph.* **Sulph.* °*Sulph. ac.* Tarax. Teucr. °*Thuj.* °*Val.* *Veratr.* Zinc.

Eyelids. **Acon.* **Ant.* **Arn.* **Ars.* Baryt. **Bell.* **Bry.* **Calc.* Carb. veg. **Caust.* **Cham.* Cinn. Cocc. °*Dig.* Euphorb. Euphr. Graph. Hep. Hyos. °*Kreas.* Lach. Lyc. Magn. art. Magn. aust. Magn. c. **Merc.* **Natr.* **N. vom.* Phosph.

Phos. ac. Puls. Rhus. Sassap. **Sep.* Spig. Spong. Staph. **Sulph.* Tarax. Thuj. Val. Veratr. Zinc.

Eyelids, margin of lids, **Ars.* **Bry.* Caust. **Cham.* **Clem.* *Dig. **Euphr.* Kal. °Kreas. Lyc. **Merc.* Natr. Phosph. **Puls.* °*Spig.* **Staph.* **Sulph.* °*Val.*

Canthi, *Acon.* Agar. Alum. Ars. Bell. *Calc.* Cham. Clem. °*Euphr.* Ign. Merc. *Petr.* Phosph. Puls.

External ear, **Acon.* **Bell.* *Borax.* Bry. *Calc.* Canth. **Cham.* °*Hep.* Kal. Kreas. **Lyc.* Magn. aust. Magn. c. *Merc.* Nitr. °*N. vom.* °*Phos. ac.* **Puls.* °*Sil.* Spong.

—, internal, **Acon.* Bell. *Borax.* Bry. Calc. Canth. *Hep.* °*Merc.* **Puls.*

—, lobe, Nitr.

—, parotid gland, **Amm.* **Bell.* °*Calc.* °*Carb. veg.* °*Cham.* °*Kal.* °*Merc.* °N. vom. °*Rhus.* Sassap.

—, margins, Sil.

Nose, Agar. **Aur.* **Aur. m.* **Calc.* Canth. °Con. Corall. Croton. °Hep.? *Merc.* *Natr. m.* Nitr. Phosph. Plumb. **Sep.* **Sulph.*

Lips, Canth.

—, eruptions, inflamed, Amm. m. Berb. Nitr.

Chin, Caust.

Buccal cavity, °*Acon.* Alum. Amm. Arg. °Ars. **Bell.* Berb. Bism. °*Borax.* **Calc.* *Canth.* °Caps. °*Carb. veg.* **Cham.* Chin. Colch. Crotal. Cupr. °Dulc.? Electr. °*Gran.?* Grat. *Hep. *Hydroc.* Hyos. **Ign.* Jod. Kal. °*Lach.* *Lyc.* °*Merc.* Mez. Mur. ac. Natr. °Natr. m. *Natr. s.* Nicc. Nitr. *Nitr. ac.* °*N. vom.* Ol. an. Oph.

Phosph. Phos. ac. Plumb. **Puls.* Ran. sc. Sabad. Sang. *Sep.* Sil. Stront. °*Sulph.* Veratr.

Buccal cavity, palate, **Calc.* Hydroc. °*Lach.* °N. vom.

—, velum palat., °*Bell.* °Lach.

—, mouth, Amm. Crotal. °Ign. °*Merc.* °*N. vom.* Oph. Veratr.

—, stomacace, °Ars. °Borax.? °Caps. °*Carb. veg.* °Dulc.? °Gran.? Hyos. °*Lach.* °*Merc.* Natr. m. °*N. vom.* °*Sulph.*

—, fauces and throat, °*Acon.* Alum. Amm. Arg. **Bell.* Bism. **Calc.* *Canth.* Carb. veg. °Cham. Chinin. Colch. Cupr. Electr. °Gran. Hydroc. **Ign.* Jod. °*Lach.* Lyc. **Merc.* Mez. Natr. *Natr. s.* Nicc. Ol. an. Phos. ac. °*Puls.* Sabad. °Sang. *Sep.* Stront. °*Sulph.*

—, tonsils, **Bell.* Berb. *Canth.* °Cham. °Gran.? °*Ign.* °*Lach.* °Merc. Natr. Natr. s. Nicc. Nitr. ac. Sep.

—, gums, Borax. Grat. Hep. Jod. Kal. Mur. ac. °Natr. m. °N. vom. Nitr. *Phosph.* *Sil.*

—, uvula, °Bell. Berb. Carb. veg. Natr. s. °*N. vom.*

—, tongue, Canth. Plumb. Ran. sc.

Abdomen, inguinal glands, Graph. **Sil.*

—, hernia, Baryt. Jod.

—, teguments, °Graph.

Anus, varices, °*Cham.* Kal.

Sexual parts, °*Acon.* *Ars.* Calc. Cann. Canth. Con. Magn. aust. **Merc.* Merc. ac. Mur. ac. Natr. Natr. m. Nitr. ac. N. vom. Phos. ac. Plumb. Puls. Sep. Spong. Staph. Thuj.

—, glans, Magn. aust. Natr.

—, urethra, **Cann.* **Canth.* Cop. Gran. Sabin.

—, orifice of urethra, Hep. Merc. Sulph. Sabin.

Sexual parts, testicles,° Acon. °Aur. °N. vom. °Spong. ? Staph. ?
—, scrotum, °Ars. ? Natr. m. Phos. ac. Plumb.
—, prostate gland, °Puls. °Thuj.
—, penis, Canth. Merc. ac. Plumb. Sep.
—, labia, Calc. Nitr. ac. °N. vom. ? °*Sep* Sulph.
—, vagina, Nitr. ac.
—, prepuce, Calc. Cann. Con. **Merc.* Mur. ac Natr. Nitr. ac.
Mammæ and nipples, °Arn. °*Bell.* °Bry. Calc °Carb. an. °Carb. veg. Con. °*Sil.*
—, nipples, Calc. Sil.
Dorsal region, axillary glands, Magn. aust. Nitr ac.
—, cervical glands, *Sulph.*
Arms, **Arg. Petr. Ran.*
Hands, Bry. Cupr. Natr. m.
—, fingers, *Ran. Sil.*
—, finger-joints, **Lyc.*
—, thumbs, Natr. Sassap.
Lower limbs, Borax. Natr. Sabad.
—, hip, °Coloc. °Sulph.
—, knee, Calc. °*Cocc.* °*Jod.* **N. vom.* Phosp °*Puls.* °*Sil.* °*Sulph.*
—, legs, Borax. Natr. Sabad.
—, tendo Achilles, Zinc.
Feet, ankles, *Mang.*
—, feet, °Rhus. Cinc.
—, dorsa of feet, Calc. **Puls.* Thuj.
—, toes, *Berb.* Carb. an. Caust. Lach. *Nitr.* Phosph. *Phos. ac. Puls.* Sulph. Teucr. *Thuj.*
Bones, periosteum, Acon. ? Ang. ? Ars. ? °*A* °*Aur.* °*Bell.* Bry. ? °*Calc.* °*Chin.* Clem. ? Co Cupr. ? Euphorb. ? °*Hep.* °*Jod.* °*Lach.* °*L*

Magn. m.? °*Mang.* °*Merc.* °*Mez.* °*Nitr. ac.* °*Phosph.* °*Phos. ac.* °*Puls.* Rhus.? Sep.? °*Sil.* °*Staph.* °*Sulph.* Thuj.? Veratr.?

Nails, Con. Hell. Kal. Lyc. Natr. m. Phos. ac. Teucr.

Glands, °Acon. °*Arn.* Ars. Aur. **Baryt.* **Bell.* Berb. °*Bry.* Calc. Camph. Canth. °*Carb. an.* °*Carb. veg.* Cham. *Con.* Dulc. °Gran.? **Graph.* Hep. Kal. Lach. Laur. Lyc. Magn. aust. Magn. m. **Merc.* **Nitr. ac.* N. vom. Petr. **Phosph.* Phos. ac. Plumb. Puls. Rhus. Samb. Sassap. **Sil.* Spig. Squill. Staph. **Sulph.* Sulph. ac. Thuj. Veratr. Zinc.

Injuries, Wounds.

ı general, °*Acon.* °Alum. °Amm. °*Arn.* °Bell. Borax. °*Bry.* °*Calc.* Carb. veg. °*Caust.* **Cham.* Chinin. °*Cic.* °*Con.* Croc. Dulc. Eugen. °*Euphr.* °*Hep.* Hyos. Jod. Kal. Kreas. °*Lach.* Laur. Lyc. Merc. Natr. Natr. m. °*Nitr. ac.* °*N. vom.* Par. °Petr. °*Phosph.* Phos. ac. Plat. Plumb. °*Puls.* °*Rhus.* °*Ruta.* Samb. Sec. Seneg. Sep. °*Sil.* °*Staph.* °*Sulph.* °*Sulph. ac.* Veratr. °*Zinc.*

ıating, °*Bell.* °*Cham.* Clem. °*Hep.* °*Merc.* °*Puls.* °*Sulph.*

ıdsores, °*Arn.* °Carb. veg. °Chin. Chinin.? Euphr.? °Puls. °*Sulph. ac.*

tes, °*Arn.* °*Sulph. ac.*

poisonous, °*Amm.* °*Ars.* °*Bell.* °Caust. Chinin.? °Lach. Natr. m. Puls. *Seneg.*

ıeding, profusely, °*Acon.* °*Arn.* **Carb. veg*

°*Chin.* Crotal. °Diad. **Lach.* Magn. arct. Natr. m. Oph. **Phosph.* Phos. ac. Puls. °*Sulph.* °*Sulph. ac.* Vip. torv. Zinc.

Bleeding, in general, °*Acon.* **Arn.* Ars. Asa. Borax. °*Carb. veg.* Caust. Chin. Clem. Con. **Croc.* °*Crotal.* °*Diad.* Eugen. °*Euphr.* Galv. °*Hep.* **Lach.* Magn. art. °*Merc.* Mez. °*Natr.* Natr. m. °*Nitr. ac.* °*N. mosch.* °*N. vom.* Oph. °*Phosph.* °*Phos. ac.* Plumb. °*Puls.* °*Rhus.* °Ruta. °Sep. °Sil. °*Staph.* °Sulph. °*Sulph. ac.* Tart. Vip. torv. Zinc.

From a blow, °*Arn.* °Cic. °Con. °*Euphr.* °Jod. °Lach. °*Puls.* °*Rhus.* °Sulph. °*Sulph. ac.* (Comp. Contusions.)

Burning, °*Acon.* Arn. °*Ars.* °*Carb. veg.* °Caust. Bry. Merc. Mez. Natr. m. Rhus. **Sulph.* °*Sulph. ac.*

Burns, °*Acon.* Agar. Alum. Ant. °*Ars.* Calc. °*Carb. veg.* °*Caust.* Euphorb. °Lach. Magn. c. Rhus. Ruta. °*Sec.* °*Stram.* °*Urtic.* (Comp. BURNT, PAIN AS IF.)

Contusions, °*Arn.* °*Cic.* °*Con.* Croc. °*Euphr.* Hep. °*Jod.* Mez. °Petr. °Phosph. °*Puls.* °*Ruta.* °Sulph. °*Sulph. ac.*

Ecchymosed, °*Arn.* °*Bry.* °*Con.* Crotal. °*Dulc.* °Hep. °*Lach.* °*N. vom.* °*Puls.* °*Rhus.* °Sulph. °*Sulph. ac.*

As if from a fall or concussion, °Arn. °Bry. °*Cic.* °*Con.* °Puls. °*Rhus.* °Sulph. ac.

Former injuries, already healed, becoming malignant again, **Carb. veg.* Caust. Con. Croc. Eugen. Galv. **Lach.* Magn. art. Natr. **Natr. m.* °*Nitr. ac.* °*N. vom.* **Phosph.* °*Sil.* °*Sulph.* (Comp. Inveterate.)

Gangrenous, °Acon. °Amm. °*Ars.* °*Bell.* °Carb. veg. °*Chin.* Euphorb. °*Lach.* °*Sil.*

Glandular, °Arn. °*Cic.* °*Con.* °Dulc. °Jod. °*Merc.* °*Phosph.* °Puls. °*Rhus.* °Sil. °*Sulph.*

Hernia, °Acon. °*Cocc.* °*N. vom.* °*Sulph.*

With inflammation, °*Acon.* °*Arn.* °*Cham.* Lach. Mez. Natr. m. Plumb. °*Puls.* °*Rhus.* °Sulph. °*Sulph. ac.*

Incisive wounds, °*Arn.* °*Natr.* °Plumb. °Sil. °*Staph.* °*Sulph.* °Sulph. ac.

Injuries of bones, °*Arn.* °Calc. °*Calend.* Phosph. °*Phos. ac.* °*Puls.* Rhus. °*Ruta.* Sil. Staph. Symphit. officinale.

Inveterate, which will not heal, Alum. Amm. *Baryt. Borax. Calc.* Carb. veg. Caust. **Cham.* Chel. Clem. Con. Croc. **Graph.* Hell. **Hep.* Kal. **Lach.* Lyc. Magn. c. Mang. **Merc.* Mur. ac. Natr. **Nitr. ac.* N. vom. **Petr.* Phosph. Phos. ac. Plumb. *Rhus.* Sep. **Sil.* Squill. °*Staph.* **Sulph.*

Itching, Chin. °*Sulph.* Tart.

Luxations, dislocations, °*Arn.* °Natr. Natr. m. Phosph. °*Rhus.*

Muscular distortions, °*Arn.* °*Natr.* Natr. m. Phosph. °*Rhus.*

Painful, becoming again, Con. Croc. Eugen. *Magn. art. Natr. m. °*Nitr. ac.* °*N. vom.* °Staph. °Sulph.

Painful as if sore, °Amm. °Bell. °*Hep.* °*N. vom.* **Phos. ac.* **Sulph.*

Wounds from the blow of a sabre, °*Arn.* °Euphr. °Lach. °*Puls.* °Staph. °*Sulph.* °*Sulph. ac.*

Shot-wounds, °*Arn.* °*Euphr.* *Plumb.* °Puls. °Ruta. °Sulph. °*Sulph. ac.*

Splinter, from, *Acon.* °*Arn.* °*Carb. veg.* °Cic. °*Hep.* Lach. **Nitr. ac.* °*Sil.* Sulph.

Sprains or Strains, °Agn. °*Amm.* Ang. °*Arn.* °Bry. °Calc. °Carb. an. °Carb. veg. °Ign. °Lyc. °Magn. aust. °Natr. °Natr. m. °Nitr. ac. °N. vom. °Petr. °Phosph. °Puls. °*Rhus.* °*Ruta.* °Sep. °Sulph. (Comp. SPRAINED, PAIN AS IF.)

Stab-wound, °*Arn.* °*Carb. veg.* °*Cic.* Con. Eugen. Hep. °*Lach.* Natr. m. °*Nitr. ac.* Plumb. Sep. °*Sil.* Sulph.

Stinging, °*Acon.* °*Arn.* Bell. °*Bry.* °*Caust.* Chin. Clem. °*Merc.* Mez. **Nitr. ac.* Sep. Sil. °*Sulph.*

Stings of insects, °*Acon.* °*Arn.* °*Bell.* °Calad. Lach. Merc. Seneg. Sep.

Straining or sprained, Amb. °Arn. Baryt. °Bry. **Calc.* °Carb. an. °Carb. veg. Caust. Chin. **Cocc.* Con. Croc. °Graph. Jod. °Kal. °Lyc. Magn. c. Mur. ac. **Natr.* °Natr. m. **N. vom.* Phosph. Phos. ac. Rhod. **Rhus.* °Sep. *Sil. Stann. °*Sulph.* Val.

—, in most cases, **Rhus.*

—, with hernia, °Cocc. °*N. vom.* °*Sulph.*

—, with prolapsus uteri, °Bell. °*N. vom.* °Sep.

Suppurating, *Asa. °*Bell.* Caust. °*Chin.* Croc. °*Hep.* °Lach. °*Merc.* Plumb. °*Puls.* °*Sulph.*

With swelling of the affected parts, °*Arn.* Bell. °*Bry.* N. vom. °*Puls.* °*Rhus.* °*Sulph.* °Sulph. ac. (Comp. SWELLING.)

Ulcerated, **Cham.* **Graph.* *Hep. *Lach. **Merc.* *Nitr. ac. **Petr.* **Sil.* °Staph. **Sulph.* (Comp. Inveterate.)

Inodorous and Insipid.

Blennorrhœa and expectoration, Amm. m. *Calc.* Carb. an. Corall. Kreas.

Insects, stings of.

In general, °*Acon.* °*Arn.* °*Bell.* °Calad. °Lach. °*Merc.* Seneg.? °Sep. Appearances like stings of insects, Ant. Ars. Caust. Coloc. Sil. Sulph. Rhus v.
Blotches, as if from stings, *Ant.*
Blisters from stings, Ant.
Pimples, Ant. Ars.
Spots, Lyc.

Face, Ant.
Arms, Ant.
Hands, Spong.
Lower limbs, Ant. Lyc.

Insensible (Comp. Painless).

Herpes, °Lyc.
Ulcers, Anac. °Ars. °Calc. Camph. °Carb. an. °*Carb. veg.* °*Con.* Dulc. °*Euphorb.* Jod. Lach. °*Laur.* °*Lyc.* Mur. ac. *Nitr. ac.* Oleand. °*Op.* °*Phos. ac.* Plumb. *Sep.* °*Sil.* °*Sulph.*

Bedsoress, s. Soreness.

Interstitial distention.

Bones, periosteum, °*Asa.* °*Calc.* °Lyc. °*Merc.*

°*Mez.* Nitr. ac.? °*Phosph.* °*Phos. ac.* Puls.? Rhus.? Ruta.? Sep.? °*Sil.* °*Staph.* °*Sulph.*
Mucous membrane, °*Bell.* °*Dulc.* °*Merc.* °*Puls.* °*Seneg.*

Inveterate, Malignant.

Ulcers, Ars. *Baryt.* Calc. *Carb. veg.* Caust. °*Cham.* °*Chel.* Clem. Con. Croc. °*Graph.* **Hep.* Kal. °*Lach.* °*Lyc.* Magn. c. Mang. °*Merc.* Mur. ac. Natr. °*Nitr. ac.* °*Petr.* *Phosph.* *Phos. ac.* °*Rhus.* °*Sep.* °*Sil.* Squill. °*Staph.* °*Sulph.*
Blotches, Ars.

Itch.

In general, Amb.? Ant? °*Ars.* Calc.? *Carb. an.?* °*Carb. veg.* °*Caust.* *Clem.?* *Coloc.?* Con.? Cupr.? *Dulc.?* Graph.? Guaj.? Heracl.? °*Kreas.* °*Lach.* Led.? Lyc.? *Mang.?* °*Merc.* Mez.? °*Natr.* Oleand.? Oph.? Petr.? *Phos. ac.?* °*Puls.* °*Selen.* °*Sep.* °*Sil.* Squill. Staph. °*Sulph.* °*Sulph. ac.* Tarax.? Tart.? Val.? °*Veratr.* Zinc.
Bleeding, *Calc.?* Dulc.? °*Merc.* °*Sulph.*
Dry, Ars.? *Calc.?* °*Carb. veg.* °*Caust.* Cupr.? *Dulc.?* Graph.? °*Lach.* Led.? °*Merc.* °*Natr.* Petr.? Phos. ac.? °*Sep.* *Sil.?* Staph.? °*Sulph.* Val.? °*Veratr.*
Greasy, suppurating, Ant.? °*Caust.* Clem.? Cic.? °*Kreas.* °*Merc.* Selen.? °*Sep.* Squill.? °*Sulph.*
Humid, Calc.? °*Carb. veg.* °*Caust.* Clem.?

Dulc. ? °*Kreas. Graph.* ? *Lyc.* ? °*Sep.* Staph.? °*Sulph.*
Rash-like, °*Carb. veg.* °*Merc.* °*Sulph.*
Suppressed, °*Amb.* °*Ars.* °*Carb. veg.* °*Caust.* Graph. ? Natr. m. ? °*Selen.* °*Sep.* °*Sulph.* Zinc. ? (Comp. SUPPRESSED, THAT WHICH IS.)

Abdomen, °Natr.
Chest, Squill.
Lower limbs, nates, **Phos. ac.*
—, thighs, Galv.
Feet, toes, °*Phos. ac.*

ITCH-LIKE.

In general, eruption, *Amb. Ant.* *Ars. Bry. **Colc.* Canth. *Carb. an.* **Carb. veg.* **Caust. Clem. Coloc.* Con. *Cupr. Dulc.* Electr. Graph. Guaj. Heracl. **Lach.* Led. Lyc. Magn. art. *Mang.* **Merc. Merc. corr. Mez.* **Natr.* Oleand. Oph. Petr. **Phos. ac.* Puls. Sabad. °*Selen.* **Sep. Sil. Squill. Staph.* **Sulph. Sulph. ac.* Tarax. *Tart.* Val. **Veratr.* Zinc.

Arms, pimples, Tart.
—, herpes, Grat.
Hands, eruption, Ant. *Lach. Rhus. Selen.* Squill. °*Sulph.*
—, fingers, °Lach. °*Sulph.*
Lower limbs, pustules, Hyos.
Feet, vesicles, Lach. Squill.

ITCHES, THAT WHICH.

Blisters, vesicles, *Amm. m.* **Bry.* Bruc. **Calc.* *Canth.* Carb. veg. *Caust.* Clem. Daph. *Kal.* Kal. chl. Kal. hdr. Kreas. **Lach.* *Magn. c.* Magn. m Mang. *Natr.* Natr. m. Nitr. ac. Ol. an. Petr. Phell. Phosph. Plumb. Ran. Rhus. v. Sassap. Seneg. Sep. *Sil.* Spong. *Sulph.*

Blisters, phagedænic, Graph. Sil.

Blotches, tubercles, Aur. Canth. Carb. an. Cham. Cocc. Dulc. Graph. Kal. Lach. Lyc. Magn. c. Magn. s. Mur. ac. Natr. m. Nitr. Nitr. ac. Op. Rhus. Staph. Stram. Stront. Zinc.

Bloodvessels, swelling of, Berb. Bruc. *Caps.* Carb. veg. Caust. Graph. Lach. Magn. art. Magn. aust. N. vom. Plumb. Puls. *Sep.* Sil. **Sulph.* Sulph. ac. Tart.

Chilblains, *Agar.* Asar. Aur. *Berb.* Borax. *Cocc.* *Colch.* Croc. **Lyc.* Magn. art. **Nitr. ac.* **N. vom.* Spig. **Sulph.*

Eruption, **Acon.* **Agar.* *Agn.* Alum. Amb. **Amm.* Amm. m. Anac. **Ant.* Arg. Arn. **Ars.* Asa. Baryt. Bell. Bov. **Bry.* *Calad.* **Calc.* Canth. Caps. Carb. an. Carb. veg. **Caust.* Cham. Chel. Cic. Cin. **Clem.* Cocc. Coff. Con. Cupr. Dig. Dulc. Graph. Hep. Heracl. *Ign.* Ipec. **Kal.* Kreas. *Lach.* Laur. *Led.* Lyc. Magn. art. Magn. arct. Magn. aust. Magn. c. Magn. m. Mang. **Merc.* Mercurial. **Mez.* Natr. Natr. m. Nitr. **Nitr. ac.* N. vom. **Oleand.* *Par.* Petr. Phosph. Phos. ac. Plumb. Puls. *Ran.* Ran. sc. **Rhus.* Sabad. Sabin. Sassap. *Selen.* **Sep.* *Sil.* Spig. Spong. *Squill.* Stann. **Staph.* Stram. Stront. **Sulph.* Tarax.

Tart. Tax. Teucr. Thuj. Val. * *Veratr.* *Viol. tr.* Zinc.

Erysipelas, Euphorb. **Rhus.*

Figwarts, Euphr. Thuj.

Herpes, Alum. Amb. °Amm. °*Ars.* °*Bov.* °Bry. *Caps.* **Caust.* Clem. °Con. Cupr. **Graph.* Ipec. Kal. hdr. **Led.* **Lyc.* Magn. s. Mang. **Merc.* Nicc. **Nitr. ac.* *Petr. Plumb. **Rhus.* °Sep. Staph. **Sulph.* Tax.

As if from lice, Arg. Canth. Magn. m. Plat. Zinc.

Nails, on the, Hep.

Pimples, **Acon.* *Amb.* *Amm.* Amm. m. *Ant.* Ars. *Baryt.* Bell. Bov. *Bry.* *Calc.* Canth. *Carb. veg.* *Caust.* *Cham.* Cin. Cinn. Clem. Cocc. Con. Dulc. Gins. Graph. *Hep.* Jod. *Kal.* Kreas. Lach. Lam. *Laur.* Led. *Lyc.* *Magn. art.* *Magn. arct.* Magn. aust. Magn. c. Magn. m. Magn. s. *Merc.* *Merc. ac.* Mill. Mur. ac. *Natr.* *Natr. m.* *Natr. s.* Nitr. *Nitr. ac.* N. vom. Ol. an. Phosph. *Phos. ac.* Poth. Puls. Ratanh. Rhus. Sabad. Sabin. Sassap. *Selen.* *Sep.* *Sil.* Squill. Stann. *Staph.* Stront. Sulph. Tab. Tarax. Tart. Tax. Veratr. Zinc.

Pustules, Anthrok. Berb. Dulc. Graph. Hydroc. °*Merc.* N. vom. Petr. Rhus. Sassap. Sulph. Tart.

Rash and the like, Alum. ***Bry.*** °***Calad.*** Daph. °***Euphr.*** °***Led.*** ***Merc.*** ***Mez.*** Natr. m. °***N vom.*** Rhab. °***Selen.*** Sep. Sil. ***Sulph.*** Tart. Teucr. Zinc.

Rhagades, Merc.

Scurfs, crusts, Caust. Merc. Phos. ac. *Rhus. Sassap. *Sil.

Spots, Agn. Amm. m. Arn. ***Berb.*** Calc. Carb.

veg. Caust. Cinn. °*Con.* Cupr. Dros. Electr. *Graph.* Hep. *Jod.* °*Kal.* Kal. hdr. *Lach.* **Led.* *Lyc.* Merc. Mur. ac. *Natr. m.* Nitr. *Nitr. ac.* Op. Phosph. Par. Ratanh. Sassap. °Sep. **Sil.* Spong. Squill. Sulph. **Sulph. ac.* Tax. *Zinc.

Swelling, Ant. Canth. Caust. Cocc. Lach. Nitr. ac. *Phosph.* Phos. ac. Puls. Rhus. Rhus v. Stram. Sulph.

Tumors, Electr. *Magn. c.* Natr. Natr. m. Nitr. ac. Op. *Rhus v.* Sassap. Sep. Stann. Stram. Sulph.

Ulcers, Agn. °*Alum.* °*Amb.* Amm. Anac. *Ant.* Arn. **Ars.* Baryt. *Bell.* °*Bov.* Bry. *Calc.* *Canth.* Carb. veg. °*Caust.* *Cham.* Chel. °*Chin.* *Clem.* Con. Dros. °*Graph.* **Hep.* Ipec. Kreas. Lach. Led. **Lyc.* *Merc.* Mez. Natr. Natr. m. Nitr. *Nitr. ac.* N. vom. Petr. *Phosph.* °*Phos. ac.* **Puls.* *Ran.* **Rhus.* Ruta. Sabad. Sassap. Selen. °*Sep.* **Sil.* Squill. °*Staph.* °*Sulph.* Tart. *Thuj.* Veratr. Viol. tr. Zinc.

Warts, Euphr. Kal. Nitr. ac. Phosph. Thuj.

Head, eruptions. **Alum.* Baryt. Bov. Graph. **Merc.* °Mez. °Nitr. ac. Oleand. Phosph. Sep. Sil. Staph.

Ears, eruption, Mosch. Mez. Natr. m. Petr. Sassap.

—, pimples, Amm. m. Magn. arct. Mur. ac.

—, herpes, Merc.

—, Scurfs, Sassap.

Buccal cavity, swelling, Phosph.

Anus, eruptions, Ign. Ipec. Lyc. Staph.

Sexual parts, eruptions, Amb. Arn. Graph. Lach. *Nitr. ac.* Sep. Sil.

Thoracic region, pimples, Bov. Staph.
—, herpes, Staph.
—, spots, °*Led.* Nitr. ac.

Dorsal region, eruption, Caust. Cinn. Led. °Sep.
—, blisters, Natr.
—, pimples, Baryt. Calc. °Carb. veg. Cinn. Clem. Kal. Led. Magn. art. Magn. aust. Mill. Natr. m. Phosph. Puls. Selen. Sil. Squill. Staph.
—, herpes, Caust.
—, spots, Carb. veg. Cinn. °Sep. Zinc.
—, swelling, Sulph.
—, blotches, Lyc.

Arms, eruptions, *Agar.* Berb. Bov. Canth. Carb. an. Carb. veg. *Caust.* Cupr. Dulc. Euphorb. Kal. Kal. hdr. ***Laur.*** Lyc. Magn. c. Mang. ****Merc.*** Mez. Mur. ac. Natr. Natr. m. Natr. s. Phosph. ***Puls.*** Ratanh. Sabad. Sabin. Staph. ***Sulph.*** Tart. Zinc.
—, herpes, Cupr. Mang. ****Merc.***

Hands, eruptions, *Agar.* Amb. Amm. m. Ant. Baryt. Berb. Canth. Carb. an. ****Carb. veg.*** Caust. Dros. Electr. Hep. Ipec. Jod. Kal. Kal. chl. Laur. Led. ***Lyc. Magn. c.*** Mur. ac. Natr. m. *Nitr. ac.* ***Rhus. Rhus v.*** Sabad. Sassap. Selen. ***Sulph.*** Tarax. Zinc.
—, herpes, Amb. Caust.
—, blisters, phagedænic, Graph. Sil.
—, swelling, Canth. Lach. Sulph.
—, ulcers, Dros. Ran.

Lower limbs, eruption, Anac. Caust. ***Kal.*** Led. Mang. ***Merc. Natr.*** Nitr. N. vom. Petr. Ratanh.
—, blotches, Electr. Lach.

Lower limbs, blisters, Kal.
—, pimples. ***Hep. Petr. Phos. ac.*** Selen. ***Sep.*** Stann. Staph.
—, herpes, Merc. Nicc. Plumb.
—, spots, Electr. Graph. Mur. ac. Sassap.
—, rash, Daph. Natr. m. N. vom. Sil.
—, ulcers, Lyc. ***Merc.*** °***Phos. ac.*** °***Sil.***
—, nettlerash, Caust.
Feet, eruption, Calc. *Con.* Electr. Sep. ***Sil.***
—, swelling, Caust. Cocc. Puls.
—, ulcers, °***Sil.***
—, scurfs, ***Sil.***
—, blister, phagedænic, Sil.

Itching.

In general, **Acon.* Agar. Agn. Alum. ****Amb.*** ****Amm.*** ****Amm. m.*** Anac. Ang. Anthrok. **Ant.* Arg. Arn. ****Ars.*** ****Asa.*** Asar. Aur. Baryt. Bell. Berb. Bism. Bov. ***Bry.*** **Calad.* Calc. Calc. ph. Camph. Cann. ***Canth.*** Caps. Carb. an. Carb. veg. Caust. Cham. *Chel. Chin.* **Cic.* Cin. Cist. *Cocc.* Coff. Colch. Coloc. *Con. Croc. Crotal. Croton. **Cycl.* Dig. °***Dros.*** Dulc. Electr. Euphorb. Euphr. Evon. Ferr. magn. Gins. Graph. Grat. Guaj. Hep. Heracl. Hydroc. Hyos. *Ign.* °***Ipec.*** Jod. Kal. c. Kal. chl. Kreas. **Lach. Laur.* ****Led.*** Lupul. **Lyc.* ***Magn. art.*** Magn. arct. *Magn. aust.* **Magn. c.* Magn. m. Magn. s. Mang. Meph. *Merc. Mercurial. *Mez. Mosch. Mur. ac. Natr. c. Natr. m. Nicc. Nitr. Nitr. ac.**N. vom.***Oleand.* Ol. an. ***Op. Par.*** Petr. Phell. Phosph. Phos. ac. Plat. ***Plumb.***

Prun. ***Puls.** ***Ran.** ***Ran. sc.*** Ratanh. Rhod. ***Rhus.** Rhus v. ***Ruta.** **Sabin.* Sassap. Sec. ***Selen.** Seneg. Sep. **Sil.* ***Spig. Spong.*** Squill. Stann. **Staph.* Stram. Stront. ****Sulph.*** ****Sulph. ac.*** Tab. Tarax. *Tart.* Tax. Teucr. Thuj. Val. ***Veratr. Viol. tr.*** Vinc. min. Zinc.

As if from ants, Lach. Phosph. °Puls. Sec.

Bitings, Amm. m. Ant. ***Berb.*** Bov. ***Bry.*** Calc. Camph. Carb. veg. Chel. *Chin.* Cocc. °***Colch.*** Coloc. Con. Euphorb. Grat. Hell. Ipec. °***Lach.*** ***Led.*** Lyc. ***Magn. arct.*** Magn. aust. Mang. ***Merc.*** Mur. ac. Natr. c. Nitr. ***N.*** *vom.* °***Oleand.*** Ol. an. Op. Phosph. °*Puls.* Sil. Staph. Stront. Tart.

Burning, **Agar.* Alum. *Amb. Amm. Anac. *Arg.* Arn. **Ars.* Aur. Baryt. Berb. Borax. Bov. °*Bry.* ***Calad.*** Calc. Calc. ph. Canth. *Caps.* Carb. veg. Chin. °*Cic.* Cocc. Coff. Colch. Dulc. ***Euphorb.*** Grat. Guaj. Hell. *Hep. Ign.* Kal. Led. Lyc. ***Magn. art.*** Magn. c. Mang. ***Merc.*** Mez. Natr. °***N.*** *vom.* Oleand. Ol. an. Op. Phell. Petr. Phosph. Phos. ac. Puls. *Ran.* °***Rhus.*** ***Sabad.*** Sassap. Seneg. Sep. *Spig.* Spong. Squill. Stann. *Staph.* Stram. Stront. *Sulph.* *Veratr. Viol. od.*

As if from congelation, **Agar.*

Corrosive itching, Rhus v.

Crawling, Arg. Ars. Dulc. Magn. c. Sil. Spig. Staph.

Creeping, Sil.

Dull, Hep.

As if of electric sparks, Phell.

As if from fleas, Arg. Jod. Lyc. **Magn. arct.**

Magn. Merc. Mez. Natr. Nicc. Ol. an. Puls. Sil. Spong. Staph. Tab. Teucr. Thuj. Zinc.

Gnawing, **Agn.* Alum. Amb. Anac. *Ars.* Berb. Bism. Bry. Caps. Caust. Cham. Clem. *Cocc.* Con. Cycl. *Dig.* Dros. *Euphorb.* Evon. Graph. Guaj. Hell. Hep. Kal. c. Led. °Lyc. *Magn. aust.* Men. Merc. N. vom. *Oleand.* Par. Phell. Phosph. *Plat. Puls. Rhod.* Rhus. °*Ruta.* Spig. Spong. Squill. *Staph.* Stann. Sulph. Thuj. Tarax. Veratr. Vinc. min.

Intolerable, Merc. Sil.

Itch-like, Amb. Merc. °Veratr.

Jerking, Staph.

Itching as of lice, Arg. Canth. Magn. m. Plat. Zinc.

As from mosquito-bites, Rhus v.

As of nettles, Colch. Lupul.

Painful, Alum. Ammon. Baryt. Cham. Cocc. Lupul. Nitr.

Pinching, Mosch.

Pleasant, Merc.

Prickling, Cin. Plat. Zinc.

Sore, Berb. Cann. Led. Magn. art. Magn. aust. Mez. Plat. Ruta. Staph. Sulph. Zinc.

Stinging, *Agn.* Alum. Anac. Ang. Ant. *Arg. Arn. Asa.* Aur. Baryt. Berb. **Bry.* Calad. Calc. Camph. Cann. Canth. Caps. Carb. veg. Caust. Cham. Chin. Cocc. Colch. *Con.* Crotal. *Cycl.* Dig. **Dros.* Dulc. Euphorb. Euphr. *Graph.* Hep. Hyos. *Ign.* Jod. Kal. Lach. Laur. *Led.* Lyc. Magn. art. *Magn. arct. Magn. aust.* Mang. *Merc.* Mez. Mosch. Mur. ac. Natr. Natr. m. Nitr. Nitr. ac. N. vom. *Oleand.* Op. Petr. Phell. Phosph. Phos. ac. Plat. Plumb. Prun. *Puls.* Ran. *Ran. sc.* Rhab. °*Rhus. Ruta.* Sabad. *Sabin.* Samb. Sassap. Sil. °*Spig.* **Spong.*

Squill. *Stann.* **Staph.* Stram. Sulph. Tab. Tarax. Teucr. °*Thuj.* *Veratr.* °*Viol. tr.* Zinc.
Tearing, Bell. Bry.
Tickling, *Agar.* Arg. Bry. Calc. Cocc. Euphorb. Euphr. Ign. *Merc.* Mur. ac. Plat. Puls. Ruta. Spong. Squill. Tart.
Titillating, Acon. Amb. Arg. Arn. Asa. Baryt. *Bell.* Bry. Calc. Camph. Canth. *Chel.* *Chin.* Cin. Euphr. Ferr. magn. Led. Magn. arct. Magn. aust. N. vom. Op. Phos. ac. *Plat.* °*Puls.* **Rhod.* *Sabad.* Sec. Sil. Spig. Spong. *Squill.* Staph. Sulph. Thuj. Veratr.
Troublesome, Coloc. Op. Stram.
Violent, *Agar.* Alum. Ammon. Cin. °*Dros.* °Dulc. Heracl. Hyos. °*Ipec.* Kal. chl. Kreas. **Lach.* Lyc. Magn. Magn. m. Merc. Natr. Nitr. ac. *Op.* Par. Phosph. Rhus v. Seneg. Zinc.
Voluptuous, Anac. Magn. arct. *Merc.* Mur. ac. Sep. Sil. Spong. Sulph.
Wandering, Cham. Graph. Kal. c. Magn. m. Mez. Ratanh. Rhus v. Spong. Staph. Zinc.
Of wounds, Chin. Tart.

Head, Agar. Agn. Alum. **Amm.* **Amm. m.* Anac. °Ant. Arn. Arg. *Ars.* Asar. *Baryt.* *Berb.* *Bov.* **Calc.* Calc. ph. Caps. Carb. an. *Caust.* *Cham.* Chin. Coff. Con. *Crotal.* Cycl. Dros. **Graph.* Grat. *Kal.* Lach. *Laur.* *Lyc.* Magn. arct. Magn. c. Magn. m. Mang. Meph. **Merc.* Mez. Mur. ac. *Natr. m.* Nitr. °Nitr. ac. *Oleand.* *Ol. an.* Par. Petr. Phell. **Phosph.* Phos. ac. Puls. Ran. sc. Ratanh. *Rhod. *Rhus.* Ruta. Sabad. **Sassap.* **Seneg.* **Sep.* **Sil.* Spig.

Staph. Stront. Sulph. Sulph. ac. *Thuj. Veratr.

Eyes, *Agar.* *Alum.* Amm. Ars. ***Asa.*** ***Baryt.*** Bell. Bov. **Calc.* Canth. Carb. an. Carb. veg. ***Caust.*** ***Chel.*** Con. Coloc. Cupr. *Cycl.* Ferr. ***Ign.*** Lach. Laur. Magn. art. Magn. arct. Magn. aust. Magn. c. *Magn. m.* *Merc.* Mosch. ***Mur. ac.*** *Natr.* ***Natr. m.*** Oleand. Petr. Phosph. Plat. ****Puls.*** Ran. Rhod. Sep. **Sil.* *Spig.* Squill. Stann. Stront. **Sulph.* Zinc.

Eyebrows, Agar. Agn. Alum. Caust. Chin. Laur. Magn. arct. Par. Selen. Sil. Spig. Sulph. Viol. tr.

Eyelids, Agn. Alum. Amb. Amm. m. Ang. Ars. Baryt. **Bell.* **Bry.* **Calc.* Camph. Carb. an. Carb. veg. Caust. Chin. Cin. Cocc. *Croc.* *Cycl.* Dros. **Euphorb.* Euphr. Ferr. Graph. Jod. Kal. Kal. hdr. Kreas. Laur. Lyc. Magn. art. *Magn. arct.* *Magn. aust.* Magn. m. ***Mez.*** Mosch. Mur. ac. *Natr.* Natr. m. Nicc. **N. vom.* Oleand. Par. Petr. ***Phosph.*** Plat. Puls. ***Rhus.*** ***Ruta.*** Sep. **Sil.* Spong. Staph. **Sulph.* Sulph. ac. *Veratr.* Zinc.

Canthi, Alum. Ant. Arg. Arn. ***Bell.*** Berb. Borax. Bruc. Bry. *Calc.* Carb. veg. *Caust.* Cin. *Con.* Crotal. Euphorb. Ferr. magn. Hell. Hyos. Ign. Jod. Lam. Laur. Led. *Lyc.* ***Magn. arct.*** *Magn. c.* Magn. m. Mur. ac. ***Natr. m.*** Nitr. ac. N. vom. Phell. Prun. ***Puls.*** Rhus. ***Ruta.*** Sep. Squill. *Staph.* ***Stront.*** Sulph. Tax. Tong.

Ears, region of, Aeth. *Agar.* *Alum.* Amb. **Amm.* Amm. m. °*Anac.* *Arg.* ***Baryt.*** Bell. Berb. Borax. ***Bov.*** *Caps.* Carb. veg. Cast. Caust. ***Con.*** Cupr. Ferr. magn. Gran. Graph. Hep. ***Ign.*** ***Kal.*** Kal. hdr. Kreas. Lach. ***Laur.*** *Lyc.* ***Magn.***

art. Magn. m. Mang. Men. Meph. Merc. Mez. Mill. Mosch. Mur. ac. Natr. m. Nitr. Nitr. ac. *N. vom.* Ol. an. Petr. Phell. ***Phosph.*** Phos. ac. ***Puls.*** Ratanh. Raph. Rhab. Rhod. ***Rhus.*** Sabad. ***Sassap. Sep. Sil. Spig.*** Stann. ****Sulph.*** Tong. Veratr. Zinc.

Ears, external, Agar. Carb. veg. Con. Hep. Kal. Sil. Spig. Sulph.

—, meatus, Alum. Caust. Ign. Nitr. Sassap.

—, lobules, Alum. Caust. Kal. Laur. Natr. m. Phos. ac. Sabad.

—, internal, Anac. Caps. Puls. Ratanh. Rhab. Ruta. Samb. Sep.

—, behind the ears, Agar. Alum. Carb. veg. Graph. Mosch. Natr. m. Nitr. ac. Therid.

Nose, Agar. Agn. °Amm. Aur. *Aur. m. Berb. Borax. Bov. **Calc.* **Carb. veg.* Caps. ***Caust.*** Coloc. ***Con.*** Eugen. Gran. Graph. Grat. Hell. Hep. Ign. Kal. Lach. ***Laur.*** Lyc. Magn. c. ***Merc.*** Mur. ac. Natr. m. Natr. s. Nitr. *Nitr. ac.* N. vom. Oleand. Ol. an. Op. Petr. ***Phell.*** Phosph. Samb. Sassap. Selen. Seneg. **Sil.* Spig. Staph. Stront. Sulph. Therid. Zing.

Face, *Agar.* Agn. **Alum.* Amb. **Amm.* Anac. °Ant. Arg. Ars. Asa. Baryt. **Bell.* Berb. **Calc.* *Cann. Caps. Caust.* °Chel. Colch. *Con. Dig. Dulc. Euphorb. Ferr. magn. Gins. Gran. Graph. Grat. Hep. Kal. Lach. Laur. *Lyc. Magn. c. Meph. Natr. *Natr. m. Natr. s. Nicc. *Nitr. N. vom.* Oleand. Ol. an. Op. Petr. Phell. ***Phosph.*** Phos. ac. Plumb. ***Rhus.*** Ruta. ***Sabad. Sassap.*** Sep. Sil. Spong. Squill. Stann. Staph. ***Stront.*** Sulph. Tab. Thuj. *Veratr.* Viol. tr. Zinc.

Face, eyes, region of, Agn. Alum. **Con.* Caust. Lach. Oleand. Spong.

—, cheeks, Agar. *Agn.* Alum. Ant. Asa. **Bell.* Berb. Bov. Caust. Chel. **Con.* Cycl. Dig. Dulc. Graph. Hep. ***Lach.*** Laur. Magn. m. Natr. m. *O'eand.* ***Rhus.*** Sabad. Sil. *Spong. Staph.* Stront. Thuj.

—, whiskers, Agar. Amb. **Calc.* Natr. Natr. m. Sil.

—, mouth, region of, Agar. Amm. m. Anac. Con. Hep. Ol. an.

—, forehead, Agar. Alum. Amb. Amm. m. Anac. Berb. Canth. Caps. Carb. an. Carb. veg. Caust. Cham. Chel. Croc. Laur. Led. Natr. m. N. vom. Oleand. Ol. an. Phell. Rhus. Samb. Sil. Spig. Squill. Veratr.

Lips and mouth, region of, Alum. Amm. Arn. Berb. Bry. Calc. Caust. Chel. Con. Ferr. magn. Graph. Hell. Kal. Laur. Magn. c. Mang. Natr. Nitr. ac. Ol. an. Phosph. Sabad. Sulph. Thuj. Zinc.

—, itching of eruptions, °Baryt. ***Bell.*** Bry. Carb. veg. Chin. Hep. ***Kal.*** Magn. m. Mang. *Nitr. ac.* Seneg. *Sil.* Squill. Staph.

Chin, Alum. Amm. Berb. Calc. Con. Dig. Grat. Hydroc. ***Kal.*** Laur. *Lyc.* Magn. aust. Magn. c. Meph. Natr. c. Natr. m. Oleand. Ol. an. Op. Phosph. Plat. Sassap. Spig. Squill. ***Stront.*** Sulph. Tarax. Thuj. ***Zinc.***

—, itching of eruptions, Bell. Dulc. Lyc. Natr. Natr. m. N. vom. Par. Sassap. Sep. Thuj. Zinc.

Lower jaw, Laur. Natr. Oleand. Par. Squill.

Buccal cavity, Amm. Bell. Calc. Caust. Cist.

Ferr. magn. Graph. *Kal.* Lach. Magn. arct. Magn. c. Merc. Nitr. ac. Phosph. Phos. ac. Prun. Rhod. Samb. *Sil.* Spig. Spong. Tong. Zinc.

Buccal cavity, palate, Ferr. magn. Kal. Phosph. Sil.

—, velum palati, Sil.

—, mouth, Magn. c.

—, fauces and throat, Cist. Samb. Spig.

—, gums, Amm. Bell. Calc. Caust. Graph. Kal. Lach. Merc. Nitr. ac. Phosph. Prun. Rhod. Spong. Tong. Zinc.

—, tongue, Alum. Magn. arct. N. vom. Phos. ac.

Abdomen and stomach, region of, Agar. Alum. Arn. Aur. Baryt. **Bell.* Berb. Bov. Cann. Coloc. Con. Ign. Kal. Kal. hdr. Laur. Led. Magn. arct. Magn. c. Mang. ***Merc. Natr.*** N. vom. ***Ol. an. Petr.*** Phosph. ***Puls.*** Sassap. Sep. Spig. Stront. Sulph. Tereb. Zinc.

—, hernia, Baryt.

—, inguinal, Berb. Laur. Magn. c. Magn. m. Magn. s. Sep. Spig.

—, umbilical region, Ign. Kal. Kal. hdr. Magn. arct. Ol. an. Phosph. ***Puls.***

Anus, Agar. **Alum.* Amb. **Amm.* Amm. m. **Anac.* Ant. Ars. Bell. Berb. Borax. Bruc. Bry. **Calc.* Canth. Caps. **Carb. veg.* **Caust.* Cham. Chin. Cin. Cocc. Coloc. Con. Croc. Ferr. magn. Gran. Graph. Grat. Ign. Jod. ***Kal.** Lach. Led. ***Lyc.** Magn. art. Magn. aust. Magn. m. ***N. vom.*** Ol. an. Petr. Phell. ****Phosph.*** Phos. ac. Plat. Prun. Rhus. ***Sabad.*** Sassap. ****Sep.***

°*Sil.* *Spig.* Squill. Stann. Staph. **Sulph.* Tereb. Teucr. Zinc.

Anus, nates, between the, Alum. Con. Gran. Seneg.

—, perinæum, Agn. Alum. Ars. Carb. veg. Gran. Ign. Mur. ac. N. vom. Plumb. Tarax.

Sexual parts, Acon. Agar. Agn. Alum. ***Amb.*** ***Amm.*** Anac. Ang. Ant. Arn. Ars. Aur. Baryt. ***Berb.*** Bry. **Calc.* Camph. ***Cann.*** *Canth.* Carb. an. ****Carb. veg.*** ***Caust.*** Cham. Chin. Cinn. ***Cocc.*** *Coff.* ****Con.*** Croc. Dig. Dulc. Euphorb. Euphr. Ferr. magn. ***Graph.*** ***Hep.*** Heracl. ***Ign.*** Ipec. Jod. ****Kal.*** ***Kreas.*** Laur. Led. ****Lyc.*** ***Magn. art.*** ***Magn. arct.*** Magn. aust. ***Magn. m.*** Mang. Meph. **Merc.* Mez. Mur. ac. Natr. **Natr. m.* Natr. s. Nicc. *Nitr. ac.* *N. vom.* Ol. an. ****Petr.*** Phos. ac. Prun. ***Puls.*** Ratanh. Rhod. ***Rhus.*** Sabin. Sassap. Selen. **Sep.* **Sil.* Spong. Staph. ****Sulph.*** *Thuj.* Viol. tr. Zinc.

—, frænulum, Cann. Caust. Hep. Merc.

—, glans, Alum. Amb. Arn. Ars. Calc. Chin. Cinn. Coff. Con. Dig. Hep. Ign. Ipec. Jod. Kal. Led. Magn. aust. Mang. ***Merc.*** Mez. ***Natr.*** ***Natr. m.*** Natr. s. *Nitr. ac.* ***N. vom.*** Petr. Sabin. ***Sep.*** Sil. Spong. *Thuj.*

—, testicles, Merc.

—, scrotum, Agar. Alum. Anac. Ang. Ant. Aur. Baryt. ***Berb.*** Calc. ***Carb. veg.*** ***Caust.*** Cham. Chin. ***Cocc.*** Coff. Croc. Ferr. magn. ***Graph.*** Hep. Heracl. Kal. *Lyc.* Magn. aust. Magn. m. Mang. Meph. Mur. ac. Natr. Natr. s. Nicc. *Nitr. ac.* *N. vom.* **Petr.* Phos. ac. Prun. Puls. Ratanh. Rhod. Selen. Staph. Thuj. Zinc.

—, clitoris, Sulph.

Sexual parts, penis, Agar. Ant. Ars. Caust. Coff. Con. Hep. Natr. s. *Nitr. ac.* Ol. an. Phos. ac.

—, mons veneris, Agar. Carb. an. Carb. veg. *Kal.* Natr. s. Sulph.

—, labia, Agar. Amb. *Amm.* ****Calc.*** ****Carb. veg.*** ****Con.*** Graph. °*Kal.* Kreas. Lyc. Magn. c. ***Merc.*** **Natr. m.* Nicc. *Nitr. ac.* **Sep.* **Sil.* *Staph.* ****Sulph.*** Thuj.

—, vagina, Canth. ****Con.*** Kreas. ****Sulph.***

—, prepuce, Acon. Agar. Ang. Ars. Bry. Calc. Camph. ***Cann. Carb. veg.*** Caust. Con. Euphorb. Euphr. Ing. Laur. ***Lyc. Magn. arct.*** Merc. Natr. *Nitr. ac. N. vom. Puls.* Rhus. Sep. Thuj. Viol. tr.

Thoracic region, Agar. Alum. Anac. Ang. *Ant.* Arn. Baryt. Berb. ***Bov.*** Calc. Canth. *Carb. veg.* Con. Kal. ***Lyc.*** *Natr. m.* Nicc. Phell. ***Phosph.*** Sabad. *Sep.* Spong. Squill. *Stann.* ***Staph.*** Sulph.

Mammæ and nipples, °Alum. Caust. ***Con.*** Hep. Magn. arct. Petr. Puls. ***Rhus.*** Sassap. Sep. °*Sulph.*

—, nipples, Con. Hep. Magn. arct. Petr. Puls. Sassap. Sep. Sulph.

Dorsal region, axilla, Anac. Asar. Carb. veg. Dig. Grat. Kal. Nitr. ac. ***Phosph.*** Sep. ***Spig.*** Spong.

—, neck, *Alum.* Anac. Ant. Calc. Carb. veg. Cinn. Mez. Nicc. Nitr. ac. ***Puls.*** Rhus. Squill. Stront. Sulph. Tab. Teucr. Thuj.

—, small of the back, Berb. Grat. Kal. Magn. m. Merc. Natr. m. Phell.

—, lumbar region, Alum. Dig. Puls.

—, nape of neck, Alum. Amm. m. Berb. Carb.

veg. Mez. Nitr. ac. Ol. an. Phell. *Sep.* Staph. Therid.

Dorsal region, back, *Agar.* Alum. Amm. m. Anac. *Ant.* Baryt. Berb. *Calc. Caust.* Daph. Eugen. Graph. Guaj. Jod. Kal. °Lach. Laur. Lyc. Magn. aust. Magn. m. Magn. s. Merc. Mill. Mur. ac. *Natr.* Natr. m. Natr. s. Nicc. *Nitr. ac.* N. vom. Ol. an. Phosph. *Phos. ac.* Seneg. Sep. Sil. Spig. Therid. Thuj. Zinc.

—, scapulæ, Alum. Arn. Baryt. Calc. Crotal. Laur. Merc. Oleand. Phell. Ratanh. Ruta. Seneg. Sil. Stront. Therid. Zinc.

—, os sacrum, Agar. Alum. Borax. Bov. Graph. Laur. Led. Par. Plumb.

Arms, Agar. Ang. Ant. Ars. Aur. *Bov.* Calc. Carb. veg. **Caust.* Chin. Con. Cupr. Graph. Hell. Kal. *Lach.* Lam. Led. °*Lyc.* Natr. N. vom. Ol. an. Op. Phell. *Phosph.* Phos. ac. Plat. *Puls.* Rhus. Ruta. Sep. Sulph. Tab. Tart. Teucr. Thuj. Veratr. Zinc.

—, elbow, Agar. Amm. m. Berb. Canth. Coloc. Dulc. Hep. Lach. *Laur.* Merc. Natr. Nitr. ac. *Oleand.* Petr. Phosph. Puls. Rhus. Sep. *Spig.*

—, upper arm, Ant. *Berb.* Bov. Carb. veg. Dig. Dulc. Euphorb. Kal. hdr. Lach. *Laur.* Led. Lyc. Magn. arct. Magn. aust. Mang. N. vom. Oleand. Phell. Phos. ac. Ran. sc. Ruta. Stront. Thuj.

—, forearm, Amm. Amm. m. Berb. Bov. Carb. an. Carb. veg. *Caust.* Con. Dulc. Euphorb. Hyos. *Laur.* Magn. c. Magn. m. Magn. s. Merc. Mill. Nitr. Puls. *Ran. Ratanh.* Sassap. Spig. Stront. *Sulph.* Tax. Verbasc.

Hands, Agar. Alum. Amb. Amm. m. Anac. Arg.

Aur. Baryt. *Berb.* Borax. Calc. ***Carb. an. Carb. veg.*** *Caust.* Cin. *Colch.* Dig. Euphorb. Calv. *Gran.* Graph. *Grat. Hep.* Ipec. Kal. Kal. hdr. ***Kreas.*** Lach. Lam. Lupul. ***Lyc.*** Magn. c. Magn. s. Mang. ***Merc.*** Mur. ac. Natr. ***Natr. m.*** *Nitr. ac.* Ol. an. Petr. ***Phell. Phosph.*** Phos. ac. Plat. Ran. ***Rhus.*** Rhus v. Ruta. ***Sassap.*** Sep. *Sil. Spig.* Staph. ***Stann.*** Stram. ***Sulph.***

Hands, wrists, Agar. Amm. m. Arg. Berb. Kal. Led. Plat. Plumb. Selen. Veratr.

—, fingers, **Agar.* Alum. Amb. Amm. m. ***Anac.*** Ant. Ars. ***Berb.*** Borax. Calc. Carb. an. Carb. veg. Caust. ***Cocc. Con.*** *Cycl.* Euphorb. Grat. *Lach.* Lact. Laur. ***Lyc.*** Magn. arct. Magn. c. Mang. ***Merc. Natr. m.*** Natr. s. N. vom. Oleand. Ol. an. Petr. Phos. ac. Plat. ***Plumb.*** Prun. ***Ran.*** Ran. sc. ***Rhod. Spig.*** Sulph. Therid. Veratr. Verb. ***Zinc.***

—, finger-joints, Alum. Arn. Camph. Caust. Crotal. Ign. Natr. m. N. vom. Petr.

—, thumb, Ant. Carb. veg. Cocc. Grat. Natr. Oleand. Ol. an. Plumb. Spong. Staph.

Lower limbs, Caust. Daph. **Lach.* **Lyc.* Merc. Natr. Natr. m. Nitr. Nitr. ac. Ol. an. Phosph. Sec. Sil. Staph. Teucr. Thuj.

—, nates and hips, Amm. Amm. m. Ant. Ars. Baryt. Calc. *Caust.* Chel. Coloc. Con. Evon. Kal. Kal. hdr. Lach. Laur. Led. Lyc. Magn. aust. Magn. c. Magn. m. Mur. ac. Natr. Nicc. Nitr. ac. Ol. an. Oleand. Petr. Phosph. Phos. ac. *Prun.* Sep. Sil. Stann. Staph. Stront. Sulph. Tarax. *Therid.* Teucr. Zinc.

—, thighs, Agar. Alum. Anac. Ang. Ant. Arn. Ars. Baryt. Berb. Bry. *Calc.* Canth. Caust.

Chel. Cic. Cocc. Con. Croton. Dig. Dulc. Electr. Euphorb. Euphr. *Graph.* Grat. Guaj. Kal. *Lach.* Laur. Led. Magn. arct. Magn. Magn. m. Mang. *Merc.* Mosch. Mur. ac. Natr. Natr. m. *Nitr. ac.* N. vom. *Oleand.* Phell. *Phosph. Prun.* Ran. sc. Ratanh. *Rhod.* Sassap. Sil. *Spig.* Spong. *Stann.* Staph. Stront. *Sulph.* Tarax. Zinc.

Lower limbs, knees, Amb. Ant. Asa. Aur. Berb. Bry. *Caust.* Coloc. Grat. Hep. Ign. Kal. Lach. **Lyc. Mang.* Men. Mur. ac. Natr. Nitr. Nitr. ac. N. vom. Ol. an. Phosph. Ran. Ratanh. *Rhus.* Samb. Sassap. *Spong.* Stann. *Sulph.*

—, Legs, Agar. Alum. Amb. Amm. m. Ant. Asa. Aur. Berb. Bism. *Calc. Caust. Cocc. Coloc.* Crotal. Cycl. Dulc. Euphorb. Euphr. Graph. Grat. °*Ipec. Kal. Lach. Laur.* Lyc. Magn. aust. Magn. m. Mang. Mez. Mosch. Mur. ac. Natr. Natr. m. Nitr. Ol. an. Op. *Phosph.* Phos. ac. Plumb. Rhus. *Sabin.* Sassap. Seneg. Sep. *Sil.* Spig. *Staph.* Stront. Sulph. ac. Tarax. Tart. Tax. Therid. Thuj. Veratr.

—, tibia, Ant. Asa. Bism. *Calc. Coloc.* Croton. *Grat. Kal. Lach.* Magn. m. Mang. Mosch. Nitr. *Phosph.* Plumb. *Sep.* Spig. *Stront.* Sulph. ac.

—, calves, Alum. *Caust. Cocc. Coloc. Cycl.* Euphr. °*Ipec. Laur.* Lyc. Magn. aust. Mang. *Mez.* Mur. ac. Ol. an. *Phosph. Rhus. Sabin.* Sassap. Sil. Staph. *Tarax.* Tax. Therid. Thuj. Veratr.

—, tendo Achilles, Berb. Selen.

Feet, *Bell. Berb. Bov. Calc. Caust.* Cham. Cocc. Dulc. Electr. Gins. Grat. Hep. *Ign.* Kal. hdr. *Lach.* Laur. Led. Ran. sc. Selen. Stram. Veratr. Zinc.

—, dorsa of feet, Agar. Alum. Anac. Asa. *Bell.* Bism. Calc. *Caust.* Coloc. Dig. Hep. *Ign. Led.* Natr. m. Natr. s. Ran. sc. *Rhus.* Spig. Stann. Stram. *Tarax. Thuj.*

—, joints and ankles, Agar. Ant. Asa. Aur. Borax. Calc. *Cocc.* Dig. Grat. *Kal.* Lyc. Magn. m. Ol. an. *Oleand.* Petr. *Phosph. ac.* Puls. *Rhus.* Selen. Sep. Stann. Staph.

—, heels, Calc. Caust. Cham. Ign. *Nicc.* Oleand. *Phosph. Phosph. ac.* Puls. Ran. sc. Sabin. Sil. *Staph.* Veratr.

—, soles, *Alum. Amb.* Amm. Amm. m. Aur. Cham. Chin. Con. Cupr. Euphorb. Hep. Kreas. Mur. ac. *Natr.* Natr. s. *Oleand.* Ran. sc. Ratanh. Rhab. Sassap. Sep. Spig. Sulph. Tarax. Tart. Thuj. *Zinc.*

—, toes, **Agar. Alum. Amb.* Amm. Amm. m. Ant. Ars. Asa. *Berb.* Borax. *Carb. an.* Clem. *Cycl.* Dros. *Graph. Hep. Kal.* Lact. Magn. arct. Magn. aust. Magn. s. Mang. Merc. Mur. ac. Natr. Natr. m. *Natr. s.* Nitr. ac. **N. vom.* Paeon. Plat. *Puls.* Ran. sc. Rhab. Rhus. Sep. Spig. Spong. Stann. *Staph. Sulph.* Tarax. *Zinc.*

Bones, periosteum, *Cycl.* Nitr. *Phosph. Veratr.*

Nails, on the, Hep.

Glands, Amm. Anac. Ant. Canth. Carb. an. Carb. veg. Caust. Cocc. Con. Kal. Magn. c. Merc. Phosph. Ran. sc. Rhab. Rhus. Sabin. Sep. Sil. Spong.

Jerks.

Corns, in the, Cocc. °*Magn. arct. Sep.* °*Sulph.* °*Sulph. ac.*
Bones, periosteum, Amm. m. Phosph. Rhod. Sulph. ac.

Laming Pain.

Bones, periosteum, *Aur.* Bell. Chin. *Cocc. Crotal.* Cycl. *Lach.* Led. *Mez.* Natr. m. N. vom. Petr. Puls. Rhus. Sabin. Sil. Staph. Veratr. Zinc.

Lead-coloured.

Paleness, Plumb. Sec.

Leprous.

Spots, °*Natr.*
Swelling, °Lach.
Blotches, °*Natr.* Phosph. *Sil.*

Lower limbs, Lach. ? °*Natr.*

Lice, Pityriasis.

In general, Ars. Lach. Magn. art. °*Merc.* °*Oleand.* Sabad. ? Staph. ? °*Sulph.*
Itching, as of, Arg. Canth. Magn. m. Plat. Zinc.

Head, itching as of lice, Bov. Caps. Laur. Merc. *Mez. Oleand.* Rhod. Ruta. Sabad. Staph.

Lips and Mouth, Region of.

Aphthæ, Ipec.
Black skin, **Acon.* **Ars.* Bry. *Chin. Merc. Phos. ac. °Rhus. °Squill. Tart. ac. °Veratr.
Blackish, which is, Spig.
Bleeding, Ars. °Bry. Carb. an. Gins.**Ign.* Kal. Plat. Phos. ac.
Bleeds, that which, °Bry. **Merc.* Nicc. Thuj.
Blisters, vesicles, *Alum.* Amm. Amm. m. °*Ars.* Aur. Bell. Bry. Canth. Carb. an. Carb. veg. Caust. Cic. Clem. Con. Graph. Hell. Hep. Kal. Laur. Magn. c. Magn. m. Mang. Merc. Mez. Mur. ac. Natr. °*Natr. m.* Natr. s. Nitr. Par. Phosph. Plat. Ratanh. Rhod. Rhus. Sassap. Seneg. Senn. Sep. *Sil.* Staph. Sulph. Val. Veratr. Zinc.
—, corners of mouth, Caust. Laur. Mez. Seneg.
Blisters, bloody, °*Natr. m.*
Blotches, Ars. Baryt. Bell. Bry. Caust. Con. Hep. Magn. art. Magn. m. Nicc. Sep. Sil. Stront. Sulph.
Blueness, Agar. Alum. Ang. **Ars.* Berb. Calc. Caust. Cin. Con. Cupr. °*Dig.* **Lyc.* Op. Phosph. Stram. Veratr. Vip.
Blue, that which is, Berb. Merc.
Boils, Natr. Petr.
Brown colour, Oleand. Squill. Tart. ac.
Brown streaks, *Ars.
Brown colour of eruptions, Berb. Phos. ac.
Burning, Agar. *Amm.* Amm. m. Anis. *Arn.* Asa. Baryt. Berb. Borax. °Bry. Caps. Carb. an. Dros. Gran. Graph. Hep. Kal. Kreas. Magn. c. Magn. s. **Merc.* *Mez.* *Mur. ac.* Natr. Natr.

m. Natr. s. °N. vom. Oleand. *Phosph. Phos. ac.* Puls. Rhod. *Sabad.* Selen. Sep. °Spig. *Staph.* Sulph. Tab. Tarax. Tart. ac. Thuj. Veratr. Zinc.

Burning, corners of mouth, Arn. Coloc. Dros. Mez. Natr. Zinc.

—, of eruptions, &c., Amm. Aur. Bell. Bov. Bry. Caust. Chin. Graph. Magn. m. Mur. ac. Nicc. Phell. Plat. Ratanh. Seneg. Senn. *Staph.* Sulph.

Burnt, sensation as if, Ars. Plat. Rhus v. Sabad.

Cancer, **Ars.* °Bell.? °Clem.? °Con. °*Sil.* °*Sulph.*

Chapped, Alum. Amm. Amm. m. *Arn.* °*Ars.* Baryt. Bell. Berb. Borax. **Bry.* *Calc.* Canth. Caps. Carb. an. **Carb. veg.* Cham. *Chin. Colch. Corall. Croc. Dros. Electr. Gins. Graph. Grat. Hep. **Ign.* Kal. Kal. hdr. Kreas. Magn. m. Men. Mez. **Natr. m.* °Nitr. ac. Ol. an. Par. Patr. °*Phosph.* Phos. ac. Puls. Sabad. Selen. °Squill. Staph. Sulph. Tab. Tarax. Tart. °Veratr. Zinc.

Cutting, which is, Graph. Lyc.

Eruption, **Ars.* Bov. **Calc.* Caps. Carb. veg. Cann. Chin. Chinin. Dig. Electr. Graph. °Hell. Hep. Ipec. Lach. Lyc. Mez. Mur. ac. *Natr.* Natr. m. Nicc. Nitr. ac. Petr. Phosph. *Phos. ac.* *Sep.* *Sil.* Spong. Squill. Sulph. Tab.

—, corners of mouth, Ant. **Bell.* **Calc.* Cann. Canth. Carb. veg. **Graph.* Hep. **Ign.* Magn. arct. **Merc.* Natr. °Nitr. ac. Petr. Rhod. Rhus. Sep. Tarax. °*Veratr.*

Eruptions, fine, Lyc.

Eversion, Merc. corr.

Glands, ulcers of, Ign.

—, induration of, Con. Sulph. Zinc.

Gnaws, that which, Bell. *Mang.* Nitr. ac. Plat.
Granular, *Ars.
Greasy condition, Amm. m.
Greenish humour, secreting a, Staph.
Hepatic spots, °Sulph.
Herpes, Anac. Ars. Caust. Magn. c. Natr. Par. Phosph. °Rhus. Sassap. Sep.
—, corners of mouth, Carb. veg. Phosph. Sep.
Humour, secreting a, Kal. Squill. Zinc.
Induration, °Bell. Cycl. °Sil.
Inflammation, Canth.
—, of eruptions, Amm. m. Berb. Nitr.
Itching, Alum. Amm. Arn. Berb. Bry. Calc. Caust. Chel. Con. Ferr. magn. Graph. Hell. Kal. Laur. Magn. c. Mang. Natr. Nitr. ac. Ol. an. Phosph. Sabad. Sulph. Thuj. Zinc.
—, of eruptions, Baryt. *Bell.* Bry. Carb. veg. Chin. Hep. *Kal.* Magn. m. Mang. *Nitr. ac.* Seneg. *Sil.* Squill. Staph.
Pad-shaped, which is, Mur. ac.
Pain as if ulcerated, Chin. Ign. Magn. arct.
Painful, which is, Kal. Natr. m. Phosph.
Paleness, Caust. **Ferr.* Lyc. Kal. Val.
Peeling off of the skin, Alum. Amm. m. Bell. Canth. Caps. Cham. °*Con. Kal.* Kreas. Mez. Mosch. Natr. m. Natr. s. *N. vom.* Plat. Plumb. Puls. Sen. Sulph. ac. Tart.
Pimples, Acon. Amm. m. Ant. Arn. Ars. Baryt. Bell. Bov. *Bry. **Calc.* Cann. Canth. Caps. Caust. Chin. Chinin. Coloc. Con. Dulc. Electr. °Hell. Hyos. Ign. Ipec. Kal. Kreas. Led. Magn. art. Magn. arct. Magn. m. Mang. Mur. ac. Natr. Nicc. N. vom. Par. °*Rhus.*

Samb. Spig. Spong. Squill. Sulph. Tarax. Teucr. Veratr. °Zinc.

Pimples, corners of mouth, Ant. *Baryt.* *Bell.* Calc. Cann. Canth. Carb. veg. Caust. Coloc. Graph. Hep. Ign. Magn. arct. Mang. Merc. Natr. Phosph. Petr. Rhus. Sep. Tarax, Veratr.

Pock-shaped, Lyc.

Pustules, Amm. Baryt. Berb. Carb. veg. Lach. Magn. art. Magn. arct. Mur. ac. N. vom. Par. Samb. Sep. Tarax. Thuj. Zinc.

Raised, which is, °Bry. Sulph.

Red eruptions, Arn. Berb. Caust. Hep. Magn. c. Thuj. Zinc.

With red areola, Bell. Samb.

Rhagades, Agar. Aloë. Amm. Arn. °Ars. Baryt. **Bry.* Cann. **Carb. veg.* Cham. **Chin.* Croc. **Ign.* Kal. Magn. m. Men. **Merc.* Mez. Mur. ac. Natr. **Natr. m.* Nicc. °*Nitr. ac.* N. vom. Phos. ac. *Plat.* Puls. Sabad. °Squill. Sulph. Zinc.

—, corners of mouth, Amb. Ant. Calc. Graph. *Sil.*

Roughness, Amb. Anac. Calc. Magn. m. **Merc.* Mur. ac. Natr. m. N. vom. Phos. ac. Plat. Sulph.

Scrophulous, which is, °Ars. °Aur. °Aur. m. °Bell. °Bov. °Calc. °Sil. °Sulph.

Scurfs, **Ars.* Baryt. **Bell.* Berb. °Bry. Calc. °Cann. Cham. Cic. *Ign. Kal. Mur. ac. N. vom. Petr. Phos. ac. Rhus. Sep. *Sil.* Squill. Staph. Sulph.

Smarting, Bell. Bry. Kal. Merc. Plat. Rhod. Rhus.

Smarting as if excoriated, Bry. Con. Natr. m. *Sil.*

Soreness, Canth. Caust. Cham. Cupr. Graph. *Ign. Kal. Lyc.* Magn. c. Merc. Mez. Natr. m. °*Phosph.* Sabad. °*Sep.* Zinc.

—, corners of mouth, Ant. Merc. °Phosph. Zinc.

Sore pain, Amm. Ant. Caust. Chin. Euphorb. Graph. Ign. Ipec. Kal. Kreas. Magn. art. Magn. arct. Merc. Phosph. Phos. ac. Plat. Puls. Rhus. Sabad. Sep. Sulph. ac. Teucr.

—, corners of mouth, Bell. Calc. Caust. Graph. Ipec. Magn. arct. Mang. Merc. Natr. m. Sulph. ac.

Splinter, sensation as of, Bov. Ign. Nitr. ac. Par. Phosph.

Spongy, which is, Sil.

Spots, Ars. Berb. Caust. Hep. *Merc. Mez. °*Natr.* °*Sulph.*

Stinging, Agar. Amm. m. Ant. Asa. Bell. Bov. Bry. Caust. Clem. Graph. Grat. Ign. Kal. Magn. arct. Merc. Natr. Natr. m. Nitr. ac. N. vom. Par. Phosph. Phos. ac. Sabad. Sassap. Spong. Stann. Staph. Sulph. Thuj.

Stings, which, Bell. Caust. Magn. arct. Mang. Merc. Petr. Phosph. Sil. Squill.

Streaks, Ars. Stram. Tart. ac.

Suppuration, Bry. **Merc.* Phos. ac. Staph.

Swelling, Alum. Arg. Arn. **Ars.* Asa. °*Aur.* °Aur. m. Baryt. **Bell.* °Bov. **Bry.* **Calc.* Canth. Caps. Carb. an. Carb. veg. Chin. Dig. Graph. Grat. °Hell. Hep. Kal. Kal. chl. **Lach.* Lyc. Magn. art. Mang. Merc. Merc. corr. Mez. Mosch. Mur. ac. *Natr. **Natr. m.* Nitr. ac. N. mosch. Oleand. Oph. Op. Par. Petr. Phell. Phosph. Puls. *Rhus.* Sep. Sil. °Staph. Stram. **Sulph.* Vip. Vip. torv. Zinc.

Swelling, corners of mouth, Asa. Oleand.
—, sensation of, Oleand. Rhus.
—, shining, Staph.
Tensive, which is, Arn. Bov. Magn. c. Magn. m. Mang. Nitr. ac.
Titillating, [illegible]t. Arn. Calc. Caust. Lact. Natr. m. Paeon. Phos. ac. Sabad. Stront.
—, of eruptions, Bell. Caust.
Ulceration, Amm. m. Arn. **Ars.* °Aur. °Aur. m. Bell. Bry. Caps. Carb. an.* Caust. Cham. Chin. Cic. Con. Dulc. Graph. Ign. Kal. Lyc. Magn. art. Magn. arct. Mang. Merc. Mez. Natr. Natr. m. Nitr. ac. N. vom. Phosph. Phos. ac. Puls. Sep. **Sil.* Staph. Sulph. Zinc.
—, corners of mouth, °Amm. m. Arn. *Bell. **Calc.* **Graph.* Hell. Hep. °*Ign.* Mang. **Merc.* °Nitr. ac. N. vom. Phosph. Sil. Zinc.
Ulcers, fetid, Merc.
Vesicles, watery, Bell. Bov. Clem. Merc. Plat. Rhus. Zinc.
Whitish, which is, Hell. Lyc. Magn. c. Magn. m. Mang. Merc. Mez. Natr. Phosph. Zinc.
Yellow, which is, Merc. Mur. ac. °Natr. Phos. ac. Stram. Zinc.

Livid, which is.

Spots, Crotal.
Swelling, Gran.
Scurfs, Chinin.

Face, Gran.
Hands, swelling, Gran.

Lower Extremities.

Arthritic, Ars. Asa.? °*Bry.* °*Calc.* Canth. Cham. Chinin. Crotal. Croton. *Graph.* Hep.? Lach. **N. vom.* Phosph. °*Rhus.* °*Sep.* °*Spong.* Staph.?
Beating, swelling, °Carb. veg.
Black colour, lower limbs, Vip. torv.
Black, swelling, N. vom.
—, ulcer, °*Lach.*
Bleeding ulcers, °Carb. veg. Phos. ac.
—, scurfs, Mez.
Blotches, as if from stings of insects, Ant.
Blueness, lower limbs, Bism. Con.
—, thighs, Bism.
—, legs, Con.
Blue spots, Amm. Ant. Con. °*Lach.* Phosph. *Sulph.*
—, swelling, °*Lach.* °*Sil.*
Boils, lower limbs, Nitr. ac.
—, hips and nates, Alum. Amm. Baryt. Graph. *Hep.* Lyc. Nitr. ac. **Phos. ac.* °*Ratanh.* Sabin.
—, thighs, Clem. *Cocc. Hyos. Ign. Lyc.* Magn. c. *Nitr. ac.* N. vom. Petr. Phosph. Sep. **Sil.*
—, knee, Natr. m. N. vom.
—, legs and calves, °*Magn. c.* Nitr. ac. **Sil.*
Bones, affections of, lower limbs, Amm. Ang. Asa. **Baryt. Berb.* **Caust. Chin.* Crotal. Dros. Kal. Lach. Magn. m. Mez. Nitr. Nitr. ac. Poth. Sulph.
—, hips, *Berb.* Calc. Caust. Cic. Kal. *Kreas.* Magn. c. Natr. s. *Oleand. Ruta.*
—, thigh, Aur. Baryt. Berb. Borax. *Canth.* Carb.

Rhod. Rhus. Ruta. Sabin. Samb. Sassap. Spig. Staph. Sulph. Sulph. ac. *Zinc.*

Burning, knee, Amm. Anoc. Asa. Baryt. Berb. Bry. Cann. Carb. veg. Grat. Kal. °*Lyc.* Mur. ac. Natr. Oleand. Petr. Phell. Phos. ac. Plat. Plumb. *Rhus.* Sabad. Stann. Staph. *Sulph.* Sulph. ac. Tab. *Tarax.* Tart. *Thuj.*

—, legs, calves, shins, *Agar.* Alum. *Anac.* Ang. Arg. **Ars.* Asa. Bell. Berb. Borax. Calc. Calend. Cann. Caust. *Chel.* Chin. *Crotal.* Cycl. Dig. Graph. Kal. °*Lyc.* Magn. arct. Magn. aust. Magn. c. Mang. Men. Mez. *Natr. Natr. s.* N. vom. Phell. Phos. ac. Puls. Ran. Rhus. Sabad. Sassap. Sep. Stront. *Sulph.* Sulph. ac. *Tarax.* Thuj. Veratr. Zinc.

—, tendo Achilles, Berb. Chel. Chin.

Burning, eruption, Aur. Mang. N. vom.

—, vesicles, Sabad.

—, pimples. Arg. Phos. ac. Puls. Staph. Thuj.

—, spots, Amm. *Chel.* Magn. c. *Rhus.* Sulph. ac.

—, crash, N. vom.

—, swelling, *Crotal.*

—, ulcers, **Ars.* Lyc.

—, streaks, *Rhus.*

—, callosities, °*Lach, Phosph.*

Caries, °*Lach.* °*Sil.*

Cicatrized skin, Sabin.

Cold spots, Petr.

—, swelling, **Rhod.*

Confluent, eruptions, Phos. ac.

Contraction of tendons, s. Muscles.

Contraction of muscles, Amm. m.° *Caust.* ° *Graph.* °*Natr. m.* °*Ruta.*

Contracted, sensation as if, lower limbs, *Berb.* Carb. an. Magn. m. Merc.
—, hip, °*Lach.* Prun.
—, thigh, Amm. *Kreas. Lach.* N. vom. *Sabin. Spong.*
—, knee, *Amm. m. Graph.* **Lach. Lyc.* Magn. arct. Magn. c. °*Natr. m.* Nitr. ac. N. vom. Ol. an. Phosph. Rhus. °*Ruta.* Samb. *Sulph. Veratr.*
—, calves, Caust. *Kal. Magn. art.* Natr. Natr. m. Rhus. *Sil.*
Creeping. lower limbs, Magn. art. *Sep.*
—, thigh, Berb. Natr.
—, knee, Ratanh. Merc.
—, legs, *Ol. an. Sep.* Tab. Zinc.
Dropsical swelling of knee, °Jod.? °*Sulph.*
—, leg, *Jod. Merc.*
Ecchymosed, °Con.
Elephantiasis, Lach.?
Eruption, lower limbs, Hyos, Staph.
—, hip and nates, Borax. Natr. *Sulph.*
—, thigh, Alum. Calc. Cann. Caust. Merc.
—, knee, Anac. Ars. Bry. Carb. veg. Kal. *Led.* Merc. N. vom. Tereb.
—, legs, Agar. *Petr. Rhus.*
Erysipelas, leg, Borax. *Calc. Hep. Puls.* °*Sulph.*
—, tendo Achilles, *Zinc.*
Erysipelatous, swelling, *Calc. Puls. Zinc.*
Fine eruption, Alum.
Fistulous ulcers, °*Ruta.*
Flat ulcer, Staph.
—, pimple, Ant.
Flesh as if loose, lower limbs, Sulph.
—, nates and hips, Zinc.

Flesh as if loose, thighs, Electr. Led. Mosch. Natr.
—, legs, Canth. Stann. Sulph.
Formication, Alum. *Ol. an.* *Rhod.* Tab. Zinc.
Freckles, Phosph.
Fungus, knee, °*Ant.* °*Jod.* °*Sulph.*
Fungus articularis, knee, °*Ant.* °*Jod.* °*Sulph.*
Glandular swelling, thigh, Phos. ac.
Gnawing, lower limbs, Alum. Bell. °*Lyc.* **Sulph.*
—, nates and hips, Amm. m. Berb. Euphorb. Evon. Kal. hdr. Led. Staph. Sulph.
—, thighs, Agar. Anac. Ars. Berb. Canth. Chel. Dig. Euphorb. Kal. hdr. Led. N. vom. Par. Phosph. Ran. sc. Spig. Stront. Tarax.
—, knees, Berb. Ran. sc. Zinc.
—, legs, Aur. Berb. Euphorb. Natr. Natr. m. Phos. ac. Tarax.
—, tibia, Bism. Coff. Lam. Laur.
Gangrene, lower limbs, *Sec.*
—, shins, *Sec.*
Gangrenous vesicle, Hyos.
—, spots, *Cycl.* *Hyos.*
—, ulcers, °*Lach.*
Gray, scurfy ulcer, Ars.
Hardness, knee, Led.
—, legs, Graph.
—, tibia, Rhus.
—, calves, Ars.
Hard, such as, eruption, Aur.
—, swelling, Aur. Bov. *Chin.* Graph. °*Led.* Magn. c. Mez. Rhus.
Herpes, lower limbs, °*Clem.* Kal. Lach. Merc. *Staph.*
—, hips and nates, Borax. Caust. Nicc.

Herpes, thigh, °*Graph.* **Merc.* Mur. ac. *Nitr. ac.*
—, knee, °*Ars.* °*Carb. veg.* °*Dulc.* °*Graph.* Kreas. Merc. **Natr. m.* °*Petr.* Phosph.
—, leg, Ars. Calc. °*Graph. Kal.* °*Lach.* Lyc.
Herpetic spots, Graph. Mur. ac. Sassap.
Humid, eruption, Merc. Puls. Selen.
—, spots, °*Sulph.*
Humour, between the thighs, *Hep.* °*Sulph.*
—, calves, Tarax.
Induration of muscles, Ars. Graph. Vip. torv.
Inflammation, lower limbs, Borax. Natr. Sabad.
—, hip, °Coloc. °Sulph.
—, knee, Calc. °*Cocc.* °*Jod.* **N. vom.* Phosph. °*Puls.* °*Sil.* °*Sulph.*
—, leg, Borax. Natr. Sabad.
—, tendo Achilles, Zinc.
Inflamed pimple, Petr.
—, swelling, Borax. Calc. **Chin.* Crotal. °*Cocc.* °*Jod.* °*Led. Natr.* **Puls.* Sabad. °*Sil.* °*Sulph. Zinc.*
—, ulcers, Ars. Graph. N. vom.
Itch, nates, **Phos. ac.*
—, thigh, repelled, Galv.
Itch-like pustules, Hyos.
Itching, lower limbs, Caust. Daph. **Lach.* **Lyc.* Merc. Natr. Natr. m. Nitr. Nitr. ac. Ol. an. Phosph. Sec. Sil. Staph. Teucr. Thuj.
—, nates and hips, Amm. Amm. m. Ant. Ars. Baryt. Calc. *Caust.* Chel. Coloc. Con. Evon. Kal. Kal. hdr. Lach. Laur. Led. Lyc. Magn. aust. Magn. c. Magn. m. Mur. ac. Natr. Nitr. Nicc. Ol. an. Oleand. Petr. Phosph. Phos. ac.

Prun. Sep. Sil. Stann. Staph. Stront. Sulph. Tarax. *Therid.* Teucr. Zinc.

Itching, thigh, Agar. Alum. Anac. Ang. Ant. Arn. Ars. Baryt. Berb. Bry. *Calc.* Canth. Caust. Chel. Cic. Cocc. Con. Croton. Dig. Dulc. Electr. Euphorb. Euphr. *Graph.* Grat. Guaj. Kal. *Lach.* Laur. Led. Magn. arct. Magn. aust. Magn. m. Mang. *Merc.* Mosch. Mur. ac. Natr. Natr. m. *Nitr. ac.* N. vom. *Oleand.* Phell. *Phosph. Prun.* Ran. sc. Ratanh. *Rhod.* Sassap. Sil. *Spig.* Spong. *Stann.* Staph. Stront. *Sulph.* Tarax. *Zinc.*

—, knee, Amb. Ant. Asa. Aur. Berb. Bry. *Caust.* Coloc. Grat. Hep. Ign. Kal. Lach. **Lyc. Mang.* Men. Mur. ac. Natr. Nitr. Nitr. ac. N. vom. Ol. an. Phosph. Ran. Ratanh. *Rhus.* Samb. Sassap. *Spong.* Stann. *Sulph.*

—, leg, Agar. Alum. Amb. Amm. m. Ant. Asa. Aur. Berb. Bism. *Calc. Caust. Cocc. Coloc.* Croton. Cycl. Dulc. Euphorb. Euphr. Graph. Grat. °*Ipec. Kal. Lach. Laur.* Lyc. Magn. aust. Magn. m. Mang. Mez. Mosch. Mur. ac. Natr. Natr. m. Nitr. Ol. an. Op. *Phosph.* Phos. ac. Plumb. Rhus. *Sabin.* Sassap. Seneg. Sep. *Sil.* Spig. *Staph.* Stront. Sulph. ac. Tarax. Tart. Tax. Therid. Thuj. Veratr.

—, tibia, Ant. Asa. Bism. *Calc. Coloc.* Croton. *Grat. Kal. Lach.* Magn. m. Mang. Mosch. Nitr. *Phosph.* Plumb. *Sep.* Spig. *Stront.* Sulph. ac.

—, calves, Alum. *Caust. Cocc. Coloc. Cycl.* Euphr. °*Ipec. Laur.* Lyc. Magn. aust. Mang. *Mez.* Mur. ac. Ol. an. *Phosph. Rhus. Sabin.* Sassap. Sil. Staph. *Tarax.* Tax. Therid. Thuj. Veratr.

Itching, tendo Achilles, Berb. Selen.
Itching eruption, Anac. Caust. *Kal.* Led. Mang. *Merc.* *Natr.* Nitr. N. vom. Petr. Ratanh.
—, blotches, Electr. Lach.
—, blisters, Kal.
—, pimples, *Hep.* *Petr.* *Phos. ac.* Selen. *Sep.* Stann. Staph.
—, herpes, Merc. Nicc. Plumb.
—, spots, Electr. Graph. Mur. ac. Sassap.
—, rash, Daph. Natr. m. N. vom. Sil.
—, ulcers, Lyc. *Merc.* °*Phos. ac.* °*Sil.*
—, urticaria, Caust.
Jerking, ulcers, Natr.
Leprous, Lach.? °*Natr.*
Marbled skin, *Caust.*
Miliary, pimples, Agar.
Numbness, lower limbs, *Berb.* * *Calc.* Carb. veg. Graph. Kal. Lyc. °*N. vom.* Sep. Sulph. Sulph. ac.
—, hips, Calc. °*Lach.* Staph.
—, thighs, Acon. Agar. Carb. veg. °*Euphr.* Ferr. °*Graph.* Hep. Men. Op. Plat.
—, knee, Calc. Graph. Plat.
—, legs, Acon. Alum. Anac. Berb. Borax. Bry. Dulc. Graph. Plat.
Œdematous swelling of lower limbs, °*Jod.* °*Rhod.*
Pain as if bruised, Laur.
—, hips and nates, Cic. Cin. Euphorb. *Kal.* Laur. *Ruta.*
—, thigh, *Arn.* Kreas. Lach. Lyc. Natr. s. *N. mosch.* *Plat.* Sulph.
—, knee, Arn. Bov. Magn. aust. Mez. Petr. *Plat.* Rhod. Sulph. ac.

Pain, legs, calves, shins, Ant. Arn. Caust. Cupr. Euphorb. Natr. m. Prun. Ruta. Sep.

Pain as if burnt, tibia, Lach.

Pain as if contused, Nitr. Rhod.

—, hips, Euphorb. Gins.

—, knee, Mez. Plat.

—, thigh, Acon. Murex.

Pain as if luxated, lower limbs, Amm. Berb.

—, hips and nates, Mez. Stann.

—, thigh, Lyc.

—, knee, Agar. Amm. Graph. Ipec. Lach. N Mosch. Phosph. *Staph.* Sulph.

—, calf, *Graph.*

Pain as if sprained, lower limbs, Dros. °*Rhus.* Thuj.

—, hip and hip-joints, Amm. m. Anac. Ang. *Arn.* Aspar. Baryt. Bell. Calc. **Caust.* Cham. Chin. Con. Dros. Dulc. Euphorb. *Hep.* °Ipec. *Laur.* Lyc. **Natr. m.* Nitr. ac. Petr. Phosph. Puls. Rhod. Rhus v. Stann. Sulph.

—, thigh, Amm. Caps. Euphorb. Led. Mosch. Rhod. Stann. Staph.

—, knee, Amb. Ars. Calc. Chin. Con. Gent. *Kal.* Kreas. *Lach.* Lyc. Men. Natr. *Natr. m.* Nitr. Nitr. ac. Phosph. Plat. Prun. Rhod. Sulph.

Pain as if sore, nates, Lyc. Magn. aust.

—, hip, Aspar. Berb. Cast. *Cic.* Natr. s. Puls. Sabin.

—, thigh, Arn. Aspar. Bell. Berb. Chel. Coff. Crotal. Kal. Led. Lyc. Mang. Mez. Phosph. Staph. Sulph. Thuj. Zinc.

—, knee, Anac. Asa. Aspar. Berb. *Carb. an.* Caust. Electr. *Led.* Lyc. Val. Veratr.

Pain as if sore, leg, Amb. Aspar. Berb. Chin. Dig. Mang. Plat.
—, tibia, Coff. Mang. Sep.
—, calf. Croc. Crotal.
Pain as if ulcerated, lower limbs, Sep.
Nates and hips, Berb. Calc. *Kal. Phosph.* Prun. Puls. Sulph. Verb.
—, thighs, Anac. Sep.
—, knee, Caust. Ol. an. Rhod.
—, legs, *Jod.* Puls.
—, eruption, Mang.
Painful, varix, Coloc.
—, tumors, Merc. N. vom.
—, pimples, Phosph.
—, spots, Amb. Cann. Caust. ° *Con.* Graph. Lach. *Mosch.* Petr.
—, swelling, *Lach. Oph.* Rhod. Sil.
—, ulcers, Staph.
Painless, swelling, Puls. Sep.
Pale, swelling, Op.
Peeling off, *Merc.*
—, legs, *Agar.*
Petechiæ, Phosph.
Phagedenic blisters, nates, Borax.
Phagedenic ulcers, Merc.
Rash, lower limbs, Daph. Galv. Ol. an. **Sulph.*
—, thigh, Bry. Merc. Mez. *N. vom.*
—, knee, N. vom. Zinc.
—, legs, Calc. Hyos. *Natr. m.* Sil.
Pimples, lower limbs, Bar. m. Natr. m. *Petr. Staph.*
—, hips and nates, Ant. Baryt. Berb. Bry. Canth. Graph. Magn. c. Merc. N. vom. *Petr.* Selen. *Thuj.*

Pimples, thighs, Agar. Ant. Berb. Bov. Bry. Calc. Chel. Cocc. *Kal.* Kal. chl. *Lach. Magn. c. Mang. Mez. Natr. m. Petr. Phosph. Prun. Rhod.* Sassap. *Selen. Stann.* Staph. *Sulph. Zinc.*

—, knee, Ant. Bry. Hep. Nicc. Phos. ac. Puls. Sassap. Sep. Sulph. Zinc.

—, legs, calves, shins, Agar. Arg. Bov. Bry. Natr. Puls. Sabin. Sassap. *Sep. Staph.* Zinc.

Pocks, knee, Hyos.

With pressure, eruptions, Kal.

Prickling, lower limbs, °*Lach.* Sil.

—, hip, Caust.

—, thigh, Nitr. ac. Zinc.

—, knee, Cann. Croton. Plat. Spong. Sulph. ac. Tart.

—, legs and calves, Croton. Phell.

—, tendo Achilles, Sulph. ac.

Pustules, lower limbs, °*Dulc.* Mez. Staph. Stram. *Thuj.*

—, nates and hips, Ant. Hydroc. Hyos.

—, knees, Bry. Hyos.

Raised, tibia, *Aur. Merc.*

—, knee, Electr.

Redness, nates, Hyos.

—, thighs, Electr.

—, knee, Bry. Electr. Kreas.

—, legs, *N. vom. Puls. Sabin.* Tarax.

Red, eruptions, Electr. Staph.

—, pimples, Ant. Chel. Rhod. Staph.

—, spots, Berb. **Calc. Cycl.* °*Con.* Electr. *Graph. Lyc. Petr.* Rhod. Rhus. Sassap. Sil. °*Sulph. Sulph. ac.*

—, herpes, Kreas.

Red, rash, Calc. Hyos.
—, swelling, Aur. Bov. °*Bry. Calc. Chin.* Lyc. *Puls. Sabad.* Zinc.
—, ulcer, N. vom.
—, tumor, *Hep.*
—, callosities, Lach. Phosph.
—, streaks, Calc. Rhus.
Red areola, blotch, Ant.
—, vesicle, Cann. Kal.
—, pustules, Lach.
Rheumatic, lower limbs, Amb. °Bry. Chin. Graph. Jod. Meph. Ol. jec. Phos. ac. Poth. Zinc.
—, hips and nates, Cycl. °*Lach.* °*Led.* Lyc. Natr. m. Tart.
—, thighs, Agar. Carb. veg. Daph. Gin. Jod. Lach. Sabin. Tart. Veratr. *Zinc.*
—, knee, Crotal. Daph. °*Lach.* Mez. Zinc.
—, legs, calves, shins, Anac. Carb. veg. Gins. Lyc. Mez. Tart. Zinc.
Rough spots, Mur. ac.
Scaly, getting, knee, Kreas.
Scaly, herpes, °*Clem.* Kreas.
Scarlet-redness, Galv.
Scurf, leg, Ars. Calc. *Sabin.* Staph. Zinc.
Scurfy, eruption, Mang.
—, herpes, *Clem.*
—, spots, Zinc.
—, ulcers, Ars. Graph.
Shining, swelling, °*Bry. Merc.* °*Sulph.*
Smarting, legs, Lyc.
—, hips, Amm. m.
—, thigh, Alum. Amm. m. Berb. Chel. Grat. N. vom. Phell.

Smarting, knee, Berb. Bry. °*Lyc.* Nitr. Ol. an. Phell. Ran. sc. *Thuj.*
—, legs, calves and shins, Amm. m. Berb. Grat. Tart. Veratr.
Smarting, pimples, Agar.
Softening of femur, °*Sil.*
Sore, spots, Electr. Rhod.
Soreness, between legs, Ars. Aur. **Caust.* !Coff. **Graph.* *Hep.* Jod. *Lyc.* Ol. an. Phosph. *Rhod.* *Sulph.*
—, hip, Bov. Mang. *Petr.* Sep.
—, nates, Kal. Natr. m. *Nitr. ac.* Selen.
Spots, lower limbs, Ant. Bry. *Hyos.* °*Natr.* Nitr. °*Sulph.*
—, hips, Rhus.
—, thighs, Amm. Ant. Berb. Cann. Cycl. Electr. *Graph.* Mur. ac. Rhod.
—, legs, **Calc.* *Chel.* Con. *Lyc.* N. vom. *Phosph.* *Stann.* *Zinc.*
—, calves, °Con. Graph. *Sassap.*
—, tibia, Amb. Ant. *Caust.* Electr. *Lach.* Magn. c. Nitr. *Phosph.* *Sil.* *Sulph. ac.*
—, tendo Achilles, Chel.
Spots, as if from stings of insects, Lyc.
Stigmata, s. spots.
Streaks, Calc. *Rhus.*
Stinging, varices, Graph.
—, eruption, Ant. N. vom. Petr. Sabin.
—, spots, Chel.
—, swelling, Graph. **Led.* °*Puls.*
—, ulcers, °Ars. Natr.
Swelling, lower limbs, *Ars.* *Con.* *Jod.* *Lyc.*? *Merc.* *Oph.* Sep. °*Sulph.* *Vip. torv.*
—, nates, Croton. Vip. red.

Swelling, thighs, Bov. *Chin.* Crotal. Ol. jec.
—, knee, Berb. °*Bry.* **Calc.* **Chin.* °*Cocc.* Ferr. Hep. °*Jod.* Lach. **Led.* **Lyc.* Magn. c. Mur. ac. **N. vom.* Phosph. **Puls.* Rhod. Sassap. Sep. °*Sil.* °*Sulph.*
—, legs, Amb. Ars. *Aur.* Borax. **Bry.* Calc. *Colch. Crotal.* Dig. *Dulc.* Graph. °*Kal.* **Lach.* Led. *Lyc. Merc.* Natr. °*N. vom. Oph.* °*Puls.* Rhod. **Sep. Sil.* Stront. *Vip. torv.*
Swelling, tibia, Graph. Lach. Rhus. Stann. Sulph. ac.
—, calves, Carb. veg. *Chin.* Hyos. Mez. Sulph.
—, tendo Achilles, Berb. Zinc.
Swollen, sensation as if, lower limbs, Prun.
—, knee, Alum. Ammoniac. Berb. Canth. Carb. veg. Lach. *Nitr. ac.*
—, legs, Lam. Lyc.
Suppurating, tumors, Sassap.
—, swelling, Chin. Jod.
—, ulcer, °*Sabin.*
Suppuration, hip-joint, Hep. ? Spong. ? Staph. ?
—, calves, Chin.
Tearing, varices, Sulph. ac.
—, ulcers, Lyc.
—, swelling, *Puls.* °*Rhod.*
Tendo Achilles, Kreas.
Tight, eruption, Nitr. ac.
—, swelling, °Carb. veg. **Led.* Sep.
Tickling, lower limbs, Carb. veg. Coloc. Corall. Ign. Laur. Petr. Sep. Spong.
Titillation, lower limbs, Ars. Baryt. Bov. Caps. Caust. Cic. Euphorb. Guaj. Hep. Kal. Magn. art. Magn. c. Nicc. Nitr. ac. Plat. Rhod. *Sec.* Sep, Staph.

Titillation, hips, Baryt. Evon. Kal.
—, thigh, Arg. Chin. Gins. Guaj. Hep. Plumb. Sep. Spig. Sulph. Sulph. ac. Tax.
—, knee, Carb. an. Electr. Gent. Kal. Merc. Rhus. Zinc. ox.
—, legs, calves, Alum. Ant. Baryt. Bell. Calc. Cast. Caust. Graph. *Ign.* Ipec. *Lach. N. vom. Ol. an.* Phos. ac. *Plat. Rhod.* Rhus. Sep. Spig. *Sulph. Sulph. ac. Veratr.* Zinc.
—, tendo Achilles, Sabin.
Transparent, swelling, *Merc.* Sulph.
Tumors, lower limbs, Ant. Spig.
—, nates, Ant. Sassap.
—, thighs, Crotal. Merc. Zinc.
—, knee, Ant.
—, legs, Carb. veg. Lach.
Ulcers, thighs, Crotal. Kal. Merc. °*Sil.*
—, tibia, *Graph.* Lach. *Sabin.* Vip. torv.
—, legs, Ars. Baryt. Bry. Calc. Canth. Carb. veg. Caust. Clem. Ipec. Lach. Lyc. Merc. Mur. ac. Natr. N. mosch. Phosph. Phos. ac. Puls. Ruta. Sabin. Sil. Staph. Sulph. Vip. torv.
—, calves, °Lach.
—, nates, Borax.
Ulcerated, swelling, Graph.
—, rhagades, *Merc.*
—, spots, *Sabin.*
Urticaria, hips, *Sulph.*
—, thighs, Caust. Zinc.
—, legs, *Aur.*
Varices, thighs, °*Calc. Zinc.*
—, legs, **Caust.* *Coloc.* Ferr. Graph. Puls. Sulph. °*Zinc.*
—, knee, aneurisms, °*Carb. veg.*

Vesicles, lower limbs, Ant. Hyos. Vip. torv.
—, hips and nates, Borax. Calc. Oleand. Phos. ac.
—, thighs, Cann. Caust. Sassap.
—, knee, Ant. Carb. veg. Caust. Phosph. Rhus. Sabad.
—, leg, calves, Bell. *Caust. Kal.* Mang.
Vesicles, watery, *Phos. ac.*
White, blotches, tumors, Ant.
—, vesicles, Cann. Sabad.
—, pimples, Chel. Staph. Thuj.
—, swelling, Arn. ? Ars. ? Bell. ? °*Calc.* °*Jod.* °*Lyc.* Merc. ? N. vom. ? Ol. jec. °*Puls.* °*Rhod.* Rhus. ? Sil. ? °*Sulph.*
Yellow eruption, Ant. Aur.
—, spots, °Con. Stann.
—, scurfs, Mez.

Lupia.

In general, Agar. Ant. °*Baryt.* °*Calc.* °*Graph.* °*Hep.* Kal. Magn. arct. °*Nitr. ac.* **Sabin.* Sil. Spong. °*Sulph.*
Burning, °Baryt.
Suppurating, °*Calc.* °*Sulph.*
Sarcomatous, °Baryt.
Stinging in them, Magn. arct.

Head, °Calc. °Lyc. ? (Compare : Abscesses.)
Ears, lobes, °Nitr. ac.
Dorsal region, °Baryt.
Arms, elbows, °*Hep.*

Lymphatic.

Swelling, *Berb. Carb. veg.* Oph.

Arms, swelling, *Berb.*

Lumpy.

Pustules, Anthrok. Cham.
Swelling, Calc. Dulc. Hep. °*Ign.* Jod. Lyc. Nitr. ac. Phosph. Rhus. Thuj.

Mammæ, glandular indurations, Bry. * *Carb. an.* Cham. Lyc. °Nitr. ac. °*Phosph.*

Maculæ Letales, of Old People.

In general, Ars. Baryt. °*Con.* Lach. °Oph. ? Vip. red.

Malignant, that which is.

Suppurations and discharges of pus, °Ars. °*Asa.* °*Calc.* °Cham. °*Hep.* °Lach. °Merc. °*Phosph.* °Rhus. °*Sil.* °Sulph. °Vip. torv.
Ulcers, Crotal. °Lach.

Mammæ and Nipples.

Abscesses, °*Phosph.* (Comp. Suppuration.)
Bleeding of the nipples, Sep. °Sulph.
Burning, *Laur.* Mez. °Sulph.

Burning, of the nipples, °Sulph.
Cancerous ulcers, °Bell. °Clem.? °Con. °*Hep.* °*Lach.* °Sil.? °Sulph.?
Distended, sensation, as if, Zinc.
Drawing, Kreas.
Dwindling, *Con. Jod.* °Nitr. ac.
Erysipelas, °*Cham.* **Phosph. Sulph.*
Fistulous ulcers, °Phosph. °Sil.
Glandular indurations, Bry. **Carb. an.* Cham. Lyc. °Nitr. ac. °*Phosph.*
Griping sensation, Borax.
Heat, Calc.
Herpes, °Caust. °Dulc.
Induration, °Bell. °Bry. **Cham. Clem.* °*Con.* °Merc. °Ol. jec.? °Sil. °Sulph.
—, nipples, °Bry.
Inflammation, °Arn. °*Bell.* °Bry. Calc. °Carb. an. °Carb. veg. Con. °*Sil.*
—, nipples, Calc. Sil.
Itching, °Alum. Caust. *Con.* Hep. Magn. arct. Petr. Puls. *Rhus.* Sassap. Sep. °*Sulph.*
—, nipples, Con. Hep. Magn. arct. Petr. Puls. Sassap. Sep. Sulph.
Pain, as if ecchymosed, Calc.
Painfulness, Amm. Berb. Borax. Calc. Con. **Graph. Merc.* Murex. N. vom. Rhab.
—, nipples, **Graph.* N. vom. Rhab.
Pressure, Berb. Sabin. Zinc.
—, nipples, Berb. Sabin.
Rhagades, nipples, °Caust.
Scaly covering on the nipples, Petr.
Scarlet-spots, Lach.
Scurfs, °Lyc.
—, phagędænic, °Lyc.

Soreness, Nitr. ac.
—, nipples, °Arn. °Calc. °Caust. **Cham.* °*Graph.* °Lyc. °Merc. °N. vom. °Sep. ? °Sil.
Sore, as if excoriated, °*Merc.* Tab. °*Sulph.* Zinc.
—, nipples, °*Sulph.* °Zinc.
Spots around the nipples, Kal.
Stinging, Alum. Baryt. Berb. Borax. Carb. an. Cocc. Con. Grat. Kal. Kreas. Laur. Lyc. Magn. aust. Mez. Murex. Natr. m. Ol. an. Phell. Phosph. Plumb. Prun. Rhab. Sabin. Sang. Sep. Zinc.
Suppuration, °Hep. °*Merc.* °Phosph. °*Sil.*
Swelling, °Bell. Calc. °Graph. **Merc.* Merc. corr. **Puls.* Sabin.
—, nipples, Merc.
Tearing, Baryt. Grat. Kal. Ol. an. Phell.
Titillation, Sabin.
Ulcers, °*Hep.* °*Phosph.* °*Sil.*
Vesicles around the nipples, °Graph.

Marbled.

Eruption, Phosph.
Spots, *Berb.* °*Carb. veg.* °*Caust.* Crotal. Lyc. *Natr. m.* Plat. **Thuj.*
Swelling, Chin. Gran. Lyc. Rhus v. Sep.

Face, Phosph.
Arms, *Berb.*
Hands, spots, Natr. m.
—, swelling, Gran.
Lower limbs, skin, *Caust.*
Feet, redness, *Caust.*

Mealy Herpes.

See: Herpes furfuraceous.

Measles, Morbilli.

In general, °*Acon.* °Ars. °Bell. °*Bry.* °*Coff.* °Dulc. °Jod. °N. vom. °*Phosph.* °*Puls.* °Rhus. Stram. ? °Sulph.
Previous to the eruption, °*Acon.* °*Bell.* °*Puls.*
During the eruption, °*Acon.* °Bell. °Coff. °Phosph. °*Puls.*
After-ailments, °*Ars.* °*Bry.* °Dulc. °Jod. °N. vom. °*Phosph.* °*Puls.* °*Rhus.*
Suppressed measles, °*Phosph.* °*Puls.* °Rhus.

Measle-shaped.

In general, **Acon.* **Ars.* **Bell.* **Bry.* *Carb. veg.* Cham. Chin. Coff. Dros. Electr. Hyos. Ign. Ipec. Magn. c. **Merc.* N. vom. **Phosph.* **Puls.* **Rhus.* Stram. **Sulph.*

Spots, Ars.
Rash, Merc. N. vom.

Mercurial, after abuse of Mercury.

Rhagades, °*Hep.* °*Sulph.*
Herpes, °Aur. °Mosch. ? °Nitr. ac.
Swelling, °Staph.
Ulcers, °Alum. °Amm. °Arn. °*Asa.* °*Aur.* °*Bell.*

°Calc. °Carb. an. °*Carb. veg.* °Cham. °Chin. °Clem. °Graph. °*Hep.* °*Lach.* °*Lyc.* °Natr. m. °*Nitr. ac.* °Phosph. °*Phos. ac.* °Sassap. °*Sep.* °*Sil.* °Staph. °*Sulph.* °*Thuj.*

Nose, °Asa. °Aur. °Con. °Lach.
Face, °Aur. °Nitr. ac.
Buccal cavity, °Arg. °*Aur.* °*Bell.* °*Lach.* °Lyc. °*Nitr. ac.* °*Staph.* °Sulph. °Thuj.
Sexual parts, °*Thuj.*
Bones, pain, °Asa. °Aur. Calc.? Carb. veg.? Caust.? °*Chin.* °*Guaj.* °*Hep.* °*Lach.* °*Lyc.* °*Mez.* °Nitr. ac. °Phosph. °*Phos. ac.* °Staph. °*Sulph.*
Glands, affections of, °*Aur.* °*Carb. veg.* °*Nitr. ac.* °Thuj.

Miliary.

Eruption, Amm. **Ars.* °*Carb. veg.* Graph. *Hep.* Natr. m. Phosph. Tab. Zinc.
Spots, Thuj.
Skin, Bov. **Calc.* *Sassap.*

Face, eruptions, Alum. Natr. m. Phosph. Tab.
Lips, **Ars.*
Chin, pimples, Ant.
Sexual parts, eruption, Thuj.
Hands, eruption, °*Carb. veg.* Graph. Hep.

Millet-shaped.

Eruption, **Agar.* Amm. Ars. Cocc. Kreas. *Led.* N. vom. Par. Val.

Pimples, Agar. Amm. Ant. Ars. Cocc. Grat. Kal. Kreas.
Tubercles, Natr. m.

Face, Amm. Kreas. Par. (Comp. RASH.)
Hands, eruption, *Agar.*
Lower limbs, pimples, Agar.

MOLES, LIKE.

Spots, °*Calc. Carb. veg. Graph.* Nitr. ac. *Petr. Phosph. ac. Sil.* °*Sulph. Sulph. ac.* **Thuj.*

MOUTH AND FAUCES, AND THEIR PARTS.

Abscess, Amm. Canth. °Caust. Natr. *Sulph.* (Comp. TUMORS, SUPPURATION and SWELLING.)
Tonsils, Bar. c. **Bell.* Berb. °Gran. ? °Ign. °*Lach.* **Merc.* Nicc. Sep. (Comp. °*Hep.* °*Sulph.*)
—, gums, Amm. Canth. °Caust. °Sulph.
—, tongue, Natr.
Aphthæ, Agar. **Borax.* °*Cham.* °Hell. Jod. **Merc.* N. mosch. ? °*N. vom.* °Sulph. °*Sulph. ac.* Sassap. Thuj. Zinc.
Black vesicle, Petr.
—, swelling, Vip. torv.
—, ulcers, Mur. ac.
Black-brown and swollen, Vip. torv.
Bleeding, Agar. *Alum.* Amm. Anac. Ant. °*Arn.* °Ars. Arum. Baryt. **Bell.* Borax. Bov. **Calc. Canth.* °*Carb. an.* **Carb. veg.* Caust. *Chin.* °Chinin. **Cist.* Con. Crotal. Croton. Euphr. Ferr. magn. °Gran. ? Graph. °*Jod.* Kal. Kal.

chl. Lach. °*Led.* Lyc. *Magn. m.* **Merc. Merc. d.* Natr. *Natr. m.* Nitr. °*Nitr. ac.* N. mosch. N. vom. Oph. *Phosph. Phos. ac.* Ran. sc. Ruta. Sec. *Sep.* °*Sil.* Staph. **Sulph.* Sulph. ac. °Tereb. *Tong.* **Zinc.*

Bleeding, hæmoptysis, °*Arn.* **Bell.* Canth. Chin. °Chinin. Lach. °Led. Merc. N. vom. Oph. Sec.

—, gums, Agar. *Alum.* Amm. Anac. Ant. °*Ars.* Arum. Baryt. Bell. Borax. Bov. * *Calc.* ° *Carb. an.* * *Carb. veg.* Caust. * *Cist.* Con. Crotal. Croton. Euphr. Ferr. magn. °Gran. ? Graph. °*Jod.* Kal. Kal. chl. Lach. Lyc. *Magn. m.* **Merc. Merc. d.* Natr. *Natr. m.* Nitr. °Nitr. ac. N. mosch. *Phosph. Phos. ac.* Ran. sc. Ruta. *Sep.* °Sil. Staph. **Sulph.* Sulph. ac. °Tereb. Tong. **Zinc.*

Bleeding, eruptions and ulcers, Alum. Bov. Canth. Graph. *Merc.* Phosph. Zinc.

Bleeding tumor, °N. vom. Ran. sc. Sep.

Blisters and ulcers, smarting, Merc. Natr. Natr. m. Phos. ac.

Blisters and vesicles, Amb. *Amm. Amm. m.* Anac. Ant. Aur. *Baryt.* Bell. Berb. Borax. Bry. *Calc. Canth. Carb. an.* Carb. veg. Caps. *Caust.* Cham. Chen. Electr. *Graph.* **Hell.* Jod. *Kal. Lyc.* Magn. c. Magn. s. Mang. Merc. Mez. Mur. ac. Natr. **Natr. m.* Natr. s. *Nitr. ac. N. vom.* Petr. Phell. Phos. ac. Sabad. *Sep. Sil.* Spig. *Spong.* Squill. Staph. **Sulph.* Sulph. ac. *Thuj. Zinc.*

—, palate, Baryt. Carb. veg. Electr. Natr. s. Phosph. Spig. Sulph.

—, buccal cavity, Amb. Anac. Baryt. Calc.

Canth. Caps. Carb. an. °Hell. Jod. Kal. *Merc.* Natr. Natr. m. *Phosph.* Spig. Spong. Staph. **Sulph.* Sulph. ac.

Blisters, fauces, *Calc.* Phos. ac.
—, gums, Aur. Bell. Calc. Canth. Caps. Carb. veg. Kal. Magn. c. Natr. s. Petr. Sep. Sil. Staph.
—, tongue, *Amm. Amm. m.* Ant. *Baryt.* Berb. Borax. Bry. Calc. Canth. *Carb. an. Caust.* Cham. Chen. Electr. *Graph.* **Hell. Kal. Lyc.* Magn. c. Magn. s. Mang. Mez. Mur. ac. Natr. **Natr. m.* Natr. s. *Nitr. ac. N. vom.* Phell. Phosph. Sabad. *Sep.* Spig. *Spong.* Squill. *Thuj. Zinc.*
Blisters, watery, Graph. Natr. Petr.
—, white, Amb. Berb. Merc. *Thuj.*
Blotches, Alum. Berb. **Calc.* Canth. Caust. Jod. Lyc. N. mosch. °Phos. ac. **Staph.* °*Sulph.*
—, buccal cavity, Jod. Lyc. **Staph.* N. mosch. Phosph.
—, gums, Alum. Berb. **Calc.* Canth. **Caust.* °Phos. ac. Plumb. **Staph.* °*Sulph.*
—, tongue, Graph. Lyc.
—, under the tongue, Amb.

Blueness, Oleand. °*Dig.* Plumb. Sabin.
—, gums, Oleand. Plumb. Sabin.
—, tongue, °*Dig.*

Bluish herpes, °Zinc.
Blue-red and swollen, Canth. Con.
—, gums, Con. Lach.
Bubbling (throbbing) in swelling, N. vom.
Burning, **Acon.* Alum. Amm. Amm. caust. Ang. Arn. **Ars.* Asa. Asar. Baryt. **Bell.*

Berb. *Bism.* Borax. Bov. *Calc.* Calc. ph. *Camph.* Cann. *Canth.* Carb. an. **Carb. veg.* *Cast.* *Caust.* °Cham. Chel. Chen. Chinin. *Cinn.* Cocc. *Coff.* *Colch.* Con. Croc. Dig. Euphorb. Galv. *Grat.* *Hydroc.* *Indig.* Jod. *Kal.* Kal. chl. Kal. hdr. **Lach.* Lact. *Laur.* Led. Lob. °Magn. arct. Magn. aust. *Magn. c.* Magn. m. **Merc.* *Mez.* Mosch. Mur. ac. Natr. *Natr. s.* Nitr. **Nitr. ac.* *N. vom.* Oleand. *Ol. an.* Par. Petr. Phell. **Phosph.* *Phos. ac.* Poth. Plumb. Prun. °*Puls.* Ran. Ran. sc. Raph. *Ratanh.* Rhod. Rhus. **Sabad.* Sec. Seneg. Sep. Sil. Spig. Squill. Staph. Stront. **Sulph.* **Tereb.* Tong. *Veratr.* Zinc.

Burning, palate, Camph. *Caust.* Chen. *Cinn.* *Cocc.* Euphorb. *Grat.* *Hydroc.* *Indig.* Lach. *Laur.* Magn. c. Mur. ac. *Natr. s.* Par. Phosph. Rhod. Sabad. Seneg. Spig. Squill. Sassap. Tong.

—, velum palati, Phos. ac. Ran.

—, buccal cavity, Asa. Baryt. Bov. Calc. Kal. *Lach.* Merc. Mez. Natr. s. *Op.* Plumb. **Sabad.* Sulph. *Tereb.* *Veratr.*

—, fauces and parts, **Acon.* Alum. Amm. Amm. caust. Arn. **Ars.* Asa. Baryt. **Bell.* *Bism.* Borax. Bov. Calc. Calc. ph. *Camph.* Cann. *Canth.* **Carb. veg.* Cast. Caust. Chel. Chen. Chinin. Cycl. Dig. Galv. Hydroc. Jod. **Lach.* Lact. Laur. Led. Lob. Magn. aust. Magn. c. **Merc.* *Mez.* Mosch. Mur. ac. Nitr. **Nitr. ac.* *N. vom.* Oleand. *Ol. an.* **Phosph.* Poth. °*Puls.* Ran. Ran. sc. Raph. Rhod. Rhus. Sabad. Sec. Seneg. Sep. *Sulph.* Veratr. Zinc.

Burning, gums, Cast. Con. °Cham. Lach. °Magn. arct. *Merc.* Mur. ac. 'Natr. s. N. vom. Petr. Phell. Phosph. Puls. Rhus. Sep. Sil. Stront. °Tereb.

—, tongue, *Acon.* Amm. Ang. Asar. Bell. Berb. Bov. *Calc.* Carb. an. *Cast. Caust. Coff. Colch.* Croc. Hydroc. Ign. *Indig. Kal.* Kal. chl. Kal. hdr. *Lach. Laur. *Magn. c.* Magn. m. Mez. Natr. Natr. s. Ol. an. Phosph. *Phos. ac.* Plumb. Prun. Ran. sc. Ratanh. Rhod. **Sabad.* Seneg. Sulph. Tereb. Veratr.

Burning, eruptions, Amb. Amm. Amm. m. Arg. *Baryt.* Bry. Calc. *Caps.* Carb. an. Graph. Kal. hdr. Magn. c. Merc. Mez. Mur. ac. Natr. m. Natr. s. Nitr. ac. Phosph. *Spig.* Spong. *Sulph.*

Burning swelling, *Bell. °Cham. Lach. Sil.

Burning ulcers, *Merc.* Natr. N. vom. Sep.

Caries, palate, °*Aur. Merc.*

Chancrous ulcers, °Lach. **Lyc.* **Merc.* °*Nitr. ac.* °*Thuj.*

After a cold, °Calc. °Crotal. °Dulc.

Creeping, *Acon.* Alum. *Arn.* **Baryt.* Carb. veg. Caust. Colch. Ign. Lach. Merc. Natr. m. Petr. Plat. Rhus. Samb. *Sec.* Seneg. Sep. Tab.

—, palate, Caust. Colch. Sabad.

—, mouth, Alum.

—, fauces and throat, *Acon.* Carb. veg. Colch. Ign. Lach. Petr. Samb. Sec. Sep. Tab.

—, gums, Acon. Arn. **Baryt.* Rhus.

—, tongue, *Acon.* Alum. Merc. Natr. m. Plat. *Sec.* Seneg.

Creeping in ulcer, °Lach.

Dark-red swelling, °Cham. Sep.
Drawing-painful, vesicles, Staph.
—, ulcers, Calc.
Eruptions, which peel off, Electr. Merc.
Excrescences, mouth and gums. Merc. **Staph.* °*Thuj.?*
Fistulous ulcers, gums, Canth. °*Caust.* Lyc. °*Natr. m.* Sulph.
Flesh loose, Lach.
—, gums, Ant. **Carb. veg.* °Cist. °Gran. °*Merc.* Phosph. **Phos. ac.* Rhus. Sep.
Formication, gums, Sec.
Gangrenous, that which is, **Ars.* Chinin. Lach.
Gnawing, Kal. *Merc.* Puls.
Hard swelling, Ign. Merc. Par.
Herpes, bluish, °Zinc.
Inflamed eruptions, Baryt. Spig.
Inflamed gums, Borax. Bov. Petr.
Inflammation, **Acon.* Alum. Amm. Arg. °Ars. **Bell.* Berb. Bism. **Borax.* °*Calc.* *Canth.* °Caps. °*Carb. veg.* **Cham.* Chin. Colch. Crotal. Cupr. °Dulc.? Electr. °*Gran.?* Grat. **Hep.* *Hydroc.* Hyos. **Ign.* Jod. Kal. °*Lach.* Lyc. °*Merc.* Mez. Mur. ac. Natr. °Natr. m. *Natr. s.* Nicc. Nitr. *Nitr. ac.* °*N. vom.* Ol. an. Op. Phosph. Phos. ac. Plumb. **Puls.* Ran. sc. Sabad. °Sang. *Sep.* Sil. Stront. °*Sulph.* Veratr.
—, palate, **Calc.* Hydroc. °*Lach.* °N. vom.
—, velum palati, °*Bell.* °Lach.
—, mouth, Amm. Crotal. °Ign. °*Merc.* °*N. vom.* Op. Veratr.
—, stomacace, °Ars. °Borax.? °Caps. °*Carb. veg.* °Dulc.? °Gran.? Hyos. °*Lach.* °*Merc.* Natr. m. °*N. vom.* °*Sulph.*

Inflammation, fauces and throat, °*Acon.* Alum. Amm. Arg. **Bell.* Bism. **Calc.* *Canth.* Carb. veg. °Cham. Chinin. Colch. Cupr. Electr. °Gran. Hydroc. **Ign.* Jod. °*Lach.* Lyc. **Merc.* Mez. Natr. *Natr. s.* Nicc. Ol. an. Phos. ac. °*Puls.* Sabad. °Sang. *Sep.* Stront. °*Sulph.*

—, tonsils, **Bell.* Berb. *Canth.* °Cham. °Gran. ? °*Ign.* °*Lach.* °*Merc.* Natr. Natr. s. Nicc. Nitr. ac. Sep.

—, gums, Borax. Grat. Hep. Jod. Kal. Mur. ac. °Natr. m. °N. vom. Nitr. *Phosph. Sil.*

—, uvula, °*Bell.* Berb. Carb. veg. Natr. s. °*N. vom.*

—, tongue, Canth. Plumb. Ran. sc.

Inflammatory swelling, °*Acon.* **Bell.* Berb. Borax. Carb. veg. **Hep.* °Ign. Jod. °*Lach.* °*Merc.* Natr. m. Natr. s. °*N. vom.* Nitr. *Nitr. ac.* Sil.

Itching, Amm. Bell. Calc. Caust. Cic. Ferr. magn. Graph. *Kal.* Lach. Magn. arct. Magn. c. Merc. Nitr. ac. Phosph. Phos. ac. Prun. Rhod. Samb. *Sil.* Spig. Spong. Tong. Zinc.

—, palate, Ferr. magn. *Kal.* Phosph. Sil.

—, velum palati, Sil.

—, mouth, Magn. c.

—, fauces and throat. Cist. Samb. Spig.

—, gums, Amm. Bell. Calc. Caust. Graph. Kal. Lach. Merc. Nitr. ac. Phosph. Prun. Rhod. Spong. Tong. Zinc.

—, tongue, Alum. Magn. arct. N. vom. Phos. ac.

Itching swelling, Phosph.

Lardaceous ulcer, °Hep.
From abuse of mercury, °Arg. °*Aur.* °*Bell.* °*Lach.* °*Lyc.* °*Nitr. ac.* °*Staph.* °Sulph. °Thuj.
Pain as from a fistula, Aur. **Calc.* Petr.
Pain as if ulcerated, Alum. *Amm.* Bell. Bov. Carb. an. Carb. veg. *Caust.* Graph. Kal. hdr. °Magn. c. Mang. Natr. *Nicc.* Nitr. Ol. an. Phell. Phos. ac.
—, palate, Amm. Caust.
—, fauces and throat, Kal. hdr. *Nicc.* Nitr. ac. Phos. ac.
—, gums, Alum. Amm. Bell. Bov. Carb. an. Carb. veg. Caust. Graph. Kal. hdr. °Magn. c. Mang. Natr. Nicc. Nitr. Ol. an. Phell.
Pain as if ulcerated, in swollen parts, Bor. Kal. hdr. N. vom. Phell.
—, of eruptions, Staph.
Painful eruptions, blisters, Anac. Arg. Bell. Berb. Borax. Chen. Graph. *Kal.* Mur. ac. Natr. m. Natr. s. Nitr. ac. *N. vom.* Phosph. Puls. Sulph. *Zinc.*
—, swollen parts, Amb. Amm. Baryt. Bov. Calc. Carb. an. **Caust.* **Cham.* Chin. Con. *Graph.* Hep. Kal. Lach. Lyc. ***Magn. art.*** Magn. arct. Magn. m. **Merc.* Natr. m. Nitr. N. vom. Phos. ac. ***Plat.*** Ran. sc. Sabin. **Sep.* ***Sil.*** Spong. Staph. Stront. **Sulph.* Thuj.
—, ulcers, Merc. Natr. m. Phosph. Rhod.
Painless and swollen, Natr. s. Par.
Paleness, Agar. Carb. an. ***Chinin.*** ***Merc.*** Natr. Nitr. ac. Raph. Staph.
—, gums, Carb. an. ***Merc.*** Nitr. ac. Staph.
—, tongue, Agar. Natr. Raph.

Pale and swollen, Nitr. ac.
Pale-red and swollen, *Baryt.
Peeling off of skin, Amm. Euphorb. Electr. Lach. Merc. Ran. sc. Sulph.
—, palate, Amm. Euphorb. Electr.
—, mouth, Lach. Sulph. Merc.
—, tongue, Ran. sc.
Peeling off, sensation as if, Agar. Phosph.
Pimples, Arg. Berb. Caps. Dulc. Hell. Kal. ***Mur. ac.*** Natr. Nitr. ac. ***N. vom.*** Plumb. Sep.
—, palate, Dulc. ***Mur. ac.*** N. vom.
—, mouth, Caps.
—, tongue, Arg. Berb. Caps. Hell. Kal. Natr. Nitr. ac. Plumb. Sep.
Prickling, Caust. Lach. Ol. an. Phell. Phosph. Rhod.
—, palate, Caust. Ol. an.
—, gums, Lyc.
—, tongue, Lach. Phell. Phosph. Rhod.
Prickling swelling, Lyc.
Pustules, Amm. Aur. Calc. Carb. veg. °***Ign.*** Magn. c. Petr. Phosph.
—, mouth, Amm. Magn. c. Phosph.
—, tonsils, °Ign.
—, gums, Aur. Calc. Carb. veg. Petr.
—, tongue, Amm.
Putrid swelling, °*N. vom.*
Ranula, °***Thuj.***
Redness, °***Acon.*** Agn. Alum. ***Amm.*** Amm. caust. ****Bell.*** Berb. Canth. Carb. an. °***Cham.*** Chen. ***Con.*** Electr. ****Hyos.*** ****Ign.*** Kal. Kal. chl. °***Lach.*** Magn. c. ****Merc.*** Nitr. Nitr. ac. N. mosch. °***Puls.*** Raph. Ran. sc. °Rhus. Sep. °Stann. Sulph.

Redness, palate, Amm. Caust. Canth. Chen. °*Puls.*

—, velum palati, Agn. °*Acon.* ****Bell.*** Berb. N. mosch.

—, tonsils, °*Acon.* Amm. caust. ****Bell.*** Berb. °Cham. °Lach. ****Merc.*** Nitr. ac. °***Puls.*** Raph. Sulph.

—, mouth, Amm. °Ign.

—, fauces and throat, °*Acon.* Alum. Amm. ****Bell.*** Ign. Natr. N. mosch.

—, uvula, Agn. °Bell. Berb. °Puls.

—, gums, *Carb. an. Con.* Jod. Kal. Kal. chl. *Lach.* Magn. c. Nitr. Ran. sc. **Sep.*

—, tongue, Ant. *Electr.* **Hyos.* Ran. sc. °Rhus. °Stann. Sulph.

Red spots, Canth.

—, inflamed parts, °*Acon.* °*Bell.* Carb. an. °*Cham.* Con. Lach. Magn. c. Nitr. Nitr. ac. Phell. Ran. Sep. Sulph.

Scurfs, tongue, Chinin.

Smarting, fauces, Amb. Dros. Ran. sc. Sep. Teucr.

—, gums, Asar. Calc. Carb. veg. Cocc. Phell. Rhod.

—, tongue, *Acon. Arn.* Ars. Asar. Bell. Cham. Chin. Ipec. Mez. Natr. Ol. an. Sulph.

Smarting, *Acon. Amb. Arn.* Ars. Asar. Bell. Calc. Carb. an. *Cham.* Chen. *Chin.* Cocc. *Dros. Ipec. Kal.* Mez. Natr. Ol. an. Phell. Ran. sc. Rhod. Seneg. *Sep.* Sulph. Teucr. Zinc.

—, palate, Cham. Chen. *Chin. Kal.* Ran. sc. Seneg. Sep. Zinc.

—, buccal cavity, Amb. Carb. an. Dros. *Ipec.*

Soreness, Agar. °*Amb. Carb. veg.* Chinin. *Dig.*

Electr. Ferr. *Graph.* Kal. **Lach.* Lyc. *Merc. Mez. Mur. ac.* Natr. m. Nitr. ac. Op. Phosph. Phos. ac. **Sabad.* Sep. **Sil.*

Soreness, palate, **Lach. Mez. Mur. ac.* Nitr. ac. Phos. ac.

—, mouth, Dig. Electr. Kal. **Lach.* Merc. Natr. m. Op. °*Phosph.* Sabad.

—, fauces and throat, °*Amb. Dig.* Ferr. *Graph. Mez.*

—, gums, *Carb. veg.* Chinin. Dig. Kal. **Lach.* Merc. Nitr. ac. Sep. Sil.

—, tongue, Agar. Carb. veg. Dig. Kal. °*Lach.* Lyc. Mur. ac. Nitr. ac. **Sabad.* **Sil.*

Soreness, Agar. Alum. Amb. Amm. Ant. Arn. Ars. Aur. Bism. Bry. *Calc. Caps. Carb. an.* **Carb. veg. Cast. Caust.* °*Cist.* Clem. Cocc. Corall. Dig. Electr. **Graph.* Hell. **Ign.* Jod. *Kal.* Kreas. **Lach.* Magn. arct. Magn. aust. Magn. c. *Magn. m.* Mang. *Merc.* Mur. ac. Natr. Natr. m. **Nitr. ac.* N. vom. Petr. *Phosph.* Phos. ac. **Puls.* Ratanh. Rhod. Rhus. Ruta. Sabad. Sassap. *Seneg.* **Sep.* Sil. Staph. Stram. Tereb. Teucr. Thuj. **Zinc.*

—, palate, Agar. Alum. Caust. Ign. *Mang.* Puls. Thuj.

—, velum palati, Ruta.

—, tonsils, Raph. Rhus.

—, mouth, Agar. Alum. Amm. Electr. Ign. Natr. Phosph. Stram.

—, fauces and throat, Alum. Amm. Aur. Calc. *Caps. Carb. an. Carb. veg. Cast. Caust.* °Cist. Corall. Dig. Hell. **Ign. Kal.* Kreas. **Lach.* Magn. aust. Magn. c. *Magn. m.* **Merc.* **Nitr.*

ac. Petr. *Phosph.* Phos. ac. **Puls.* Rhus v. Sabin. Seneg. **Sep.* Staph.

Soreness, gums, Alum. Ars. Asa. Aur. Bism. Bry. **Carb. veg.* Clem. Cocc. **Graph.* Jod. Magn. arct. Mur. ac. Natr. m. Nitr. ac. N. vom. Petr. Phosph. Phos. ac. Puls. Ratanh. Rhod. Ruta. Sassap. Sep. Sil. Staph. Tereb. Thuj. **Zinc.*

—, uvula, Caust.

—, tongue, Alum. Amb. Amm. Ant. Arn. *Calc. Caust.* Graph. *Ign.* Laur. *Merc.* Natr. Natr. m. *Nitr. ac.* Sabad. Sep. Staph. Teucr. Thuj. Zinc.

Sore, eruptions, blisters, Arg. Electr. Lyc. Magn. c. Sil.

—, swollen parts, Aur. Bism. Graph. Natr. m. Sassap. Sep. Sil. Thuj. Zinc.

—, ulcers, Amm. Bov.

Sore, as if corroded, Ars. Kal. Merc.

Splinter, sensation as from, Laur. Nitr. ac.

Spots, as if ecchymosed, Con.

Stinging in blisters, vesicles, Berb. Caps. Cham. Hell. Natr. Natr. s. Spong. Staph.

—, in swollen parts, Laur. Lyc. Merc. Natr. m. N. vom. Petr. Ran.

—, in ulcers, Amm. m. Nitr. ac. Staph.

Suppurations, Amm. Baryt. **Bell.* Berb. Canth. °*Caust.* °Gran. ? °Ign. °*Lach.* Lyc. **Merc.* °Natr. m. °Nicc. Sep. **Sulph.* Sulph. ac.

—, mouth, Canth.

—, tonsils, Baryt. **Bell.* Berb. °Gran. ? °Ign. °*Lach.* **Merc.* Nicc. °Sep.

—, gums, Canth. °*Caust.* Lach. Lyc. °Natr. m. Sulph. Sulph. ac.

Suppurations, tongue, Canth.
Swelling, reddish-yellow, Canth.
—, gums, Canth.
Swelling, in general, Agar. Alum. Amb. *Amm. Amm. m.* Anac. Aur. **Baryt.* Bar. m. **Bell.* Berb. Bism. Borax. Bov. Bruc. **Calc.* Canth. Carb. an. Carb. veg. Cast. Caust. **Cham. Chin.* **Cist.* Coccin. Cocc. Coff. Con. Crotal. Croton. Dig. Dros. Dulc. Electr. Ferr. **Graph.* Hell. °*Hep.* °*Ign.* Jod. Kal. Kal. hdr. **Lach.* Laur. Lyc. Magn. art. Magn. arct. Magn. c. Magn. m. **Merc. Mercurial. Mur. ac.* Natr. Natr. m. *Natr. s.* Nicc. Nitr. *Nitr. ac.* *N. vom. Par. Petr. Phell. *Phosph. Phos. ac.* Plat. Plumb. Poth. Puls. Ran. sc. Raph. Sabad. Sabin. Sassap. Sec. **Sep.* Sil. Spig. Spong. **Staph.* Stram. Stront. **Sulph.* Sulph. ac. Tab. *Thuj.* Veratr. Vip. *Zinc.*
—, palate, Bar. m. °*Calc. Chin.* °*N. vom.* Par.
—, velum palati, °Bell. Coff. °Lach.
—, tonsils, Alum. Amm. **Baryt.* **Bell.* Berb. **Calc.* °Cham. *Graph.* °*Hep.* °Ign. °*Lach.* **Merc.* Natr. Natr. s. Nicc. *Nitr. ac.* N. vom. *Phosph.* Plat. Ran. sc. Sep. **Staph. Sulph.* Tart. *Thuj.* Zinc.
—, mouth, Amm. °Bell. Calc. Canth. Caust. Ferr. °*Merc.* °*N. vom.* Sep.
—, fauces and throat, Ant. Arg. **Bell.* **Calc.* Carb. veg. Caust. *Lach. Nitr. ac.* °Op. Petr. Phos. ac. Poth. Sep. Spig. Sulph. ac. Thuj.
—, salivary glands, Bar. m. *Merc.* Thuj.
—, gums, Agar. *Alum.* Amb. Amm. Amm. m. Anac. Aur. Baryt. **Bell.* Bism. Borax. Bov. **Calc.* Caps. Carb. an. Carb. veg. Cast. *Caust.

Cham. Chin. **Cist.* Coccin. Cocc. Con. Croton. Ferr. **Graph.* Hep. Jod. Kal. Kal. hdr. Lach. Lyc. Magn. art. **Magn. arct.* Magn. c. Magn. m. **Merc.* *Mercurial.* Mur. ac. Natr. Natr. m. Natr. s. Nicc. Nitr. Nitr. ac. **N. vom.* Petr. Phell. Phosph. Phos. ac. Plumb. Puls. Ran. sc. Sabin. Sassap. **Sep.* Sil. Spong. **Staph.* Stront. **Sulph.* Sulph. ac. Thuj. Veratr. Zinc.

Swelling, uvula, °Bell. Berb. Carb. veg. Chin. Coff. Jod. Lyc. Merc. Natr. s. **N. vom.* *Sabad.* *Sil.*

—, tongue, Calc. Con. *Crotal.* Dig. °*Dulc.* Electr. Hell. Kal. **Lach.* Laur. Lyc. Merc. Mercurial. Natr. m. Phosph. Phos. ac. Sec. Sil. Stram. Thuj. *Vip. red.* Zinc.

—, lingual glands, *Staph.* Tab.

Swelling, sensation of, in general, Alum. Amm. Anac. Baryt. °*Bell.* Bry. Chin. Cocc. Daph. *Hep.* Ign. Lach. Lyc. Nitr. N. vom. Plumb. Puls. Rhod. *Sabin.* Sang. Spong. Stront. Sulph. Thuj. *Zinc.*

—, palate, Ign. N. vom. Puls.

—, mouth, Amm. Lyc.

—, fauces and throat, Alum. Baryt. **Bell.* Bry. Chin. *Hep.* **Lach.* *Nitr. ac.* **N. vom.* Plumb. **Puls.* Rhus. *Sabin.* Sang. **Sulph.* Thuj. *Zinc.*

—, gums, Amm. Chin. Daph. Hyos. Nitr. N. vom. Puls. Rhod. Sabin. Spong. Stront.

—, uvula, **Puls.*

—, tongue, Anac. Cocc. Lyc. Magn. aust.

Syphilitic ulcers and eruptions, °Lach. °*Merc.* °Thuj.

Tearing, Calc. Dulc. **Merc.*

—, eruptions, Dulc.

Tearing, swelling, **Merc.*
—, ulcers, Calc.
Throbbing swelling, Calc. Lach. Magn. m. Sep. **Sulph.*
Transparent vesicles, Phosph.
Ulcers, Agar. **Agn.* Alum. Amm. **Aur.* Berb. Borax. Bov. **Calc.* Canth. **Caust.* Cic. Dig. Dulc. Graph. Gran. °*Hep.* °*Jod.* Kal. °*Lach.* **Lyc.* **Merc.* **Natr. m.* *Nitr. ac.* **N. vom.* Op. Petr. Phosph. Plumb. Sabin. *Sil.* *Staph.* **Sulph.* Sulph. ac. Thuj. Zinc.
—, palate, °*Aur.* Dulc. °*Lach.* Op. *Sil.*
—, tonsils, Calc. **Lyc.* °Ign.
—, mouth, Agn. Alum. Borax. Canth. °Gran.? °*Hep.* °Jod. **Merc.* *Mercurial.* *Nitr. ac.* °N. vom. Op. Petr. Plumb.
—, fauces and throat, Jod. °Lach. *Nitr. ac.* N. vom.
—, gums, °*Agn.?* Alum. Aur. Berb. Bov. **Calc.* Hep. °Jod. Kal. Lyc. **Merc.* *Natr. m.* N. vom. Phosph. Sabin. *Sil.* *Staph.* Sulph. ac. Zinc.
—, fistula dentalis, Canth. °*Caust.* Lyc. °*Natr. m.* °*Sulph.*
—, tongue, Agar. Amm. Bov. Cic. °Dig. Graph. Lyc. *Merc.* Mur. ac.
Ulceration, Alum. Kal. hdr. Natr. *Natr. m.* Sep.
—, mouth, **Merc.* Natr. *Natr. m.* Rhod.
—, gums, Alum. Kal. hdr. Natr. *Natr. m.* Sep.
—, tongue, Cic. Natr. m.
Ulcers, phagedænic, *Merc.* Nitr. ac.
Ulcers, yellow, Calc. Plumb. Zinc.
Vesicles, which break, Phosph.

Vesicles, painful as if burnt, Amb. Bell. Carb. an. Lyc. Sep. Sulph.
White swelling, Sabin.
—, ulcers, Calc. Dros. Graph. °*Merc.*
Worse after chagrin, Calc.

Nails, diseases of.

In general, *Alum.* Amm. m. **Ant.* *Ars.* Aur. Baryt. Bell. *Borax.* Bov. *Calc.* *Caust.* Chel. Chin. Cocc. Colch. *Con.* Dig. Dros. **Graph.* *Hell.* **Hep.* Jod. Kal. **Lach.* Lyc. Magn. art. Magn. arct. **Magn. aust.* **Merc.* Mosch. Mur. ac. **Natr. m.* *Nitr. ac.* *N. vom.* *Par.* Petr. Phos. ac. Plat. **Puls.* *Ran.* **Rhus.* Ruta. *Sabad.* Sec. **Sep.* **Sil.* *Squill.* **Sulph.* *Sulph. ac.* Thuj.
Beating, *Amm. m.* Con. Magn. aust. Sep.
Bleeding, Crotal.
Blue, Amm. °*Aur.* Carb. veg. Chel. **Chin.* Cocc. °*Dig.* Dros. Lyc. °*Natr. m.* **N. vom.* Petr. Phos. ac. Sassap. °*Sil.*
Boring, Colch.
Breaking off, decayed, Alum. **Graph.* *Merc.* Sabad. Sep.? *Sil.* °*Sulph.*
Brittle, **Alum.* Calc. °*Graph.* Merc. Sabad. Sep. **Sil.* °*Sulph.*
Burning, Alum. Calc. *Caust.* Con. Kal. Merc. Nicc. Nitr. ac. Vinc.
Dirty, discoloured, *Ant.* Ars. °*Graph.* Mur. ac. °*Nitr. ac.* Sil. Sulph.
Distorted, Alum. Calc. °*Graph.* Merc. Sabad. °*Sep.* °*Sil.* °*Sulph.*

Falling off, Ant.? Ars. Hell. **Graph.* *Merc.* *Sec.* Sep. Squill.? Thuj.?

Furrowed, Sabad. Sil.

Gnawing, Alum.

Growing into the flesh and sensation of, Colch. Graph. Kal. **Magn. aust.* Sil. °*Sulph.* Teucr.

Growing slowly, Ant.

Hang nails, **Calc.* Lyc. Merc. Natr. m. **Rhus.* Sabad. Stann. **Sulph.*

Inflammation, Con. Hell. Kal. Lyc. Natr. m. Phos. ac. Teucr.

Itching, Hep.

Jerking pain, Calc. Caust. Graph. Magn. aust. Merc. Natr. m. N. vom. Puls. Rhus. Sil.

Pain as if contused, Nitr.

Pain as if ulcerated, **Amm. m.* *Bell.* Berb. Caust. Chin. *Con.* **Graph.* Hell. **Hep.* **Kal.* Magn. art. Magn. aust. **Merc.* Mur. ac. Natr. m. Natr. s. Nicc. °*Nitr. ac.* N. vom. Ol. an. **Puls.* Ran. °*Rhus.* Sep. Sil. *Sulph.* *Sulph. ac.* Thuj.

Painfulness, Amm. m. *Ant.* Bell. Carb. veg. **Caust.* **Graph.* **Hep.* Kal. Lyc. Magn. art. **Magn. aust.* *Merc.* Natr. m. *Nitr. ac.* N. vom. Par. Petr. Phos. ac. Puls. Ran. Rhod. Rhus. Sabad. Sep. *Sil.* *Squill.* Stann. *Sulph.*

Pressure, Calc. Caust. Magn. art. Magn. aust. Sassap. Sulph.

Roughness, Sabad. Sil.

Sore, Alum. Graph. Hep. Kal. Magn. aust. Merc. Mez. Natr. m. N. vom. Puls. Sep. Sulph.

Splitting, **Sil.* Squill.

Splinter, pain as from, Bell. Carb. veg. Colch. Hep. *Nitr. ac.* Petr. *Sil.* *Sulph.*

Spotted, Alum. Ars. Natr. m. *_Nitr. ac. Sep._ °_Sil._ Sulph.

Stinging, Amm. m. Bell. Carb. veg. Colch. Con. Graph. Hep. _Kal._ Lyc. Magn. aust. Natr. s. Nicc. _Nitr. Nitr. ac._ Phos. ac. Sep. _Sil. Sulph._

Suppuration, Calc. Kal. Phos. ac. Sep.

Swelling around, Natr. m.

Tearing, around, Amb. Baryt. Bism. Camph. _Carb. veg._ Colch. _Coloc._ Jod. Lyc. Nitr. Ol. an. Sulph. ac.

Thickened, Alum. Calc. *_Graph._ Merc. Sabad. Sep. *_Sil._ °_Sulph._

Ulceration, panaritia, °_Alum._ Ant. °_Ars. Baryt._ Bell. ? Borax. ? Bov. _Calc._ Caust. _Con._ °_Crotal._ Ferr. magn. °_Graph._ *_Hep._ Jod. °_Kal._ *_Lach._ Lyc. Magn. aust. *_Merc._ Natr. m. ? °_Nitr. ac._ Petr. _Phosph._ °_Puls._ °_Rhus._ *_Sep._ *_Sil._ Squill. *_Sulph._ Sulph. ac.

Yellow, Amb. Ant. Ars. Aur. Carb. veg. Chel. *_Con._ Ign. °_Merc._ °_Nitr. ac._ °_N. vom._ Phos. ac. *_Sep._ *_Sil._ Spig. °_Sulph._

Nettlerash, like.

Eruption, °_Acon._ Amm. Amm. m. _Ant._ Anthrok. *_Ars._ Baryt. _Bell._ *Bry. *_Calc._ Carb. an. *_Carb. veg._ *_Caust._ Chin. Cic. Cocc. *_Con._ Cop. *_Dulc._ Fragar. Graph. *_Hep._ °_Ign._ Ipec. Kal. Kreas. Lach. Led. _Lyc._ Magn. c. Merc. _Mez._ Natr. _Natr. m._ Nitr. ac. N. vom. °_Petr._ Phosph. Phos. ac. _Puls._ *_Rhus._ Ruta. Sec. Selen. _Sep._ Sil. Staph. Stram. _Sulph._ Tart. Thuj. °Urt. Veratr. Zinc.

Blotches, Berb. Kreas. Lach. Sassap. Veratr.
Spots, Berb.

Head, itching, Ant. Calc.
Face, Ant.
Sexual parts, Tart.
Dorsal region, Sil.
Arms, itching and eruption, Berb.
Hands, eruption, *Berb.* Euphorb. °*Hep.* Natr. *Natr. m.* Natr. s. *Sulph.*
—, finger, °*Hep.*
Lower limbs, hip. *Sulph.*
—, thigh, Caust. Zinc.
—, legs, *Aur.*

Nodosities, arthritic.

In general, °Acon. ? °*Agn.* °*Ant.* °Arn. °Aur. °*Calc.* °*Carb. an.* °*Caust.* °*Clem.* °Cic. °Colch. ? °Dig. °*Graph.* Hep. Led. °*Lyc.* °*Merc.* Nitr. °Nitr. ac. °*Puls.* Ran. °Rhod. ? °*Rhus.* °*Sabin.* °*Staph.* °*Sulph.*
Wrists, °*Calc.*
—, finger-joints, °*Agn.* °*Calc.* °*Clem.* °*Graph.* °*Lyc.* °Staph. ?

Nose and Nostrils, Region of.

Acne punctata, °Dros. Graph. Selen. °*Sulph.*
Black skin, °Merc.
Bleeding, **Acon.* Agar. Amb.**Amm.* *Anac. Ant. Arg. **Arn.* *Ars.* *Baryt.* *Bell. Berb. Borax. **Bry.* **Calc.* **Cann.* Canth. Caps. *Carb. an.* **Carb. veg.* *Caust.* **Cham.* **Chin.* Chinin.

Coff. Colch. Con. Corall. **Croc.* Crotal. Cupr. ac. Diad. Dig. **Dros.* Dulc. Electr. °Euphr. Ferr. Galv. *Graph.* Hep. Hyos. *Ign. *Jod.* Ipec. *Kal.* Kal. chl. Kal. hdr. Kreas. Lach. Led. *Lyc.* Magn. art. Magn. arct. *Magn. c.* Magn. m. Magn. s. Meph. **Merc.* Merc. d. Mosch. Mur. ac. Natr. *Natr. m.* Natr. s. **Nitr. ac.* N. vom. Oph. Par. *Petr.* **Phosph.* Phos. ac. **Puls.* Ratanh. Rhod. **Rhus.* **Ruta.* Sassap. Sec. **Sep.* **Sil.* Spong. Stann. **Sulph.* Sulph. ac. Tarax. Thuj. Veratr. Zinc.

Bleeds, that which, Amm. m. Ferr. Stront.

Blisters, bloody, Sep.

Blotches, **Bell.* Jod.

Blueness of the wings, Hydroc.

Boils, Amm. Carb. an. Magn. m.

Bone-pain, Ars. **Aur.* Corall. Hep. Indig. Laur. *Merc.* Natr. m. Nitr. Thuj.

Brown-red, Aur. Tax.

Burning, Agar. Alum. **Ars.* **Bell.* Bov. Caps. Carb. an. Chen. Cin. Cist. Gran. Graph. Jod. Kal. Led. Magn. art. **Magn. m.* Natr. m. Nicc. Nitr. Nitr. ac. Petr. Phosph. Phell. Sulph. ac. Tab.

Cancer, °*Ars.* °Aur. °Carb. an. ? °Sep. °*Sulph.*

Caries, °Aur.

As if from chilblains, Zinc.

As of drunkards, °Lach.

Eruption, in general, Calc. Carb. veg. Croton. Nicc. Sassap. Spong.

—, BY the nose, Alum. Canth. Caps. Chin. Magn. art. Natr. Rhus. Spig. Tarax.

—, ON the nose, Ant. °*Aur.* Caust. Graph.

Eruption, near the wings, Carb. veg. Con. Dulc. Euphr. Laur. Natr. Petr. Rhus. Sil. Thuj. Veratr.

—, IN the nose, Ant. Arn. Canth. Carb. an. Cic. Cocc. Guaj. Lach. Magn. c. Phell. Ran. Selen. **Sil.* Spig.

—, at the tip, Carb. an. Carb. veg. °*Caust.* Nitr. ac. Phos. ac. *Sep.* Sil. Spong.

—, in the canthi, Anac. Dulc. Euphr. Mang. Plumb. Rhus. Thuj.

—, below the nose, Arn. Baryt. Bov. Caps. Squill. Teucr.

Erysipelas, Canth. Plumb.

Falling off of the hair of the nostrils, Calc. *Caust.* *Graph.* Sil.

Figwarts, °Nitr. ac.

Freckles, Phosph. °*Sulph.*

Gangrenous, becoming, Sec.

Hardness, Alum. Canth. Rhus. Thuj. Zinc.

Herpes, Nitr. ac. Spig.

Herpes on the nose, Aur. Calc. Jod. Phos. ac. Rhod. Tax. Veratr.

Herpes furfuraceous, °Ars.

Humour, secreting a, Graph.

Inflammation, Agar. **Aur.* **Aur. m.* **Calc.* Canth. Con. Corall. Croton. °Hep.? *Merc. Natr. m.* Nitr. Phosph. Plumb. **Sep.* **Sulph.*

Itching, Agar. Agn. °Amm. Aur. *Aur. m. Berb. Borax. Bov. **Calc.* **Carb. veg.* Caps. *Caust.* Coloc. *Con.* Eugen. Gran. Graph. Grat. Hell. Ign. Kal. Lach. *Laur.* Lyc. Magn. c. *Merc.* Mur. ac. Natr. m. Natr. s. Nitr. *Nitr. ac.* N. vom. Oleand. Ol. an. Op. Petr. *Phell.* Phosph.

Samb. Sassap. Selen. Seneg. **Sil.* Spig. Staph. Stront. Therid. Zing.

Abuse of mercury, from, °Aur. °Asa. °Con. °Lach.

Pain as if sore, Amb. Amm. Ang. *Ant.* Aur. Bov. Camph. Caust. Chin. Cic. Cin. Coff. Colch. Con. Hep. Ign. Lyc. Magn. art. Magn. c. *Magn. m.* Mang. *Mez.* Nitr. m. Nitr. ac. **N. vom.* Phosph. *Rhod.* Rhus. *Sep.* Sil. Spig. Squill. *Staph.* Sulph. Zinc.

Pain as if ulcerated, Amm. m. Arn. Bry. Camph. Canth. Cocc. Dulc. Graph. Ign. Kal. Mur. ac. Nitr. **N. vom.* Petr. Puls. Rhus. Staph. Veratr.

Painful, which is, **Alum.* Amm. Amm. m. Arn. Ars. **Bell.* Borax. **Bry.* Calc. Canth. Caps. *Carb. an.* Clem. Coff. Colch. Corall. Dulc. °Euphr. *Graph. Guaj. **Ign.* *Kal.* Lach. Lam. Led. *Lyc.* **Magn. m.* Merc. Natr. *Natr. m.* Nitr. *N. vom.* Petr. Phos. ac. Poth. Puls. Rhus. *Sep.* *Sil.* Spig. Squill. Sulph. Tart. Zinc.

Peeling off of the skin, °Ars. °Aur. *Aur. m. Canth. Carb. an. Croton. Natr. Tax.

Pimples, **Amm.* *Anac.* Arn. Baryt. Bell. Bov. **Calc.* Canth. Carb. veg. **Caust.* Clem. Dulc. Euphorb. *Graph.* Guaj. Kal. Kal. hdr. Lach. Lam. Magn. arct. Mang. *Natr.* Natr. m. Nitr. Ol. an. Petr. *Phosph.* Phos. ac. Ratanh. *Sep.* *Sil.* Stront. Sulph. Tarax. Tax. Teucr. Thuj.

Pocks, Canth. **Merc.*

Polypus, °Calc. °*Phosph.* °*Puls.* °Teucr. ?

Pustules, *Amm. *Anac.* Arn. Bell. Bov. Clem. Cocc. Euphr. Mang. Natr. Nitr. *Petr.* Plumb. Tarax.

Rash-pimples, Sil.
Red nose, **Alum.* **Aur.* **Aur. m.* **Bell.* Borax. Bov. **Calc.* *Canth.* *Carb. an.* Chin. Croton. *Graph.* *Hep.* Jod. Kal. °*Lach.* Magn. arct. Magn. c. **Magn. m.* *Merc.* Natr. *Natr. m.* Nicc. *Nitr.* Nitr. ac. Phosph. Poth. Rhod. Rhus. **Sil.* Sulph. Vinc.
Red, which is, Calc. Crot. Jod. Lach. Phos. ac. Rhod. Sil. Stront. Teucr. Thuj. Veratr. Zinc.
With red areola, Anac. Natr. Petr. Sil.
Rhagades, **Ant.* Carb. an. Merc.
Saddle, yellow, Sep.
—, swollen, Poth.
Scurfs, crusts, **Ant.* °Baryt. Bell. Bov. *Carb. an.* Carb. veg. Croton. Natr. m. Nitr. ac. Petr. **Phos. ac.* Ratanh. *Rhus.* Sep. *Staph.* °Sulph.
—, in the nostrils, **Alum.* Amm. m. **Aur.* Borax. Bov. **Calc.* Carb. an. Cham. °Cic. Ferr. °*Graph.* Hep. Jod. **Kal.* Lach. °Lyc. Magn. c. **Magn. m.* Merc. Natr. Nitr. ac. Petr. *Phosph.* *Puls.* *Sep.* **Sil.* °*Sulph.* *Thuj.
—, at the tip, *Carb. an.* Carb. veg. *Sep.*
Scrofulous, which is, °Aur. °Calc. °Phosph.
Shines, that which, Borax. Calc. *Canth.* *Merc.*
Skin, shining as if from oil, Calc.
Smarting, Arn. Berb. Chen. Chin. Euphorb. Grat. Hell. Lyc. Nitr. Plat. Sabad. °Spig. Teucr. Thuj.
Soreness, Agar. **Alum.* Caps. Carb. an. ?Euphr. Galv. °*Graph.* **Kal.* Lach. °Magn. m. Mez. *Natr. m.* *Nitr. ac.
Suppuration, discharge of pus, °Alum. Arg. n. °Asa. ! °Aur. ? °Aur. m. Cic. Cin. °*Con.* **Lach.* *Merc.* °Petr. *Puls.* Sulph.

Swelling, **Alum.* Amm. m. *Arn. Ars. *Aur. **Aur. m.* *Bell. Borax. **Bry.* **Calc.* *Carb. an.* Caust. Cist. Cocc. Corall. °Graph. *Hep.* °Ign. *Kal.* Lyc. Magn. c. **Magn. m.* *Merc.* *Natr. m.* Nicc. °*Petr.* **Phosph.* Phos. ac. *Rhus.* **Sep.* **Sulph.* Thuj. **Zinc.*

—, wings, Alum. Calc. Carb. an. Magn. m. Merc, Sulph. Thuj. Zinc.

—, nostrils, Bell. Canth. Cocc. Lach. Zinc.

—, dorsum, Phos. ac. Poth.

—, tip, Calc. Kal. Lyc. Merc. Nicc. Sep. Sulph.

—, root, Calc.

Syphilitic, °Lach. °Merc. °Nitr. ac. °Thuj.

Tuberous swelling, °Ars. °Merc.

Tubercle, Natr.

Ulceration of the nostrils, Alum. Amm. m. **Ant.* *Aur. **Aur. m.* Borax. **Calc.* Caps. Corall. °*Graph.* Hyos. Ign. Kal. °Lyc. **Magn. m.* **Merc.* Natr. *Nitr.* *Nitr. ac.* Phosph. *Puls.* Ratanh. **Sil.* *Staph.* Tart. **Thuj.*

—, of external nose, *Puls.*

Vesicles, Amm. Carb. an. Croton. Lach. Magn. m. Natr. *Natr. m.* Nitr. ac. Petr. *Phell.* Phosph. **Sil.* Veratr.

Warts, °Caust.

White, which is, Carb. veg. Kal. Natr. Natr. m.

Wrinkles of the skin, Cham.

Yellow, which is, **Aur.* Croton. *Sep.*

Numbness of the skin.

In general, **Amb.* **Anac.* Ang. Cham. *Con.* Cycl. Lach. °*Lyc.* Magn. art. N. vom. °*Oleand.*

Phosph. °*Phos. ac.* Plat. Plumb. °*Puls.* **Sec.* Stram. *Sulph.* Tart.

Ears, °*Mur. ac.*

Arms, Acon. **Amb.* Calc. ph. *Cham.* °*Ign.* *Kal. Meph.* Natr. m. °*Nitr.* Phosph. Puls. °*Rhus.* Sec.

—, elbow, Sulph.

—, forearm, Berb. Casp. Nitr. *Stront.* Sulph.

Hands, Acon. Ars. Bov. Bry. Cann. Carb. an. *Carb. veg.* Cocc. Graph. Lach. Lam. °*Lyc.* Nitr. Puls °*Ruta.* Sep. Sil. Zinc.

—, wrists, Bov. Plumb.

—, fingers, Anac. Ang. Calc. Cann. Caust. Cic. Cin. Coff. Colch. Con. Crotal. Cupr. Dig. *Electr.* *Euphr.* Ferr. Kal. Kreas. *Lach.* Lyc. Magn. m. Mur. ac. Nicc. *Ol. an.* **Phosph.* Phos. ac. Plat. Rhod. Rhus. *Sec.* *Sep.* *Sil.* Spong. Staph. Stront. *Sulph.* Tart. Thuj. Verb. Zinc.

—, finger-joint, Anac.

—, thumb, Cin. Kal. Plat. *Stront.* Verb. Zinc.

Lower limbs, *Berb.* **Calc.* Carb. veg. Graph. Kal. Lyc. °*N. vom.* Sep. Sulph. Sulph. ac.

—, hips, Calc. °*Lach.* Staph.

—, thighs, Acon. Agar. Carb. veg. °*Euphr.* Ferr. °*Graph.* Hep. Men. Op. Plat.

—, knees, Calc. Graph. Plat.

—, legs, Acon. Alum. Anac. Berb. Borax. Bry. Dulc. Graph. Plat.

Feet, Acon. Amb. Ang. Ant. Ars. *Carb. veg.* *Con.* Electr. Graph. Hep. Lyc. Op. Par. Phos. ac. *Plat.* Rhus.

Feet, heels, Alum. Caust. Clem. *Ign.* N. vom. Sep. Stront.
—, soles, Bry. *Puls.* Sulph.
—, toes, Arn. Chel. Crotal. Cycl. Lach. °*Plumb.* Puls.

Pain, as if contused.

In general, *Acon.* Alum. Ang. *Ant.* **Arg.* **Arn.* *Asa.* Berb. Borax. Calc. Canth. Carb. an. Carb. veg. **Caust.* Cham. Chel. **Cic.* Cin. Clem. **Con.* Cupr. *Cycl.* Dig. **Dros.* Dulc. Euphorb. **Euphr.* Hep. Hyos. *Ign.* *Jod.* *Ipec.* *Kal.* *Lach.* *Led.* Magn. art. Natr. Natr. m. *Nitr.* Nitr. ac. **N. mosch.* **Oleand.* *Par.* Petr. *Phosph.* **Plat.* **Puls.* *Rhod.* **Rhus.* **Ruta.* Sabad. Sabin. *Sep.* Spong. **Sulph.* **Sulph. ac.* Teucr. Thuj. *Veratr.* *Verbasc.* Viol. od. Zinc.
—, as after a blow or push, *Acon.* °*Alum.* *Amm.* *Amm. m.* Anac. **Arn.* Baryt. Bov. Bry. *Cann.* Caust. Cic. **Cin.* Cocc. **Con.* Croc. Cupr. Dros. Dulc. Graph. *Kal.* *Lach.* *Laur.* *Led.* Magn. art. Magn. arct. **Magn. aust.* Magn. c. Magn. m. Mang. *Mez.* Mosch. **Natr.* *Natr. m.* **N. mosch.* N. vom. **Oleand.* **Phosph.* Phos. ac. **Plat.* *Plumb.* **Puls.* Ran. *Ruta.* Sabad. *Sassap.* Staph. Sulph. *Sulph. ac.* Tarax. Thuj. Val. Zinc.

Ears, Arn. Cic. Ruta.

Anus, Alum. Lact. Staph.
—, perinæum, Alum.

Sexual parts, Acon. Arg. *Calc.* Dig. Cal. °Lach. Natr. c. Nitr. ac. Rhod. Sabad. Sabin. Thuj.
Arms, *Dros. Dulc.*
—, shoulder, Acon. Berb. Dros.
—, elbow, Dros. Plat.
—, upper arm, Cycl. Merc.
—, fore arm, Dros. Hep.
Hands, Dros. Spig.
—, finger, Caust. Prun. *Ruta.* Verbasc.
—, thumb, Plat.
Lower limbs, Nitr. Rhod.
—, hip, Euphorb. Gins.
—, knee, Mez. Plat.
—, thigh, Acon. Mur.
Feet, toe, Berb. Daph. Mez. Ruta.
Bones, Ign. Ruta.
Nails, Nitr.
Glands, Arg. Arn. Ars. Carb. an. Caust. Chin. Cic. Con. Cupr. Jod. Kal. Magn. arct. Natr. m. Phosph. Plat. Puls. Rhod. Rhus. Ruta. Sep. Staph. Sulph. Sulph. ac.

SPLINTER, PAIN AS IF FROM A.

Pimples, Arn.
Swelling, Stann.
Splinters, stitches as if from, *Carb. veg.* Cic. *Colch. Hep.* **Nitr. ac.* *Petr.* Plat. Ran. **Sil.* Sulph.

Lips, Bov. Ign. Nitr. ac. Par. Phosph.
Buccal cavity and throat, Laur. Nitr. ac.

Hands, fingers, **Arn.* Bell. Carb. veg. Colch. °*Hep.* °Lach. **Nitr. ac.* Petr. Puls. Ran. *Sil.* Sulph.
Feet, Petr.
Nails, Bell. Carb. veg. Colch. Hep. *Nitr. ac.* Petr. *Sil. Sulph.*

Pain as if luxated.

Dorsal region, Natr. m. Sulph.
Arms, Coloc. Merc.
—, elbows, Lach.
—, upper arm, Caust.
Hands and joints, *Amm. Amm. m. **Arn.* Berb. Bry. **Calc. Carb. veg. Caust.* Hep. *Lach. Laur.* Lyc. Petr. *Puls. Rhod.* Sabin. Sil. *Stann. Verb.*
—, fingers and joints, Ang. Berb. Camph. Cham. Cupr. *Kreas. Phosph.*
—, thumb, Camph. *Kreas. Magn. art. Phosph.* Prun.
Lower limbs, Amm. Berb.
—, hips and nates, Mez. Stann.
—, thighs, Lyc.
—, knees, Agar. Amm. Graph. Ipec. Lach. N. mosch. Phosph. *Staph.* Sulph.
—, calf, *Graph.*
Feet, Agn. *Anac.* Ang. Ant. Ars. *Baryt. Berb.* **Bry.* Camph. Chel. Cupr. Gran. Laur. *Led. Magn. art.* Magn. aust. *Merc.* Mur. ac. Natr. m. Natr. s. *Phosph.* Phos. ac. Plat. Puls. Ran. Rhus. *Sulph.* Veratr. Zinc.
—, heel, *Merc.*
—, toe, Zinc.

Pain as if sprained or strained by lifting.

In general, Alum. **Amb.* **Arn.* Baryt. Borax. **Bry.* **Calc.* **Carb. an.* **Carb. veg.* *Caust.* Chin. **Cocc.* Coloc. Con. Croc. Dulc. Ferr. **Graph.* *Jod. **Kal.* Lach. **Lyc.* *Magn. c.* Merc. *Mur. ac.* **Natr.* **Natr. m.* Nitr. ac. *N. vom.* Oleand. *Phosph.* *Phos. ac.* Plat. Rhod. **Rhus.* Ruta. **Sep.* **Sil.* Spig. Stann. Staph. **Sulph.* Sulph. ac. Thuj. Val.

Dorsal region, Bell. **Calc.* Canth. *Caust.* Cocc. Kal. Mur. ac. *N. vom.* Oleand. °*Rhus.* Stann. *Staph.* Val.

Pain, as if sprained or strained by wrenching.

In general, Acon. Agar. **Agn.* Alum. **Amb.* **Amm.* **Amm. m.* Anac. Ang. Ant. **Arn.* Ars. Asar. Aur. Baryt. Bell. Bov. **Bry.* *Calc. Camph. *Caps.* **Carb. an.* **Carb. veg.* **Caust.* Cham. Chel. Chin. Cin. Cocc. Con. Croc. Cycl. Dig. Dros. Dulc. Euphorb. **Graph.* Hell. Hep. **Ign.* Ipec. Kal. Led. *Lyc.* Magn. art. Magn. arct. **Magn. aust.* Magn. c. Magn. m. Mang. Men. Merc. Mez. Mosch. Mur. ac. *Natr.* **Natr. m.* Nitr. **Nitr. ac.* N. mosch. **N. vom.* Oleand. **Petr.* **Phosph.* *Phos. ac.* Plat. Plumb. **Puls.* Ran. **Rhod.* **Rhus.* **Ruta.* Sabin. Sassap. Seneg. **Sep.* Sil. Spig. Spong. Stann. Staph. **Sulph.* Tart. Thuj. Val. Veratr. *Zinc.*

Lower jaw, Hep. Ign. Magn. Magn. arct. Rhus. Spig. Spong. Staph.
Dorsal region, **Calc.* N. vom. *Puls.*
—, neck, Cinn. Sassap.
—, small of back, Agar. Lach. Magn. aust. Ol. an. Petr. Rhod. Sep. *Sulph.*
—, nape of neck, Agar. Nicc. Nitr. Sulph. Tong.
—, back, Agar. Bell. Con. Lyc. *Petr. Sulph.*
—, scapulæ, Baryt. Kal. Petr. Plumb. *Rhod.* Sulph.
Arms, Bov. Ign. Nitr. ac. Phosph. Stann.
—, shoulder and joint, Alum. Amb. Anac. Asar. Bry. Caps. Caust. Croc. Pep. Ign. Magn. arct. Magn. c. Mang. Mur. ac. Oleand. Petr. Phosph. Puls. Ruta. Sabin. Sep. Spig. Stann. Staph. Tart.
—, elbow, Alum. Mang. Tab.
—, upper arm, Alum. Euphorb. Lact. *Rhod.* Tereb.
—, forearm, Cocc. Led. Natr.
Hands and joints, Alum. **Amm. m.* Anac. *Arn.* Baryt. Bov. *Bry.* **Calc. Carb. an. Caust.* Cin. Cist. Con. Ferr. magn. Graph. *Ign.* Lach. Mez. N. vom. Phosph. Prun. *Rhod. Rhus.* °*Ruta.* Sassap. Seneg. Sil. *Stann. Sulph.* Thuj. Zinc.
—, fingers and joints, Acon. Alum. °*Graph. Ign. Laur.* Lyc. Magn. c. *Natr. m. Nitr.* N. mosch. *Phosph.* Rhod. Stann. *Sulph.*
—, thumb, Con. °*Graph. Laur. Magn. art.* Natr. m. Nitr. Petr. *Phosph.* Prun. *Sulph.* Veratr.
Lower limbs, Dros. °*Rhus.* Thuj.
—, hips and joints, Amm. m. Anac. Ang. *Arn.* Aspar. Baryt. Bell. Calc. **Caust.* Cham. Chin. Con. Dros. Dulc. Euphorb. *Hep.* °*Ipec. Laur.*

Lyc. **Natr. m.* Nitr. ac. Petr. Phosph. Puls. Rhod. Rhus. v. Stann. Sulph.

Lower limbs, thighs, Amm. Caps. Euphorb. Led. Mosch. Rhod. Stann. Staph.

–, knees, Amb. Ars. Calc. Chin. Con. Gent. ***Kal.*** Kreas. ***Lach.*** Lyc. Men. Natr. ***Natr. m.*** Nitr. Nitr. ac. Phosph. Plat. Prun. Rhod. Sulph.

—, tendo Achilles, Kreas.

Feet and joints, Ang. Arg. Arn. Ars. Bell. ****Bry.*** Calc. ***Caust.*** Chin. Cocc. Croton. ***Cycl.*** Dig. Dros. Hell. ***Ign.*** ***Lyc.*** Magn. art. Magn. aust. ***Men.*** Mosch. °*Natr.* Nitr. Nitr. ac. N. vom. Plumb. ***Prun.*** ***Rhab.*** ***Rhus.*** Ruta. Sil. Sulph. ***Val.*** ***Zinc.***

—, heel, Cycl. Euphorb. Laur. Nitr.

—, toes, °*Amm.* Arn. Aur. Carb. an. Kal. Mosch. Petr. Ratanh. Sil.

Pain as if ulcerated.

In general, Alum. Amb. *Amm.* **Amm. m.* Anac. Ang. Ars. Bell. Bov. ****Bry.*** Canth. Caps. Caust. ****Cham.*** ***Chin.*** *Cic.* Cocc. Dros. Ferr. ***Graph.*** Hep. Ign. Kal. ***Kreas.*** Lach. Laur. Magn. c. ****Magn. m.*** ***Mang.*** ***Merc.*** ***Mur. ac.*** Natr. ***Natr. m.*** Nitr. Nitr. ac. N. vom. Petr. Phosph. Phos. ac. ****Puls.*** ****Rhus.*** ***Ruta.*** ***Sang.*** Sassap. ***Sep.*** ****Sil.*** Spig. Spong. Stann. Staph. Sulph. Sulph. ac. Tarax. ****Thuj.*** Veratr. Zinc.

Pain as if from subcutaneous ulceration, in general, Agn. Amm. Anac. ****Arn.*** Ars. Asa. Aur. Baryt. ****Bry.*** Calc. Carb. veg. Chin. Colch. Con. ***Cycl.*** Dros. Euphorb. ***Graph.*** ****Hep.*** Hyos. Jod.

*_Kal._ Kreas. Led. *_Mang._ Natr. m. Nitr. ac. N. vom. Par. Petr. ***Phosph.** ***Puls.** **Ran.** _Rhod._ ***Rhus.** Ruta. Sassap. _Sec._ _Sil._ Stann. Staph. _Sulph._ Tarax. Val. Veratr. _Zinc._

Ears, Anac. Calc. Ferr. Kal. Magn. c. Mang. Mur. ac.

Nose, Amm. m. Arn. Bry. Camph. Canth. Cocc. Dulc. Graph. Ign. Kal. Mur. ac. Nitr. *_N. vom._ Petr. Puls. Rhus. Staph. Veratr.

Face, Acon. Caps. Chin. Lyc. Mang. Natr. Natr. m. Rhus. _Staph._

Lips, Chin. Ign. Magn. arct.

Chin, Euphorb. Mang. Spong.

Lower jaw, Caps. Magn. c. Natr.

Buccal cavity, Alum. _Amm._ Bell. Bov. Carb. an. Carb. veg. _Caust._ Graph. Kal. hdr. °Magn. c. Mang. Natr. _Nicc._ Nitr. Ol. an. Phell. Phos. ac.

—, palate, Amm. Caust.

—, fauces and throat, Kal. hdr. _Nicc._ Nitr. ac. Phos. ac.

Gums, Alum. Amm. Bell. Bov. Carb. an. Carb. veg. Caust. Graph. Kal. hdr. °Magn. c. Mang. Natr. Nicc. Nitr. Ol. an. Phell.

Abdomen, region of, Amm. m. _Bov._ Dig. Hell. _Kreas._ Magn. c. Mang. °Nitr. ac. **Ran.** **Rhus.**

—, umbilical region, Magn. c.

Anus, Magn. c.

Thorax, °Spig. _Staph._

Dorsal region, axillary glands, Prun.

—, lumbar vertebræ, Kreas.

—, nape of neck, Puls.

Dorsal region, spinal column, Carb. an.
—, scapulæ, Calend. Cist.
Arms, Sep. Staph. Tab. Thuj.
—, elbow, Natr. s.
—, upper arm, Baryt.
—, forearm, Stront.
Hands, Plat. Sil. Sulph. ac. Teucr.
—, wrists, Bov.
—, fingers, Berb. Bry. Carb. veg. Caust. Graph. Kal. Par. Plat. Sassap. *Sil.*
—, finger-joints, Kal.
Lower limbs, Sep.
—, nates and hips, Berb. Calc. ***Kal. Phosph.*** Prun. Puls. Sulph. Verbasc.
—, thighs, Anac. Sep.
—, knee, Caust. Ol. an. Rhod.
—, legs, *Jod.* Puls.
Feet, Amm. m. **Bry.* Caust. Hep. Indig. Lyc. **Natr. m.* Nitr.
—, soles, Amb. *Baryt.* Calc. *Canth. Graph.* °*Ign.* Kreas. Laur. Lyc. Magn. s. Nitr. °***Phosph.*** Prun. *Puls. Spig.* Sulph. Zinc.
—, heel, Amm. Amm. m. Berb. Carb. an. ***Caust.*** Euphorb. Graph. Kal. hdr. Laur. Natr. s. Zinc.
—, toes, Amm. Carb. an. Carb. veg. Caust. Con. Kal. hdr. *Natr.* Phos. ac. *Sil.* Val. Zinc.
Glands, Amm. Amm. m. Aur. Bell. Bry. Calc. Canth. Caust. Cham. Chin. Cic. Cocc. Graph. Hep. Ign. Kal. Merc. Mur. ac. Natr. Natr. m. Nitr. ac. Petr. Phosph. Puls. Rhus. Ruta. Sil. Staph. Sulph. ac. Teucr. Zinc.

Painful, which is.

Blisters, vesicles, Anac. ***Bell.*** Berb. Borax. Chen. Cic. Graph. ***Kal.*** Lach. Natr. m. Natr. s. Nitr. ac. N. vom. ***Phosph.*** Puls. Sulph. Val. Zinc.

Bloodvessels, swelling of, ****Caust.*** Coloc.

Chilblains, Arn. Bell. Chin. Hep. Lyc. Magn. c. °*Nitr. ac.* N. vom. °***Petr.*** Phosph. Phos. ac. °***Puls.*** Sep.

Cicatrices of former ulcers and wounds, Carb. veg. Lach. Natr. m. °*Nitr. ac.* °***N.*** *vom.*

—, during a change of weather, Carb. veg. °*Nitr. ac.*

Corns, Agar. Alum. Amm. ****Ant.*** °***Arn.*** °***Baryt.*** Bov. Bry. **Calc.* Camph. Carb. an. Carb. veg. Gran. Hep. **Ign.* Jod. Kal. Lach. °***Lyc.*** Magn. art. °*Magn. arct.* Magn. aust. Meph. Natr. Natr. m. **Nitr. ac.* °*N. vom.* Petr. Phosph. °***Puls.*** Ran. Rhus. ****Sep.*** °***Sil.*** Spig. °***Sulph.***

Eruption, ***Agar.*** Amb. ***Ant.*** Arg. ***Arn.*** ****Ars.*** *Asa.* Aur. Baryt. ***Bell.*** Calc. Cann. Canth. Caps. ***Chin.*** *Clem.* Cocc. *Con.* *Cupr.* ***Dulc.*** Guaj. ***Hep.*** Kal. Kal. chl. **Lach.* Led. **Lyc.* Magn. arct. Magn. aust. ***Magn. c. Magn. m. Merc.*** Natr. N. vom. Par. ***Petr.*** Phosph. *Phos. ac.* ***Puls.*** Ran. Ran. sc. Rhus. Ruta. Selen. Seneg. *Sep.* *Sil.* *Spig.* Spong. Stram. Sulph. Tart. Thuj. Val. *Veratr.* Verb.

Figwarts, Sabin.

Herpes, °Dulc.

Nails, Amm. m. ***Ant.*** Bell. Carb. veg. ****Caust.*** ****Graph.*** ****Hep.*** Kal. Lyc. Magn. art. ****Magn. aust. Merc.*** Natr. m. ***Nitr. ac. N. vom.*** Par.

Petr. Phos. ac. Puls. Ran. Rhod. Rhus. Sabad. Sep. ***Sil. Squill.*** Stann. ***Sulph.***

Pimples, Ant. Arg. Arn. Cocc. ***Con.*** Graph. Kal. Kal. chl. Kal. hdr. Lach. Mur. ac. Natr. Nitr. ac. N. vom. Phosph. Plumb. Puls. Seneg. Spong. Squill. Sulph. Veratr.

Pustules, Ars. Berb. Stram. Tart.

Rhagades, Graph. Mang. Zinc.

Scurfs, Magn. m.

Spots, Alum. Amb. Ars. Berb. Calc. Cann. Caust. °*Con.* Lach. Mosch. Nitr. ac. Petr. Rhod.

Swelling, Amb. *Amm.* **Arn.* **Ars.* *Aur.* Baryt. **Bell.* Bov. °*Bry.* Calc. Canth. Carb. an. Carb. veg. *Caust.* **Cham.* **Chin.* *Con.* Cop. Crotal. Croton. Cupr. °*Daph.* Dig. Dulc. Electr. **Ferr.* **Hep.* Kal. Kal. hdr. **Lach.* **Led.* **Lyc.* Magn. art. **Magn. arct.* *Magn. c.* *Magn. m.* **Merc.* **Merc. corr.* Mez. Mur. ac. Natr. Natr. m. Nitr. **Nitr. ac.* **N. vom.* Oph. **Phosph.* **Phos. ac.* Plat. Plumb. **Puls.* Ran. sc. Rhod. **Rhus.* Sabin. Sassap. Sec. **Sep.* **Sil.* Spig. Spong. Stann. Staph. Stront. **Sulph.* Tereb. **Thuj.* *Vip. torv.*

Tubercles, *Amm.* Ars. Bell. Bov. °*Lach.* Lyc. Phos. ac. Zinc.

Tumors, blotches, °Ars. Caust. *Lyc.* *N. vom.* Oph.

Ulcers, Alum. Amm. Anac. Ang. °*Arn.* **Ars.* °*Asa.* Aur. *Bell.* Carb. an. **Carb. veg.* Caust. Cham. Chin. Cic. Cinn. Clem. Cocc. Coff. Con. Croc. Cupr. Dig. Dulc. **Graph.* **Hep.* Hyos. Jod. Kreas. °*Lach.* °*Lyc.* °*Merc.* ***Mercurial.*** Mez. ***Mur. ac. Natr. m. Nitr. ac.*** N. vom. ***Petr.***

Phosph. °*Phos. ac.* °*Puls.* ***Ran.*** Ran. sc. Rhus. **Sabin.* Sassap. Selen. °*Sep.***Sil.* Squill. Staph. ***Sulph.*** Thuj. *Veratr. Zinc.*

Warts, ****Caust.*** Natr. Natr. m. Nitr. ac. Sabin. Sulph. Thuj.

Head, °Clem. °Daph. *Graph. Hell. Kal. Magn. c. Merc. N. vom. Par.

Nose, **Alum.* Amm. Amm. m. Arn. Ars. ****Bell.*** Borax. **Bry.* Calc. Canth. Caps. ***Carb. an.*** Clem. Coff. Colch. Corall. Dulc. °Euphr. *Graph. Guaj. **Ign.* ***Kal.*** Lach. Lam. Led. ***Lyc.*** **Magn. m.* Merc. Natr. ***Natr. m.*** Nitr. ***N. vom.*** Petr. Phos. ac. Poth. Puls. Rhus. ***Sep. Sil.*** Spig. Squill. Sulph. Tart. Zinc.

Face, Alum. Bell. Berb. Cham. Con. Eugen. Lach. Sabad. Stann. Val.

Lips, Kal. Natr. m. Phosph.

Buccal cavity, eruptions, blisters, Anac. Arg. Bell. Berb. Borax. Chen. Graph. ***Kal.*** Mur. ac. Natr. m. Natr. s. Nitr. ac. ***N. vom.*** Phosph. Puls. Sulph. Zinc.

—, swollen parts, Amb. Amm. Baryt. Bov. Calc. Carb. an. **Caust.* °*Cham.* Chin. Con. ***Graph.*** Hep. Kal. Lach. Lyc. ****Magn. art.*** Magn. arct. Magn. m. **Merc.* Natr. m. Nitr. N. vom. Phos. ac. ***Plat.*** Ran. sc. Sabin. ****Sep.*** **Sil.* Spong. Staph. Stront. **Sulph.* Tab. Thuj.

—, ulcers, Merc. Natr. m. Phosph. Rhod.

Abdomen, swelling, °Lach. Tereb. Thuj. Vip. torv.

—, inguinal glands, region of, Agar. Ant. Croton. ****Graph.*** Hep. ****Therid.***

Anus, eruptions, Lyc.
—, swelling, Aur.
—, ulcers, Sassap.
—, varices, Amm. °*Anac.* Ars. Calc. Caps. ****Carb. veg. Caust.*** Coloc. Ferr. °***Graph.*** Grat. Kal. Lach. Lyc. Magn. art. Magn. c. Magn. m. Mur. ac. °*Natr. m. Nitr.* Nitr. ac. N. vom. Phosph. Puls. Sabin. Sep. Sil. Stront. Sulph. ac. Thuj. Zinc.

Sexual parts, eruptions, Bov. Con. Nitr. ac. Sil.
—, swelling, °Arn. Ars. Cop. **Merc.* Vip. torv.

Thoracic region, eruption, °Lyc.
—, pimples, Con.
—, swelling, Rhus.

Dorsal region, eruption, Clem. °Lyc. Magn. aust.
—, blisters, Cic.
—, pimples, Ant. Arn. Puls. Spong. Squill.
—, swelling, Amm. Arn. **Bell.* Carb. veg. Cupr. Kal. Lach. Lyc. Magn. m. Natr. **Nitr. ac.* N. vom. Rhus. Sassap. Spig. Spong. Sulph.
—, blotches, °Lach. Phos. ac. Zinc.

Arms, eruptions, Ars. Kal. °Lyc. Petr.
—, swelling, N. vom. Rhus.

Hands, Amb. Ars. Borax. Calc. Led. Magn. arct. Mang. Sec. Sulph. ac. Zinc.
—, rhagades, ***Graph.*** Mang. *Merc.* ****Sulph.*** Zinc.
—, ulcers, Lyc.
—, swelling, Chin. Hep. Merc. Nitr. ac. N, vom. Phosph. Sep.

Lower limbs, varices, Coloc.
—, blotches, Merc. N. vom.
—, pimples, Phosph.

Lower limbs, spots, Amb. Cann. Caust. °*Con.* Graph. Lach. ***Mosch.*** Petr.
—, swelling, ***Lach. Oph.*** Rhod. Sil.
—, ulcers, Staph.
Feet, eruption, Lyc. Phosph. Spig. °***Sulph.***
—, swelling, °***Bry.*** Con. °*Daph.* Ferr. ***Led.***°***Merc.*** Phosph. Phos. ac. Rhus. Sabad. ***Sulph.***

PAINFULNESS, PAINFUL SENSITIVENESS.

In general, Acon. °*Agar.* Alum. °*Amm.* Anac. Ant. Arn. **Ars.* **Asa.* Aur. Baryt. Berb. ****Bell.*** Bov. *Bry.* **Calc. Camph.* Cann. ***Canth.*** Caps. **Carb. an.* **Carb. veg.* Caust. Cham. ***Chin.*** Chinin. Cinn. Cocc. *Coff.* Colch. °***Con.*** Croc. °*Ferr.* Galv. ***Hep.*** Hyos. Ign. °*Ipec.* Kal. Kal. chl. Kreas. **Lach.* **Led.* **Lyc.* Magn. arct. Magn. aust. *Magn. c.* Merc. Mez. ***Mosch.*** Mur. ac. *Natr. Natr. m.* °Nitr. ac. *N. mosch.* **N. vom.* Oleand. Oph. Par. **Petr.* ***Phosph.*** ****Phos. ac.*** Plumb. *Puls.* Ran. Ran. sc. ****Rhus.*** Sassap. Sec. ***Selen.*** Seneg. ***Sep.*** ****Sil.*** **Spig.* Spong. Squill. Stann. Staph. Stram. ***Sulph.*** Sulph. ac. Tart. **Thuj.* **Veratr.* Vinc. Vip. red. Vip. torv.

———

Scalp, Alum. Amb. Ars. **Baryt.* ***Bell.*** Borax. Bov. *Bry.* ***Calc.*** Carb. an. ***Carb. veg.*** **Chin.* Chinin. ***Ferr.*** Grat. Ign. ***Lach.*** Lyc. Magn. c. Magn. m. Mang. Natr. c. Natr. m. Nitr. *Nitr. ac. **N. vom.* Par. ***Petr.*** Phosph. Phos. ac. Rhus. Sassap. Selen. ***Sep. Sil.*** Spig. Spong. Squill. ***Sulph.*** *Zinc.

Head, Agar. Alum. Amb. Amm. Ant. ***Ars.** **Baryt.** **Bell.** **Bry.** **Calc.** **Carb. veg.** ***Chin.** Cinn. **Ferr.** Ign. Lact. Lyc. Magn. c. ***Merc.** Mez. **Mosch.** Natr. c. Natr. m. Nitr. Nitr. ac. ***N. vom.** Par. **Petr.** Phosph. Phos. ac. Rhod. Rhus. Sabin. Sassap. **Spig.** **Staph.** **Sulph.**

Chin, Mang. N. mosch.

Mammæ and nipples, Amm. Berb. Borax. Calc. Con. ***Graph.** **Merc.** Murex. N. vom. Rhab.

—, nipples, *Graph. N. vom. Rhab.

Bones, periosteum, Acon. Agn. ***Amb.** Agar. Alum. Amm. Amm. m. Anac. Ang. Ant. ***Arg.** Arn. ***Ars.** ***Asa.** ***Aur.** Baryt. Bell. Bism. Bry. ***Calc.** Camph. Cann. Canth. Caps. Carb. an. Carb. veg. Caust. Cham. Chel. ***Chin.** Chinin. Cic. Clem. °***Cocc.*** Colch. Coloc. °**Con.** ***Crotal.** ***Cupr.** ***Cycl.** °**Daph.** Dig. **Dros.** Dulc. **Euphorb.** **Ferr.** Graph. Guaj. Hell. °**Hep.** Ign. Jod. Ipec. **Kal.** ***Kreas.** ***Lach.** Led. °**Lyc.** Magn. art. Magn. arct. Magn. c. Magn. m. ***Mang.** ***Merc.** ***Mez.** ***Mur. ac.** Nat. **Natr. m.** ***Nitr. ac.** N. mosch. **N. vom.** Oleand. Op. Petr. **Phosph.** ***Phos. ac.** Plumb. Poth. ***Puls.** Ran. sc. ***Rhod.** ***Rhus.** ***Ruta.** Sabad. ***Sabin.** Samb. Sassap. Sec. Sep. ***Sil.** **Spig.** Spong. ***Staph.** Stront. ***Sulph.** Thuj. Val. **Veratr.** Viol. tr. ***Zinc.**

Nails, Amm. **Ant.** Bell. Carb. veg. ***Caust.** ***Graph.** ***Hep.** Kal. Lyc. Magn. art. ***Magn. aust.** **Merc.** Natr. m. **Nitr. ac.** **N. vom.** Par. Petr. Phos. ac. Puls. Ran. Rhod. Rhus. Sabad. Sep. **Sil.** **Squill.** Stann. **Sulph.**

Glands, ***Acon.** Alum. Amb. Amm. Ant. Arn. Ars. Aur. ***Baryt.** ***Bell.** Berb. Borax. Bry. ***Calc.** Calend. ***Cann.** Canth. ***Carb. an.** Carb.

veg. Caust. Cham. Chin. Cic. Clem. Cocc. *Coloc.* Con. Coral. Dulc. ****Graph.*** Hell. Hep. Ign. ****Jod.*** Kal. ****Lyc.*** Magn. arct. Magn. c. Magn. m. ****Merc.*** Murex. Natr. m. Nitr. ac. N. vom. Petr. ****Phosph.*** °Phos. ac. Puls. Rhab. Rhus. Selen. °Sep. **Sil.* *Spig.* *Spong.* Squill. Stann. Staph. Stram. ****Sulph.*** Sulph. ac. Tart. Thuj. Veratr.

PAINLESS, WHICH IS.

Eruption, ***Amb.*** *Anac.* Ant. Bell. Cham. *Cocc.* ***Con.*** Cycl. Dros. *Hell.* ***Hyos.*** Lach. Laur. ***Lyc.*** Nitr. ***Oleand.*** Phosph. ***Phos. ac.*** Puls. Rhus. Samb. ***Sec.*** Spig. Staph. *Stram.* *Sulph.* Tart.
Blisters, vesicles, Stront. Sulph.
Pimples, Alum. Sulph.
Pustules, Rhod.
Spots, Graph. Led. Phos. ac. Sep. Stann.
Swelling, Calc. Dros. °*Euphr.* °Lyc. Natr. s. Par. Phosph. Puls. Rhus. *Sep.* Sil. Staph.
Ulcers, ***Ars.*** Bell. *Carb. veg.* Cocc. Con. Hell. Hyos. Ign. *Lach.* Laur. Lyc. Magn. art. Merc. Nitr. ac. Oleand. Op. Phosph. °*Phos. ac.* Puls. Rhus. Sec. *Sep.* Stram. Sulph.
Blotches, tubercles, Arn. Bell. Graph. °*Ign.* Led. Oleand. Squill. Veratr.

Mouth, swollen parts, Natr. s. Par.
Sexual parts, eruptions, Arn. Bell.
—, swelling, Jod.
—, ulcers, Nitr. ac.
Dorsal region, eruption, Nitr.
—, swelling, Sep.
—, indurations (glandular), °Ign.
Hands, swelling, Euphr. Lyc.

Lower limbs, swelling, Puls. Sep.
Glands, swelling or suppuration, Ars. Asa. **Calc.* *Cocc.* *Con.* Cycl. *Dulc.* Ign. Lach. Nitr. ac. *Phos. ac.* Plumb. Rhod. *Sep.* Sil. Spig. Staph. Sulph.

Paleness, pale colour.

Of the skin in general, **Ars.* Baryt. *Bell.* **Calc.* **Camph.* Carb. an. Carb. veg. Caust. **Chin.* **Cocc.* **Con.* **Crotal.* Dig. **Ferr.* Graph. Hydroc. **Hell.* Ign. *Kal.* *Lach.* *Lyc.* Merc. **Natr. m.* **Nitr. ac.* **N. vom.* Oleand. *Oph.* **Phosph.* Phos. ac. **Plat.* Plumb. **Puls.* Sabin. *Sec.* *Sep.* *Spig.* Staph. **Sulph.* Sulph. ac. Val. *Vip. red.* Zinc.
Chlorotic, °Ars.? °*Calc.* °Chin.? °Cocc. °*Con.* °*Crotal.* °Ferr. °Graph. °Hell. °*Lyc.* °N. vom. °*Phosph.* °*Puls.* °*Sulph.*
Lead-coloured. Plumb. Sec.

Lips, Caust. *Ferr.* Kal. Lyc. Val.
Mouth, Agar. Carb. an. *Chinin.* **Merc.* Natr. Nitr. ac. Raph. Staph.
—, gums, Carb. an. **Merc.* Nitr. ac. Staph.
—, tongue, Agar. Natr. Raph.
Hands, fingers, Cic. *Kreas.* Lach. Par. Sec.

Pale, that which is.

Eruption, Ars.
Swelling. °*Arn.* Ars. **Baryt.* Bell. Bov. **Bry.* *Calc.* Chin. Cocc. Con. Dig. Euphorb. Ferr. Graph. Hell. °*Jod.* Kal. *Lach.* **Lyc.* *Merc.*

Nitr. ac. N. vom. Oph. Plumb. ***Puls.*** *****Rhus.*** *Sep.* Spig. Sulph. Vip. torv.

Face, swelling, Bov. °***Bry.*** Euphorb. Hell. N. vom. Rhus. Sep.
Buccal cavity, swelling, Nitr. ac.
Arms, swelling, Sec. Vip. torv.
Hands, swelling, ****Bry.*** *N. vom.* Sec.
Lower limbs, swelling, Op.
Feet, swelling, Ars.

PALE-RED, THAT WHICH IS.

Vesicles, Rhus.
Pimples, Bell.
Pus, Dulc.
Pustules, Ars.
Tetters, Clem. °Dulc.
Spots, Cann. Carb. an. Carb. veg. Rhod. Sassap. Teucr. Vip. red.

Face, eruptions, Bell. Carb. an. Carb. veg. Sassap. Teucr.
Buccal cavity, swelling, **Baryt.*
Sexual parts, eruptions, Cann.
Hands, eruption, ***Ars. Rhus.***

PALE TURNING.

In the cold, spots, *Sabad.*
From pressure of the finger, Bry. Ferr. magn.

PARCHMENT, LIKE.

Hard skin, **Ars. Chin.* Dulc. Kal. Led. °*Lyc.* Phosph. °*Sill.* Squill.

Pedunculated.

Figwarts, °***Lyc.***
Warts, Dulc. °***Lyc.*** Phos. ac.? °***Thuj.***

Peeling off of the skin, exfoliation.

In general, Acon. Amm. Ant. Ars. Borax. Dig. Dros. °***Dulc.*** ***Graph.*** Hell. ***Merc.*** ***Mercurial.*** ***Merc. dulc.*** Mez. Ran. Rhus. Sec. ***Sep.*** ***Sil.***
—, peeling off, sensation as if, ***Agar.*** Alum. ***Amm.*** ***Baryt.*** Calc. ***Lach.*** Merc. ***Phosph.*** ***Phos. ac.*** Sep. Sulph.

Head, Lach.
Nose, °Ars. °Aur. *Aur. m. Canth. Carb. an. Croton. Natr. Tax.
Face, Amm. Canth. Phosph. °Puls. Rhus.
Lips and mouth, Alum. Amm. m. Bell. Canth. Caps. Cham. °***Con.*** ***Kal.*** Kreas. Mez. Mosch. Natr. m. Natr. s. ****N. vom.*** Plat. Plumb. Puls. Sep. Sulph. ac. Tart.
Buccal cavity, Amm. Euphorb. Electr. Lach. Merc. Ran. sc. Sulph.
—, palate, Amm. Electr. Euphorb.
—, mouth, Lach. Merc. Sulph.
—, tongue, Ran. sc.
Arms, forearm, Merc. Stront. Tax.
Hands, Alum. Amm. Amm. m. Baryt. Eugen. Ferr. ***Merc.*** Natr. m. ***Sep.***
—, fingers, Baryt. Sabad. Sep. Sulph.
Lower limbs, ***Merc.***
—, Legs, ***Agar.***

Feet, °*Dulc.* Merc.
—, in erysipelas, °*Dulc.*

PEELING OFF, SENSATION AS IF.

Buccal cavity, Agar. Phosph.

PEELS OFF, THAT WHICH.

Eruption, °*Acon.* °*Amm.* *Amm. m.* Ars. Aur. ****Bell.*** Clem. Cupr. Dulc. Hell. Lach. ****Led.*** Magn. c. Merc. Mez. Oleand. Phell. °***Phosph.*** Phos. ac. Puls. Ran. Sec. °*Sep.* °*Sil.* °*Staph.* Sulph. Teucr. Veratr.
Erysipelas, °Dulc. Puls. Rhus.
Hard skin, Amm. Ant. Borax. °*Dulc.* ***Graph.*** ***Lach.*** Ran. *Rhus.* °*Sep.* *Sil.* Sulph.
Herpes,°*Dulc.* Magn. *Merc.* Sep. (Comp. PEELING OFF.)
Pimples, Thuj.
Pustules, Crot. Hyos.
Spots, Amm. Sep.
Rash, Ars. Stram. Sulph.
Ulcers, Merc.
Vesicles, *Bry. Puls. Rhus.
Head, Lach.
Buccal cavity, eruptions, Electr. Merc.
Thorax, eruptions, Led.
Back, eruption, Phell.
Arms, vesicles, Puls.
Hands, eruptions, Ferr. Jod.

PETECHIÆ, LIKE.

Spots, Arn. °***Ars.*** Bell. ***Berb.*** °***Bry.*** Con. ***Hyos.***

Lach. Led. **N. vom.* ***Oph.*** Phell. °***Phosph.*** ****Rhus.*** Ruta. ***Sec.*** Sil. Stram. Sulph. ac.

Spots, as if ecchymosed, **Arn.* °***Bry.*** °***Calc.*** Cham. Chin. °***Con.*** Crotal. Dulc. Electr. Euphr. Ferr. °***Hep.*** Lach. Laur. Natr. Natr. m. **N. vom.* Par. Plumb. °***Puls.*** Rhus. °Ruta. Sec. ****Sulph.*** **Sulph. ac.*

Pimples.

In general, **Acon.* Agar. Agn. Alum. Amb. Amm. Amm. m. Anac. Ang. **Ant.* Arg. Arn. **Ars.* Asa. Asar. Aur. Aur. m. Baryt. Bar. m. ****Bell.*** Berb. Bism. Borax. Bov. **Bry.* Calad. Calc. Camph. Cann. *Canth.* Caps. Carb. an. Carb. veg. ****Caust.*** ****Cham.*** Chal. Chin. Cic. Cinn. Clem. ***Cocc.*** Coff. Colch. Coloc. ***Con.*** Corall. Crotal. Croc. Cupr. Cycl. Daph. Diad. Dig. ***Dulc.*** Electr. Euphorb. Euphr. Evon. Graph. Grat. Guaj. Hell. Hep. Heracl. Hyos. Jatroph. Ign. Jod. Ipec. Kal. Kal. chl. Kal. hdr. Creas. Lach. Laur. Lyc. Magn. art. Magn. arct. Magn. aust. Magn. c. Magn. m. Magn. s. Mang. Men. ****Merc.*** Mercurial. Mez. Mosch. Mur. ac. Natr. **Natr. m.* Natr. s. Nitr. **Nitr. ac. N.* mosch. N. vom. Oleand. Ol. an. Oph. Op. Par. Petr. **Phosph.* ****Phos. ac.*** Plat. ****Puls.*** Ran. Ran. sc. Rhab. Rhod. **Rhus.* Ruta. Sabad. Sabin. Samb. Sassap. Sec. Selen. Seneg. **Sep.* Sil. Spig. ***Spong.*** Squill. Stann. ****Staph.*** Stram. Stront. ****Sulph.*** Sulph. ac. Tab. Tarax. ***Tart.*** Tereb. Teucr. Thuj. Val. Veratr. Verb. Viol. od. Viol. tr. Vip. red. Vip. torv. ***Zinc.***

Acuminated, ***Ant.*** Ars. Tart.

Acne-shaped, **Bell. Carb. veg.* Hep. Lach.
Black, Carb. veg. Spig.
Bleeding, Stront. Thuj.
Boil-shaped, Natr.
Brown, Veratr.
Burning, Alum. Amm. Arg. *Ars.* Bell. Bov. Bry. *Canth. Caust.* Cinn. Dig. Dulc. *Graph.* Grat. *Kal.* Kal. chl. Lyc. Magn. art. Magn. aust. Magn. m. *Merc. acet.* Mosch. Natr. Natr. m. Natr. s. Nicc. Nitr. Nitr. ac. Ol. an. Phell. Petr. Phosph. °*Phos. ac.* Puls. Ratanh. Rhus. Sabad. *Squill.* Stann. *Staph. Stront. Sulph.* Thuj.
Close together, Cham. Veratr.
Confluent, Mur. ac. Phos. ac.
Containing blood, **Ars.*
Cracked, Merc. acet.
Cutting, Rhus.
As in drunkards, Kreas. °Led.
Drawing, Con. Magn. m. Staph.
Dry, Bov. Kreas.
Fine, Kal.
Flat, Ant.
Gnawing-itching, Ant. *Caust.* Mang. Nitr. ac. Tarax.
Greasy, Kreas.
With green crusts, **Calc.*
Hard, *Bov.* Sabin. Veratr.
Humid, **Calc.* Graph. Kal. Natr. s. Ol. an. Puls. Sil. Sulph. Thuj. Zinc.
Inflamed, Agar. Berb. Petr.
As if from insects, Ant. Ars.
Itching, °*Acon. Amb. Amm.* Amm. m. *Ant.* Ars. *Baryt.* Bell. Bov. **Bry. Calc.* Canth. *Carb.*

veg. ***Caust.*** ***Cham.*** Cin. Cinn. Clem. Cocc. ***Con.*** Dulc. Gins. Graph. ***Hep.*** Jod. ***Kal.*** Kreas. Lach. Lam. ***Laur.*** Led. ***Lyc.*** ***Magn. art.*** ***Magn. arct.*** Magn. aust. Magn. c. Magn. m. Magn. s. ***Merc.*** ***Merc. acet.*** Mill. Mur. ac. ***Natr.*** ***Natr. m.*** ***Natr. s.*** Nitr. ***Nitr. ac.*** N. vom. Ol. an. Phosph. ***Phos. ac.*** Poth. ***Puls.*** Ratanh. Rhus. Sabad. Sabin. Sassap. ***Selen.*** ***Sep.*** ***Sil.*** Squill. Stann. ***Staph.*** Stront. Sulph. Tab. Tarax. Tart. Tax. Veratr. Zinc.

Itch-like, Ant. Bar. m. Bry. Kreas. Magn. art. Rhus. Squill. Tart.

Miliary, Agar. Amm. Ant. Ars. Cocc. Grat. Kal. Kreas.

Painful as if ulcerated, Dulc. Staph.

Painful, Ant. Arg. Arn. Cocc. *Con.* Graph. ***Kal.*** Kal. chl. Kal. hdr. Lach. Mur. ac. Natr. Nitr. ac. N. vom. Phosph. Plumb. Puls. Seneg. Spong. Squill. Sulph. Veratr.

Painless, Alum. Sulph.

Pale, pale-red, Bell.

With peeling off, Thuj.

Pock-shaped, ***Ant.*** ***Arn.*** Petr. Tart.

With pressure, Stann.

Raised, Tax.

Rash-like, Bov. Kal. chl. Rhus. Sassap.

Red, Acon. Alum. Amm. ***Ant.*** Arn. Bell. Berb. ***Bov.*** Bry. Calc. ph. Caust. Cham. Chel. Cin. Crotal. Cycl. Dros. Dulc. Jod. Kal. ***Lach.*** Led. ***Magn. c.*** Phosph. ***Phos. ac.*** Plumb. Rhod. Sassap. Spig. ***Squill.*** ***Staph.*** ***Stront.*** Sulph. Tax. Teucr. ***Thuj.*** Veratr. Zinc.

With red areola, Anac. Canth. Cycl, Samb. Tarax.

Rough, Alum.

Scaly, Dros. Merc.
Old scars, upon, Jod.
Scattered, Berb. Crotal. Kal. chl.
Scurfy, Bell. **Calc.* Carb. an. Cham. Hep. Mur. ac. *Oleand. Petr. Sabin. Staph.
Smarting, Agar. ***Bell.*** Calc. Cham. Coloc. Dig. Kal. Lyc. Merc. Nitr. Teucr. Veratr.
Sore as if excoriated, Alum. Arg. Bell. Bov. Bry. Calc. Clem. Guaj. *Hep.* Hyos. Lam. Magn. arct. Mez. Phos. ac. *Rhus. Sabin.* Selen. Spig. Stann. Teucr. Veratr. Zinc.
Sticking like splinter, Arn.
Stinging, Alum. Ant. Arn. *Bell.* Calc. ph. *Canth.* Caps. Caust. Cocc. Hell. Kal. Kreas. Magn. art. Magn. arct. Natr. Nitr. Petr. Squill. Staph.
Suppurating, Amm. m. Anthrok. Ant. **Ars.* Aur. Baryt. *Bell.* Berb. Calc. ph. Canth. Caust. Cham. **Cic.* *Clem.* Cocc. Con. Croton. Cycl. **Dulc.* Evon. Graph. Grat. Hep. Hydroc. Hyos. Kal. Kal. chl. Kreas. Lach. Lyc. Magn. art. Magn. arct. Magn. c. Magn. m. **Merc.* Mez. *Nitr. ac.* Op. °*Petr.* Phos. ac. Plumb. °*Puls.* **Rhus.* Samb. Sassap. Sec. *Sep.* Sil. Spig. **Staph.* Stram. **Sulph.* Tarax. **Tart.* Thuj. Veratr. Zinc.
Tearing, Dulc.
Tensive, *Arn. Bov.* Con. Mang. Natr. s.
Tickling, Canth.
Titillating, *Bell.* Caust. Magn. m. Veratr.
Transparent, clear, Con.
Ulcers, around the, °Sulph.
Ulcerated, **Merc.* Nitr. ac. Sabin. Sep.
Wart-shaped, Phell.
Water, full of, Coloc. Thuj.

Whitish, Ars. Bov. ***Carb. veg.*** Chel. Coloc. Con. Cycl. Dros. ***Kal.*** Magn. arct. Magn. m. Mang. Natr. m. Petr. Phos. ac. Staph. Sulph. Zinc.

With white tips, *Ant.* Puls. *Tart.*

Yellow, Ant. Grat. Magn. m. Zinc.

Head, Agar. Alum. Anac. Ant. ***Amb.*** Arg. ****Ars.*** Baryt. Bar. m. Berb. Bov. Calc. °Clem. ***Con.*** Cycl. Hell. ****Hep.*** Kal. ****Led.*** Lyc. Magn. art. Magn. arct. Mur. ac. Natr. °*Natr. m.* Nitr. N. vom. Oleand. Par. Petr. Puls. Rhus. Sil. Tarax. Zinc.

Eyes, Baryt. Chel. Guaj. Hep. Ign. Mosch. Par. Selen. **Staph.* Tarax. Thuj.

Eyelids, Alum. Canth. Chel. Hep. Lyc. Natr. m. Rhus. Selen. Seneg.

Ears, Agar. Amm. Berb. Cic. Kal. Kreas. Magn. art. Mur. ac. Natr. m. Petr. Phosph. Sabad. Selen. Spong. Staph. Verbasc.

Nose, ****Amm. Anac.*** Arn. Baryt. Bell. Bov. **Calc.* Canth. Carb. veg. **Caust.* Clem. Dulc. Euphr. *Graph.* Guaj. ***Kal.*** Kal. hdr. Lach. Lam. Magn. arct. Mang. *Natr. Natr. m.* Nitr. Ol. an. Petr. *Phosph.* Phos. ac. Ratanh. ***Sep. Sil.*** Stront. Sulph. Tarax. Tax. Teucr. Thuj.

Face, Agar. Alum. Amb. Amm. Amm. m. **Ant.* Arn. Ars. Aur. *Baryt. ***Bell.*** Berb. Borax. ***Bov. Bry. Cham.*** **Calc.* Calc. ph. ***Canth. Carb. an.*** **Carb. veg. Caust.* *Cic. Clem. ***Cocc.*** Coloc. °Con. Dros. Dulc. Eugen. ****Graph.*** °Hep. ***Kal.*** Kal. chl. Kal. hdr. ****Kreas.*** Lach. Led. ****Lyc.*** Magn. c. Magn. m. Magn. s. Meph. ****Merc.*** Mosch. °Mur. ac. Natr. ****Natr. m.*** °*Nitr. ac.* Ol. an. Petr. °*Phosph.* ****Phos. ac.*** Rhod. Rhus.

Sabin. Sassap. **Sep.* *Sil.* Stann. ***Staph.*** ***Sulph.*** Tab. Tarax. Tart. Thuj. *Veratr.* Vinc. Zinc.

Lips and mouth, region of, Acon. Amm. m. Ant. Arn. Ars. Baryt. Bell. Bov. *Bry. **Calc.* Cann. Canth. Caps. Caust. Chin. Chinin. Coloc. Con. Dulc. Electr. °Hell. Hyos. Ign. Ipec. Kal. Kreas. Led. Magn. art. Magn. arct. Magn. m. Mang. Mur. ac. Natr. Nicc. N. vom. Par. °*Rhus.* Samb. Spig. Spong. Squill. Sulph. Tarax. Teucr. Veratr. °Zinc.

—, corners of mouth, Ant. *Bar.* **Bell.* Calc. Cann. Canth. Carb. veg. Caust. Coloc. Graph. Hep. Ign. Magn. arct. Mang. Merc. Natr. Petr. Phosph. Rhod. Rhus. Sep. Tarax. Veratr.

Chin, Alum. Amb. Anac. Ant. Bell. Berb. Calc. Canth. Caust. Cic. Clem. Con. Dros. Dulc. Hep. Hyos. Laur. Lyc. Magn. art. Magn. aust. Natr. Natr. s. Nitr. ac. N. mosch. N. vom. Oleand. Par. Rhus. Sabin. Sassap. Sep. Sil. Spig. Spong. Sulph. Thuj. Veratr. Verb. Zinc.

Lower jaw, Par.

Buccal cavity, Arg. Berb. Caps. Dulc. Hell. Kal. *Mur. ac.* Natr. Nitr. ac. *N. vom.* Plumb. Sep.

—, palate, Dulc. *Mur. ac. N. vom.*

—, mouth, Caps.

—, tongue, Arg. Berb. Caps. Hell. Kal. Natr. Nitr. ac. Plumb. Sep.

Abdomen and stomach, region of, Ars. Bar. m. Bry. Cham. Dulc. Natr. Natr. m. Petr.

Anus, Carb. veg. Kal. Nitr. ac.

—, perinæum, Nitr. ac.

Sexual parts, Amb. *Con.* Graph. Kal. *Lach.* Magn. aust. *Merc.* Natr. m. *Nitr. ac.* Phos. ac. Sil. Tart. Thuj. Zinc.
—, glans, Lach. Magn. aust. Nitr. ac.
—, hairy part, Lach.
—, scrotum, Phos. ac. Thuj. Zinc.
—, penis, Phos. ac.
—, mons veneris, Amb. Kal. Sil.
—, labia, Con. Graph. Kal. Natr. m.
—, prepuce, Magn. aust. Nitr. ac. Sil.
Chest, Amm. Ant. Bell. Berb. Borax. Bov. Calc. Canth. Chin. Cocc. Con. Dulc. Gins. *Hep.* Jod. *Lach.* Magn. m. Natr.. *Plumb. Rhus.* Squill. Staph. *Stront.* Tab. Zinc.
Dorsal region, axilla, Phosph.
—, neck, Ant. Aur. Berb. Bov. *Cinn.* Clem. Gins. Hep. Magn. arct. Magn. c. Mez. Nitr. Phell. Phos. ac. *Puls.* Spig. Spong. *Squill.* Staph. Sulph. *Thuj.*
—, small of back, Calc. Tab.
—, loins, Cham. Chin.
—, nape of neck, Arn. Bar. m. Bell. Berb. Borax. Calc. °Carb. veg. Hep. Kal. Lyc. Magn. aust. Magn. c. Natr. Nitr. *Sil.* Staph.
—. back, Alum. Berb. Calc. °Carb. veg. Cocc. Con. Dig. Jod. Led. Magn. m. Meph. Mill. *Natr. m.* Phos. ac. Puls. Sassap. *Selen. Squill.* Sulph. Tab. Zinc.
—, scapulæ, Ant. Bell. Berb. Crotal. Kal. chl. Lyc. Magn. m. Mosch. *Puls.* Ratanh. Squill.
Arms, Amm. Amm. m. Ant. Baryt. Bell. Berb. Bov. Bry. Canth. Carb. veg. *Caust.* Chin. Cocc. *Dulc. Hyos. Kal.* Lach. Laur. *Magn. c.* Magn. s. Mosch. Natr. Natr. s. *Nitr.* °*Phos.*

ac. Ratanh. Rhod. Sabad. *Sabin.* Sassap.. Sep. *Staph.* Sulph. Tart. *Tax. Zinc.*

Arms, shoulder, Berb. Cocc. *Kal.* Magn. c. Nitr. *Zinc.*

—, arm, Baryt. Canth. Chin. Kal. Lach. Magn. c. °*Phosph. ac.* Tart.

—, elbow, Amm. m. Ant. Bell. Berb. Bry. *Dulc. Hyos.* Lach. Natr. Nitr. *Sabin.* Sep. *Staph.*

—, upper arm, Carb. veg. *Dulc. Kal.* Lach. *Laur.* Mosch. Tax.

—, forearm, Amm. Amm. m. Bov. *Caust.* Lach. Laur. Lyc. Magn. c. *Magn. s. Natr. s.* Nitr. Ratanh. Rhod. Sabad. Sassap. Sulph. *Tax. Zinc.*

Hands, Agar. Amm. m. Ant. Bov. Canth. *Kreas. Lyc.* Mur. ac. Par. *Rhus. Selen. Tarax. Zinc.*

—, wrists, Baryt. Bry. *Rhus.*

—, fingers, Anac. Ant. Arn. Ars. Berb. Canth. Cycl. *Kal. Lyc.* Magn. c. Mur. ac. *Phos. ac. Spig.* Squill. Tab. Tarax. *Therid. Zinc.*

—, wrist-joints, Cycl.

—, thumb, Ant. *Kal. Lyc. Therid.*

Lower limbs, Bar. m. Natr. m. *Petr. Staph.*

—, nates, hips, Ant. Baryt. Berb. Bry. Canth. Graph. Magn. c. Merc. N. vom. *Petr.* Selen. *Thuj.*

—, thigh, Agar. Ant. Berb. Bry. Bov. Bry. Calc. Chel. Cocc. *Kal.* Kal. chl. *Lach.* Magn. c. *Mang. Mez. Natr. m. Petr. Phosph. Prun. Rhod.* Sassap. *Selen. Stann.* Staph. *Sulph. Zinc.*

—, knee, Ant. Bry. Hep. Nicc. Phos. ac. Puls. Sassap, Sep. Sulph. Zinc.

Lower limbs, legs, calves, shins, Agar. Arg. Bov. Bry. Natr. Puls. Sabin. Sassap. *Sep.* *Staph.* Zinc.
Feet, Ars. *Bov.* Led. Mosch. *Selen.* *Sep.* Sulph.
—, soles, Con.
—, toes, Borax. *Sulph.* Zinc.

Pocks.

In general, °Acon. Amm. m. **Ant.* *Arn.* **Ars.* °*Bell.* *Bry.* Canth. (Cham.) Clem. Cocc. (Coff.) *Hydroc.* **Hyos.* Lach. Magn. art. **Merc.* Nitr. ac. Oph. *Puls.* **Rhus.* Sec. Sil. °*Sol. m.* Stram. *Sulph.* **Tart.* Thuj.
Variola, Ant.? °*Ars.* °Bell. °*Merc.* °*Rhus.* °Sulph. °Tart.
Burning, °Ars. Lach. Merc.
Suppurating, Ars. °Bell. °*Merc.* °*Sulph.* Thuj.
Varioloid, °Ant. °*Ars.* °*Bell.* °Bry. °Merc. °*Puls.* °*Rhus.* °Sulph. °Tart.
Varicellæ millæ, °*Led.* °*Rhus.*
Black pocks, Ant. **Ars.* **Bell.* Bry. Hyos. **Lach.* Mur. ac. °*Rhus.* *Sec.* Sep. Sil. Spig.
Varicellæ conoïdes, °*Acon.* **Ant.* Ars. Bell. °*Bry.* °*Carb. veg.* Caust. Cycl. Ipec. Natr. Natr. m. **Puls.* °*Sep.* **Tart.* *Thuj.*
Varicellæ aquosæ, Acon. Ant. *Bell.* °*Puls.* °*Rhus.* Sec. °*Sil.* °Sol. m. *Tart.* Thuj.
Whitish pocks, Jod. Lyc.

Head, Bov.
Nose, Canth. **Merc.*
Chest, Alum. °*Led.* *Tart.*
Dorsal region, Hydroc.

Dorsal region, nape of neck, Natr.
—, back, *Tart.* Zinc.
Arms, *Ars.* Hydroc.
—, upper arm, Sep.
Hands, finger, *Lach.*
Lower limbs, knee, Hyos.
Feet, Electr. Sec.

Pock-shaped.

Pimples, *Ant. Arn.* Petr. Tart.
Pustules, *Ant.* Hyos. *Tart.* Thuj.

Face, Ant. Arn. Hyos. Lach. Petr. Tart.
Lips, pocks, Lyc.
Chin, Hyos.
Abdomen, pustules, *Puls.*
Anus, black pocks, Sassap.
Sexual organs, pimple, Thuj.

Polypus.

In general, Amb.? Ant.? Aur.? Bell.? °*Calc.* °*Con.* Graph. Hep. °*Lyc.* °*Merc.* Mez.? Natr. m.? °*Nitr. ac.* Petr.? °*Phosph.* °*Phos. ac.* °*Puls.* Sep.? Sil. °*Staph.* Sulph. Sulph. ac. °Teucr.?? Thuj.
—, of every kind, °*Calc.* °*Lyc.* °*Staph.*

Ears, °*Calc.*
Nose, °Calc. °*Phosph.* °*Puls.* °Teucr.?

Pressure.

Mammæ and nipples, Berb. Sabin. Zinc.

Mammæ nipples, Berb. Sabin.

Bones, periosteum, Alum. Amm. *Anac.* Ang. Anis. **Arg.* Arn. Ars. Asa. *Aur.* **Bell. Bism.* Bry. Cann. Canth. Carb. veg. Cham. Chel. Cocc. *Colch. Coloc.* Con. ° *Cupr.* * *Cycl.* ° *Daph.* Dros. *Graph.* Guaj. Hell. Hep. Ign. **Kal.* Led. Magn. arct. Magn. aust. *Merc. Mez.* Nitr. N. mosch. N. vom. * *Oleand.* Phosph. *Plat. Puls.* Rhod. **Rhus.* **Sabin.* Sil. Spong. Stann. **Staph.* Teucr. *Thuj.* Val. *Veratr.* Viol. tr. Zinc.

Nails, Calc. Caust. Magn. art. Magn. aust. Sassap. Sulph.

Glands, Alum. Arg. *Ars. Aur. Bell. Calc.* Carb. veg. *Caust.* Chin. Cin. Cocc. Con. Cycl. *Ign.* Kal. *Lyc.* Magn. arct. Magn. m. Mang. Men. *Merc.* Natr. m. Nitr. ac. Par. Phos. ac. Puls. Rhab. *Rhus.* Sabin. *Spong.* Stann. Staph. Stram. *Sulph.* Veratr. *Zinc.*

Prickling.

On the skin, in general, Agar. Bell. Cann. Cin. Croc. Dros. Lyc. Mez. Mosch. Plat. Ran. sc. Sabad. Sep. Sulph. Tart. Zinc.

Mouth, Caust. Lach. Lyc. Ol. an. Phell. Phosph. Rhod.

—, palate, Caust. Ol. an.

—, Gums, Lyc.

— tongue, Lach. Phell. Phosph. Rhod.

Sexual parts, scrotum, Plat.

Arms, Alum. Coloc. Magn. arct. Plat.

—, arm, Magn. arct. Plat.

Arms, forearm, Alum. Coloc.
Hands, Lach. *Plat.* Seneg. Sil.
—, finger, Ferr. magn. Natr. m. *Ol. an.* Sil. *Sulph.*
—, thumb, Ol. an.
Lower limbs, °*Lach.* Sil.
—, hip, Caust.
—, thigh, Nitr. ac. Zinc.
—, knee, Cann. Croton. Plat. Spong. Sulph. ac. Tart.
—, legs, calves, Croton. Phell.
—, tendo Achilles, Sulph. ac.
Feet, Puls. Ran. sc. °*Sep.* Tart. *Zinc.*
—, heel, Ferr. magn.
—, soles, Alum. Ant. Natr. Ruta. *Sep.* Staph.
—, toes, Lach. Mez. Sulph. ac. *Zinc.*

Prolapsus.

Anus, Ant. °Asar. Canth. Dulc. Gran. Graph. **Ign.* Lach. *Lyc.* Magn. art. Magn. m. °*Merc.* Mur. ac. Natr. m. Nitr. ac. °*N. vom.* *Ruta. **Sulph.*
Sexual parts, °Bell. Ferr. °Gran.? Kreas. **Merc.* °*N. vom.* °Sep. Stann.
—, vagina, Ferr. °Gran.? *Merc. °*Sep.* Stann.
—, uterus, °Bell. °Gran.? Kreas. °*N. vom.* °*Sep.*

Proud flesh.

Ulcers, in the, Alum. Ant. **Ars.* Bell. *Carb. an.* Carb. veg. Caust. °*Cham.* *Graph.* Kreas. °*Lach.* Merc. °*Petr.* Phosph. Sabin. °*Sep.* °*Sil.* Staph. °*Sulph.* Thuj.

PUS, ACCORDING TO KIND AND QUALITY.

Black stain, leaving a, Bry. Chin. Lyc. °*Sulph.*
Bloody, Arg. Arn. **Ars.* *Asa.* Bell. *Carb. veg.* *Caust.* Con. Croc. Dros. **Hep.* Hyos. Jod. Kal. Kreas. Lach. *Lyc.* Magn. art. **Merc.* Mez. Natr. m. *Nitr. ac.* Phosph. Phos. ac. *Puls.* Rhus. Ruta. Sabin. Sec. Sep. *Sil.* Sulph. Sulph. ac. Tart. Zinc.
Brownish, Anac. Ars. Bry. Calc. Carb. veg. Con. Puls. Rhus. *Sil.*
Cheesy, Merc.
Corrosive, Amm. Anac. **Ars.* Bell. Calc. *Carb. veg.* **Caust.* Cham. Chel. Clem. Con. Cupr. Graph. *Hep.* Ign. Jod. Kreas. Lach. *Lyc.* **Merc.* Mez. Natr. Natr. m. *Nitr. ac.* N. vom. Phosph. Plumb. Puls. *Ran.* Ran. sc. **Rhus.* Ruta. Sep. **Sil.* Spig. Squill. Staph. Sulph. Sulph. ac. Zinc.
Fetid-smelling, (Comp. Stinking), °*Ars.* °Chel. *Merc.* Mur. ac. °*Puls.* °*Sil.* °Stann.
Gelatinous, Arg. Arn. Baryt. Cham. Ferr. Merc. Sep. Sil.
Gray, *Amb.* Ars. Carb. an. **Caust.* Chin. Lyc. Merc. Sep. *Sil.* Thuj.
Greenish, Ars. °*Asa.* Aur. Carb. veg. °*Caust.* Kreas. **Merc.* Natr. N. vom. °*Puls.* Rhus. Sep. °*Sil.* Staph.
Herring-brine, smelling like, Graph.
Ichorous, Amm. **Ars.* °*Asa.* Aur. Bar. m. *Bell.* Bov. Calc. **Carb. veg.* °*Caust.* *Chin. °Chinin.? *Clem. Con. Dros. Graph. Hep. Kal. Kreas. °*Lach.* °*Lyc.* Mang. **Merc.* *Mercurial.* Mur. ac. **Nitr. ac.* N. vom. Phosph. Phosph. ac. Plumb. Ran. **Ran. sc.* **Rhus.* Sec. Sep. **Sil.*

Mawworms, full of, Ars. Calc. Merc. °*Sabad.* °*Sil.* Sulph. Squill. °*Staph.* Sulph. Tart. Vip. red. Vip. torv.

Old cheese, smelling like old, Calc. **Hep.* Merc. Sulph.

Pale-red, Phosph. Plat. Puls. Rhod. Rhus.

Salt, *Amb. Ars.* Baryt. Calc. Chin. *Graph.* **Lyc.* Magn. c. Magn. m. Merc. **Natr. Petr.* °*Phosph. Puls.* **Sep. Sil.* Stann. Staph. Sulph. Zinc.

Sour-smelling, Calc. Graph. **Hep. Merc.* Natr. Sep. Sulph.

Stinking, Amm. **Ars.* °*Asa.* Aur. Bar. m. Bell. Bov. Bry. *Calc.* Caust. **Carb. veg.* Chel. *Chin.* Chinin. Cic. Con. Cycl. *Graph.* **Hep.* Kreas. **Lach. Lyc.* Mang. Mez. Mur. ac. Natr. Nitr. ac. N. mosch. N. vom. Phosph. **Phos. ac.* Plumb. Puls. Rhus. Ruta. Sabin. Sec. *Sep.* **Sil.* Staph. **Sulph.* Sulph. ac. Thuj. Vip. red.

Tallowy, **Merc.*

Tenacious, Ars. Asa. °Bov. Cham. °*Con.* Merc. Mez. Phosph. ac. Sep. Sil. Sulph.

Thin, **Asa.* Carb. veg. **Caust.* Dros. Jod. Kal. Lyc. **Merc.* Nitr. ac. Plumb. Puls. Ran. Ran. sc. Rhus. Ruta. *Sil.* Staph. *Sulph.* Thuj.

Watery, **Ars.* **Asa.* Calc. *Carb. veg.* **Caust.* Clem. Con. Dros. *Graph.* Jod. Kal. Lach. *Lyc.* **Merc. Nitr. ac.* N. vom. Plumb. Puls. *Ran. Ran. sc. Rhus.* Ruta. *Sil. Squill. Staph. Sulph.* Thuj.

Whitish, milky, Amm. Ars. *Calc.* Carb. veg. Hell. Lyc. Natr. m. Puls. Sep. Sil. Sulph.

Yellow, Acon. Amb. Amm. Anac. Ang. Arg. Ars. Aur. Bov. **Bry.* *Calc. Caps. **Carb. veg.* **Caust.*

Cic.** °*Clem.* Con. Croc. Dulc. Graph. Hep. Jod. °Kreas. Lyc. Magn. c. Mang. ***Merc. Natr. Natr. m. Nitr. *Nitr. ac.* N. vom. °*Phosph.* *Puls. Rhus. °Ruta. Sec. Selen. **Sep.* °*Sil.* Spig. **Staph.* Sulph. ac. Thuj. Viol. tr.

Pustules.

In general, Amm. m. Anthrok. Ant. **Ars.* Aur. Baryt. **Bell.* Berb. Calc. ph. Canth. Caust. Cham. **Cicc. Clem.* Cocc. Con. Croton. Cycl. *Dulc. Evon. Graph. Grat. Hep. *Hydroc.* **Hyos. Kal.* Kal. chl. Kreas. Lach. Lyc. Magn. art. Magn. arct. Magn. c. Magn. m. ****Merc.*** Mez. *Nitr. ac.* Op. °*Petr.* Phos. ac. Plumb. °*Puls.* **Rhus.* Samb. Sep. Sassap. Sec. Sil. Spig. **Staph.* Stram. **Sulph.* Tarax. **Tart.* Thuj. Veratr. Zinc.

Acuminated, Dulc. Thuj.

Black, Bry. Rhus.

Bleeding, Tart.

Brown, Tart.

Burning, *Amm.* Berb. Cic. Crotal. Graph. Mez. °*Petr.* Tart.

Confluent, **Cic.* °***Merc.*** Tart.

Cowpox, like, Tart.

Cracked, Rhus.

Dry, Evon. °***Merc.***

Greasy, Kreas.

Hard, Anac. Crotal.

Humid, Bell.

Inflamed, Rhus. Stram.

Itching, Anthrok. Berb. Dulc. Graph. Hydroc.

°***Merc.*** N. vom. Petr. Rhus. Sassap. Sulph. Tart.
Itch-like, Clem. Grat. Magn. art.
Lumpy, Anthrok. Cham.
Painful, as if sore, Baryt.
Painful, Ars. Berb. Stram. Tart.
Painless, Rhod.
Pale-red, Ars.
With peeling off, Crot. Hyos.
Pock-shaped, *Ant. Hyos. Tart.* Thuj.
Pustulous, Amm. m. *Ant.* Arn. **Ars.* Bell. Bry. Clem. Cocc. Croton, Cycl. °*Dulc.* Evon. Grat. Hydroc. **Hyos.* Kreas. Magn. m. ****Merc.*** Mez. Nitr. ac. Op. °*Petr.* °*Puls.* **Rhus.* Sassap. Sec. Sil. °*Staph.* °Sulph. **Tart.* Thuj.
Rose-coloured, Ars. Dulc.
Red, Anac. °***Ars.*** Berb. Caust. **Cic.* Crotal. Croton. Graph. Hydroc. Kal. Mez. ***Nitr. ac.*** Tart.
Red areola, with, Anac. Borax. Lach. Nitr. ac. Par. Tart. Thuj.
Scurfy, Ant. Bov. Croton. Dulc. Merc. Tart.
Scaly, Merc.
Small, Evon. Hydroc. Nitr. Tart.
Sore, °***Merc.***
Stinging, Amm. Berb. Dros. Rhus.
Tensive, Crotal. Magn. s. Nitr. Tart.
On the tetters, Kreas.
Titillating, Mez.
Ulcerated, °***Ars.*** °*Dulc.* Magn. m. °***Merc.*** Sassap. Sil. Tart.
Water, containing, Stram.
White, Cycl.
Yellow, Hyos.

Head, Arn. **Ars.* Bov. Gran. Kal. Mur. ac. N. vom. Puls. Rhus. Sil.

Eyes, **Merc.* **Sep.*

Nose, *Amm. *Anac.* Arn. Bell. Bov. Clem. Cocc. Euphr. Mang. Natr. Nitr. *Petr.* *Plumb.* Tarax.

Face, Amm. Amm. m. Anac. **Ant.* Aur. **Bell.* Bov. Calc. ph. Carb. an. Caust. **Cic.* Clem. Cocc. Coloc. Crotal. Dros. Grat. Hyos. Kal. Kal. hdr. Magn. c. Magn. m. Magn. s. °*Merc.* Nitr. °*Nitr. ac.* Par. Phosph. **Rhus.* Sassap. Tarax. Veratr.

—, whiskers, °Ars.

Lips and mouth, region of, Amm. Baryt. Berb. Carb. veg. Lach. Magn. art. Magn. arct. Mur. ac. N. vom. Par. Samb. Sep. Tarax. Thuj. Zinc.

Chin, Bell. Canth. Caust. Graph. Mang. Merc. Nitr. ac. N. mosch. Oleand. Rhus. Sabin. Sassap. *Zinc.*

Buccal cavity, Amm. Aur. Calc. Carb. veg. °*Ign.* Magn. c. Petr. Phosph.

—, mouth, Amm. Magn. c. Phosph.

—, tonsils, cervical glands, °Ign.

—, gums, Aur. Calc. Carb. veg. Petr.

—, tongue, Amm.

Abdomen, inguinal region, *Puls.*

Anus, Calc.

Sexual parts, Bov. Bry.

Chest, Aur. Cocc. Evon. Graph. *Hep.* Magn. m. Sil. Stront. Tart.

Dorsal region, neck, Ant. Aur. °Clem. *Squill.* Tart.

—, small of back, Calc. Natr.

Dorsal region, nape of neck, Bell. Natr. Nitr.
—, back, °Dulc. Evon.
—, scapulæ, Cocc. Magn. m.
Arms, Anac. Merc. Mez. *Rhod.* Rhus. *Staph.* *Sulph.*
—, elbow, Sulph.
—, upper arm, Anac. Merc.
—, forearm, *Rhod.* Rhus. *Staph.*
Hands, Cic. Natr. m. Rhus. °*Sep.* Sil.
—, finger, Anac. Baryt. Borax. *Sassap.* Spig. Zinc.
Lower limbs, °*Dulc.* Mez. Staph. Stram. *Thuj.*
—, nates and hips, Ant. Hydroc. Hyos.
—, knees, Bry. Hyos.
Feet, toes, Cycl.

Putrid, that which is.

Blisters, vesicles, Vip. torv.
Ulcers, Amm. **Ars.* *Asa.* Aur. °*Bell.* °*Borax.* Bov. *Bry.* °*Calc.* Carb. veg. Caust. °*Chel.* °*Chin.* Cic. Con. °*Cycl.* *Graph.* °*Hep.* Kreas. *Lyc.* Mang. **Merc.* Mez. **Mur. ac.* Natr. *Nitr. ac.* N. mosch. N. vom. Oph. *Phosph.*°*Phos. ac.* Plumb. **Puls.* °*Rhus.* Ruta. Sabin. Sec. *Sep.* **Sil.* Staph. °*Sulph.* Sulph. ac. Thuj.

Mouth, swelling, °*N. vom.*

Raised, that which is.

Eruption, Ars. Asa. Calc. Caust. Dulc. Lach.

Merc. Mez. N. vom. Oph. Op. Phosph. Sulph. Tab. Tax. Val.
Blisters, vesicles, Merc. Selen. Sulph.
Pimples, Tax.
Herpes, Merc.
Spots, Calc. Carb. an. Dulc. Kal. Merc. Phosph. Puls. Sassap. Teucr. Thuj.
Rash, Bruc. Selen.
Scurfs, crusts, Sabin.
Blotches, tubercles, Oleand. Rhus v. Val.

Face, Dulc. Oleand. Phosph. Sassap. Sulph. Teucr.
Lips, °Bry. Sulph.
Dorsal region, eruption, Mez. Val.
Arms, eruption, *Merc. Mez. Natr. m.* Sabin. *Staph.*
Hands, eruption, Bruc. Kal. Lach. Rhus vom. *Sulph. ac.*
Lower limbs, tibia, *Aur. Merc.*
—, knees, Electr.
Feet, spots, Puls.

Raised margin, with.

Ulcers, °*Ars.* Asa. Bry. Carb. an. Caust. Cic. Cin. °*Hep.* Lyc. **Merc.* °*Petr.* Phosph, Phos. ac. °*Puls.* °*Sep.* °*Sil.* °*Sulph.*

Ranula.

Mouth, °*Thuj.* (°Amb. °Calc. °Merc.)

RASH AND THE LIKE.

In general, **Acon.* Alum. **Amm. Amm. m.* °*Ant.* **Arn.* **Ars.* Asa. **Bell.* Bov. Bruc. **Bry.* °*Calad. Calc. Canth.* °*Carb. veg.* **Caust.* **Cham.* Chin. *Clem. Coff.* Coloc. Cupr. Daph. Dig. *Dulc.* Electr. °*Euphr.* Galv. Gins. *Graph.* °*Hell.* °*Hyos.* **Ipec.* Kal. chl. °*Lach.* °*Led.* **Merc.* **Mez.* Natr. m. °*N. vom.* Op. *Phosph.* **Phos. ac.* °*Puls.* Rhab. °*Rhus.* Ruta. *Sassap.* Sec. °*Selen.* Sep. Sil. Spong. °*Staph. Stram.* **Sulph.* **Tart.* Teucr. Val. °*Veratr.* °*Viol. tr.* Zinc.

—, skin, in the open air, °*Sassap.*

—, — in the room, °Calc.

After abuse of Belladonna, °*Hyos.*

After sting of bee, Sep.

Bleeding, Alum.

Burning, Bry. Calad. Euphr. Merc. N. vom. Phos. ac. Teucr.

Chronic, °*Amm.* Clem. Mez. °*Staph.*

Gnawing-itching, Mez. Natr. m. **Sulph.* Viol. tr.

Itching, Alum. **Bry.* °*Calad.* Daph. °*Euphr.* °*Led.* **Merc.* **Mez.* Natr. m. *N. vom.* Rhab. **Selen.* Sep. Sil. **Sulph.* Tart. Teucr. Zinc.

Itch-like, °*Merc.*

Measles, like, Merc. °*N. vom.*

With peeling off, Ars. Stram. Sulph.

Purple-coloured, °*Acon.* °Bell. °*Coff.*

Raised, Bruc. Selen.

Red, in general, **Acon.* Amm. Ars. **Bell.* Bruc. **Bry.* °*Carb. veg.* Caust. **Cham.* Coloc. °*Coff.* *Dulc.* °*Euphr.* °*Hyos.* °*Ipec.* °*Lach.* °*Led.*

**Merc. Phosph. *Phos. ac. °Rhus.* Sep. °*Staph. Stram. *Sulph. *Tart.* Teucr.
Scarlet-coloured, °*Acon.* °Amm. ? °Ars. ? °Bell. °*Bry. ?* °Carb. veg. ? °Caust. ? °*Coff.* °Dulc. ? Galv. °Hyos. °*Ipec.* °Lach. ? °*Merc.* °Phosph.? °Phos. ac. ? °Rhus ? °Sulph. ?
Scorbutic, Ars.
Shining through, Cin.
In spots, Mez.
Stinging, Mez. Natr. m. Sulph. Teucr. Viol. tr.
Suppressed, °*Ipec.*
Suppurating, Tart.
Tickling, Bry.
Titillating, Gins.
White, Agar. °*Ars.* Bov. °*Bry.* Ipec. °*N. vom. Phosph. Sulph.* **Val.*

Head, Natr. m. Spong. Tart.
Face, Sulph.
Abdomen, Bruc. Selen.
—, liver, region of, Selen.
Sexual parts, Bry. °Dulc. Rhus.
—, glans, Bry.
—, scrotum, Rhus.
—, labia, °Dulc.
Thoracic region, Amm. *Bry.* Calad. Cupr. Galv. Lach. **Led.* Merc. *Sil. Staph.* Stram. Tart.
Dorsal region, neck, Ammon. Bry. Galv.
—, nape of neck, Ant. Caust. Mez. °Sec.
—, back, Merc. Mez. Stram.
—, scapulæ, Ant. Caust.
Arms, Alum. Bry. Galv. Mez. N. vom. **Sulph.* Tart.

Arms, elbow, Zinc.
—, upper arm, Ant.
—, forearm, Amm. Bry. Calad. *Merc.* Selen.
Hands, Bruc. Bry. Cupr. Dig. *Led.*
Lower limbs, Daph. Galv. Ol. an. **Sulph.*
—, thighs, Bry. Merc. Mez. *N. vom.*
—, knees, N. vom. Zinc.
—, legs, °Calc. Hyos. *Natr. m.* Sil.
Feet, Bry.

Rash-like.

Pimples, Bov. Kal. chl. Rhus. Sassap.
Spots, Mez.
Itch, °*Carb. veg.* °*Merc.* °*Sulph.*
Scarlet-rash, °*Acon.* °Amm.? °Ars. ? °Bell.? °*Bry.* ? °Carb. veg. ? °Caust. ? °*Coff.* °Dulc. ? Galv. °Hyos. °*Ipec.* °Lach.? °*Merc.* °Phosph. ? °Phos. ac. ? °Rhus. ? °Sulph. ?

Nose, pimples, Sil.
Face, eruption, Sulph.
Hands, pimples, **Carb. veg.*
Feet, pimples, Bov.

Raw, like.

Eruption, °*Graph.*
Face, in the, °*Graph.*

Redness.

Of the skin, in general, **Acon.* **Agar.* Agn. Amm. Anthr. Ant. **Arn.* **Ars.* **Asa.* *°Bell.* Berb. Bov. **Bry.* Calc. Camph. *Canth.* Carb. veg. Caust. **Cham.* *Chin.* Cin. Clem. Cocc. Con. Crotal. Croton. Cycl. **Dulc.* Electr. **Euphorb.* Ferr. magn. **Graph.* **Hep.* Hydroc. Hyos. Ign. Ipec. Jod. Kal. Kal. chl. Kreas. Lach. Lam. Led. **Lyc.* Magn. art. Magn. c. Magn. m. *Mang.* **Merc.* Mez. Natr. m. Nitr. **N. vom.* Oleand. Op. Petr. *Phosph.* **Phos. ac.* Plumb. **Puls.* Ran. sc. **Rhod.* **Rhus.* *Ruta.* Sabad. Sassap. *Sec.* **Sep.* Sil. Spig. Spong. Squill. Stann. *Stram.* **Sulph.* **Sulph. ac.* Tarax. Tax. Teucr. Val. Vinc. Vip. red. Vip. torv. Zinc. (Comp. Inflammation, Red, which is, Erysipelas and Scarlet-red, which is.)

Eyes, **Acon.* Aeth. Agar. Alum. Amb. Amm. Amm. m. Ang. **Ant.* *°Arn.* *°Ars.* *Asa.* Aur. Baryt. **Bell.* *Bism.* Borax. Bov. Bruc. **Bry.* **Calc.* Camph. Caps. Caust. **Cham.* Chel. **Chin.* Clem. Con. Crotal. Croton. *Cupr.* Dig. Electr. Eugen. *°Euphr.* Ferr. Galv. Gent. **Graph.* Grat. Hell. Hep. Hyos. *°Ign.* Jod. Ipec. *Kal.* Kal. chl. Kal. hdr. Kreas. *°Lach.* *Led.* Lyc. Magn. c. Magn. m. *°Meph.* **Merc.* Mosch. Mur. ac. Natr. m. Nicc. Nitr. **Nitr. ac.* *°N. vom.* Op. **Phosph.* Phos. ac. Plumb. **Puls.* Ran. sc. Rhus. Sassap. **Sep.* **Sil.* **Spig.* **Spong.* Staph. Stann. *Stram.* *Stront.* **Sulph.*

Sulph. ac. Tab. Tart. Teucr. *Thuj.* Val. Veratr. Viol. od. Zinc.

Eyelids, **Acon.* Amm. m. *Ant.* **Ars.* Baryt. **Bell.* Bism. Bry. **Calc.* °*Canth.* °*Cham.* Carb. veg. Caust. **Dig.* Ferr. Graph. Jod. Kal. hdr. Kreas. Lach. **Lyc.* Merc. Mosch. Mur. ac. Natr. m. Nicc. °*N. vom.* Par. Phosph. Phos. ac. Plumb. Puls. Rhod. Sabad. Sep. Spong. Stram. Sulph. Teucr.

Canthi, °*Ars.* °*Aur.* Bell. Bism. Bov. Bruc. Bry. Calc. Eugen. Grat. *Magn. c.* Nitr. ac. Ran. Rhus, **Sulph.* Teucr. Val. Zinc.

Ears, Agar. *Alum.* *Ant.* *Camph.* Carb. veg. *Chin.* Electr. Evon. Galv. Graph. *Hep.* *Ign.* Kal. Kreas. *Magn. c.* Meph. *Merc.* Natr. m. Nitr. ac. Petr. Phosph. Plat. *Puls.* Sep. Sil. Sulph. *Tab.*

Nose, **Alum.* **Aur.* **Aur. m.* **Bell.* Borax. Bov. **Calc.* *Canth.* *Carb. an.* Chinin. Croton. *Graph.* *Hep.* Jod. Kal. °Lach. Magn. arct. Magn. c. **Magn. m.* *Merc.* Natr. *Natr. m.* Nicc. *Nitr.* Nitr. ac. Phosph. Poth. Rhod. Rhus. **Sil.* Sulph. Vinc.

Face, Alum. Amb. Amm. Anac. Ant. Arn. °Ars. °Aur. *Bell.* Borax. Bry. Calc. ph. Carb. an. Caust. Cham. **Cic.* Crotal. Dig. Dros. °Euphr. Ferr. mur. °Ipec. Kal. Kal. hdr. °Kreas. Lach. Led. *Merc.* *Nitr. ac.* Par. Phosph. Phos. ac. *Puls. °Samb. **Sep.* *Sulph.* Tab. Thuj. Teucr. Veratr.

Chin, Canth. Gins. Zinc.

Buccal cavity, °*Acon.* Agn. Alum. *Amm.* Amm. caust. **Bell.* Berb. Canth. Carb. an. °*Cham.* Chen. *Con.* Electr. **Hyos.* °Ign.

Kal. Kal. chl. °*Lach.* Magn. c. **Merc.* Nitr. Nitr. ac. N. mosch. °*Puls.* Ran. sc. Raph. °Rhus. **Sep.* °Stann. Sulph.

Palate, Amm. caust. Canth. Chen. °*Puls.*

—, velum palati, Agn. °*Acon.* **Bell.* Berb. N. mosch.

—, tonsils, °*Acon.* Amm. caust. **Bell.* Berb. °Cham. °Lach. **Merc.* Nitr. ac. °*Puls.* Raph. Sulph.

—, mouth, Amm. °Ign.

—, fauces and throat, °*Acon.* Alum. Amm. **Bell.* Ign. Natr. N. mosch.

—, uvula, Agn. °Bell. Berb. °Puls.

—, gums, *Carb. an. Con.* Jod. Kal. Kal. chl. *Lach.* Magn. c. Nitr. Ran. sc. **Sep.*

—, tongue, Ant. *Electr.* **Hyos.* Ran. sc. °Rhus. °Stann. Sulph.

Abdomen and stomach, region of, Amm. Graph. **Rhus.*

Sexual parts, Calad. *Calc.* Cann. Carb. veg. Cinn. Corall. Croton. Magn. aust. Merc. Natr. m. Sabin. **Sep.*

—, glans, Calad. Cann. Corall. Croton. Magn. aust. Sabin.

—, scrotum, Merc. Natr. m.

—, pudendum and thighs, between, *Sep.

—, labia, Calc. Carb. veg. Merc. **Sep.*

—, prepuce, Calc. Cann. Cinn. Corall. **Sil.* Sulph.

Dorsal region, neck, Bell. Jod. Veratr.

Arms, Arg. **Bell.* Lach. Ruta. Sabad.

—, upper arm, Dulc.

—, forearm, Tax.

Hands, Baryt. Carb. an. *Dulc.* Hep. Indig. *Natr. s.* N. vom. Ran. Sabad. Staph. Sulph.
—, wrist-joints, Magn. c. Merc. acet.
—, fingers, **Agar.* Berb. Borax. Gent. Laur. *Lyc.* Magn. c. Mur. ac. **N. vom.* Ran. Rhod. Therid. *Thuj.*
—, finger-joints, Gent. **Lyc.* Spong. *Sulph.*
—, thumbs, Lach.
Lower limbs, nates, Hyos.
—, thighs, Electr.
—, knees, Bry. Electr. Kreas.
—, legs, *N. vom. Puls. Sabin.* Tarax.
Feet, Ant. °*Bry.* Hyos. Lach. *Puls.* Sassap. Sil.
—, ankles, Hep. Phos. ac.
—, heel, Berb.
—, soles, *Kal.* Phosph.
—, toes, **Agar. Alum.* Amm. Arn. *Berb. Borax.* °*Carb. veg. Lyc. Mur. ac. Natr. m. Nitr. ac. Sabin.* Sep. Staph. Zinc.
Glands, see: INFLAMMATION.

RED, WHICH IS.

Blisters, vesicles, *Ant.* Cic. Cycl. Crotal. Led. Mang. Natr. *Natr. m.* Sil. Stront. Val.
Blotches, Electr. Ipec. Natr. m. Op.
Blotches, tubercles, *Amm.* Berb. Bov. Carb. an. Carb. veg. Dig. Electr. *Hep.* Kal. chl. Kal. hdr. *Lach.* °*Led.* Magn. c. Magn. m. *Merc.* Mur. ac. Natr. m. Nitr. ac. Op. Phos. ac. Puls. Sep. Spig. Sulph. Thuj. Veratr.
Bloodvessels, swelling of, **Acon.* Aeth. **Amb.* Amm. °*Ars.* **Bell.* Bruc. Electr. Eugen. *Kal.*

°*Lach.* Laur. Meph. **Merc.* Phosph. °Phos. ac. Spig. **Sulph.*

Callosities, *Sabad.*

Chilblains, *Agar.* Amb. *Ant.* °*Arn.* **Ars.* Asar. Aur. **Bell. Berb.* Borax. °*Bry.* **Carb. an.* °Carb. veg. *Cham. Chin.* Cocc. *Colch.* Croc. °*Cycl. Hep.* °*Hyos.* Kal. *Lyc.* Magn. arct. Magn. aust. **Nitr. ac.* N. mosch. **N. vom.* Op. **Petr.* **Phosph.* °*Phos. ac.* **Puls.* Rhab. **Rhus.* Ruta. Sep. Spig. Stann. *Staph.* **Sulph.* °*Sulph. ac.* **Thuj.* Zinc.

Cicatrices of former ulcers, wounds, Lach. **Merc.* Natr. m.

Eruption, **Acon.* **Agar.* Agn. Alum. Amb. **Amm.* Amm. m. Ant. **Arn.* **Ars.* Aur. Baryt. **Bell.* Bov. Bry. Calad. *Calc.* Cann. Canth. Caps. Carb. an. Carb. veg. Caust. Cham. Chin. Cist. **Clem. Cocc.* Coff. **Con.* Croc. Croton. Cupr. *Cycl.* Dros. **Dulc. Graph.* Hep. Hyos. Jod. Ipec. **Kal.* Kreas. **Lach.* Led. Lyc. Magn. art. Magn. arct. Magn. c. Magn. m. **Merc.* Mez. Natr. Natr. m. Nitr. *Nitr. ac.* N. vom. Op. Par. Petr. **Phosph.* **Phos. ac.* Plumb. Puls. Rhod. *Rhus.* Ruta. *Sabad. Sec.* **Sep. Sil.* Spong. Stann. Staph. *Stram.***Sulph.* **Sulph. ac.* Tab. Tart. Tax. Teucr. Val. Veratr. Vip. torv. Zinc.

Herpes, °Amm. °Ars. °Clem. °Dulc. Kreas. °*Lach.* Magn. Magn. s. Oleand. °Sulph. Tax.

Pimples, Acon. Alum. Amm. *Ant.* Arn. Bell. Berb. *Bov.* Bry. Calc. ph. Caust. Cham. Chel. *Cin.* Crotal. Cycl. Dros. Dulc. Jod. Kal. *Lach.* Led. *Magn. c.* Phosph. *Phos.ac.* Plumb.

Rhod. Sassap. Spig. *Squill.* ***Staph.*** ***Stront.*** Sulph. Tax. Teucr. *Thuj.* Veratr. Zinc.

Pustules, Anac. °*Ars.* Berb. Caust. **Cic.* Crotal. Croton. Graph. Hydroc. Kal. Mez. *Nitr. ac.* Tart.

Rash, rash-like, **Acon.* Amm. Ars. **Bell.* Bruc. **Bry.* °*Carb. veg.* Caust. **Cham.* Coloc. °*Coff.* *Dulc.* °*Euphr.* °*Hyos.* °*Ipec.* °*Lach.* °*Led.* **Merc.* *Phosph.* **Phos. ac.* °*Rhus.* Sep. °*Staph.* *Stram.* **Sulph.* **Tart.* Teucr.

Ridges, **Bell.* Calc. °*Carb. veg.* Euphorb. **Hep.* Phosph. *Phos. ac.* Rhus. Sabad.

—, worse in the cold, *Sabad.*

Scurfs, Amm. m.

Spots, Acon. *Alum.* *Amb.* Amm. *Ant.* **Arn.* **Ars.* **Bell.* *Berb.* **Bry.* Calad. **Calc.* Canth. Caps. Carb. an. *Carb. veg.* Caust. Cham. Chin. Cinn. Cist. Cocc. °*Con.* Croc. *Croton.* *Cycl.* *Dros.* *Dulc.* Electr. Ferr. magn. Graph. Hep. Jod. °*Ipec.* °*Kal.* Kal. hdr. **Lach.* *Led.* *Lyc.* Magn. arct. ***Magn. c.*** ***Magn. m.*** Mang. ****Merc.*** Mez. Mosch. *Natr.* *Natr. m.* Nitr. **Nitr. ac.* Op. Par. *Petr.* **Phosph.* *Phos. ac.* Plat. *Plumb.* Poth. Puls. Ratanh. Rhod. **Rhus.* **Sabad.* °*Samb.* *Sassap.* **Sep.* *Sil.* Spong. *Squill.* *Stann.* **Sulph.* **Sulph. ac.* *Tab.* Tart. Tax. Teucr. Thuj. Veratr. *Vip. torv.* *Zinc.*

Swelling, **Acon.* **Ant.* Alum. Amm. Amm. m. **Arn.* **Ars.* **Asa.* Asar. *Aur. m. Baryt. **Bell.* *Borax.* Bov. **Bry.* *Carb. an.* °*Carb. veg.* **Cham.* **Chin.* *Con.* Crotal. Electr. **Hep.* *Kal.* Lach. **Lyc.* *Magn. c.* **Merc.* *Mur. ac.* *Natr.* Natr. m. Nicc. Nitr. *Nitr. ac.* **N. vom.* Oleand. °*Oph.* Phell. **Phosph.* Phos. ac. Poth.

Puls. *Ran.* Ran. sc. *Raph.* °*Rhod.* **Rhus.* Sabin. Sassap. **Sep.* **Sil.* Spong. **Stann.* Stram. **Sulph.* Tab. Therid. *Thuj.*

Head, eruption, Agar. Amb. Anac. Ant. Ars. Bov. Kal. *Mosch.* Natr. c. N. vom.
Eyes, bloodvessels, **Acon.* Aeth. *Amb. Amm. °*Ars.* **Bell.* Bruc. Electr. Eugen. *Kal.* °Lach. Laur. Meph. **Merc.* Phosph. °Phos. ac. Spig. **Sulph.*
—, spots, Phos. ac. *Puls.*
—, lids, Camph. Sil.
—, streaks, N. vom. Sassap.
Ears, herpes, Oleand.
Nose, Calc. Croton. Jod. Lach. Phos. ac. Rhod. Sil. Stront. Teucr. Thuj. Veratr. Zinc.
Face, red-swollen, **Arn.* **Bell.* Borax. °Bry. °Coloc. Crotal. Kal. *Lach. Natr. **N. vom.* Oleand. **Rhus.* **Stram.* °Sulph.
Lips, eruptions, Arn. Berb. Caust. Hep. Magn. c. Thuj.. Zinc.
Chin, Natr. m.
Lower jaw, Stann.
Buccal cavity, spots, Canth.
—, swollen parts, °*Acon.* °*Bell.* Carb. an. °*Cham.* Con. Lach. Magn. c. Nitr. Nitr. ac. Phell. Ran. Sep. Sulph.
Abdomen and stomach, region of, spots, Bell. Lach. *Sabad.*
—, rash, Bruc.
—, swelling of glands, Lyc. **Merc.*
Sexual parts, eruptions, Bov. Kal. Lach. Merc. Petr. Phos. ac. Sep. **Thuj.* Zinc.

Sexual parts, spots, Arn. Carb. veg. Caust. Con. Lach. Natr. m. **Nitr. ac.* Petr. Sil. °Thuj.
—, swelling, °Arn. Ars. Merc.
—, ulcers, Corall.
Thoracic region, pimples, Bov. Plumb. Staph. Stront.
—, spots, **Bell.* °Ipec. Magn. c. *Mez.*
—, rash, Amm. **Led.* Staph.
Dorsal region, eruption, Ant. Bry.
—, blisters, Ant. Cic.
—, pimples, Ant. Bell. Led. Mez. Phos. ac. Spig. *Squill. Thuj.*
—, spots, Ant. Bell. Carb. veg. Cinn. Cist. Cocc. Lach. Sep. Stann. Vip. torv.
—, swelling, Amm. m. Baryt.
—, tubercles, °Lach. Mur. ac.
Arms, eruptions, Amm. Arg. Bry. Dulc. Magn. c. *Merc.* Natr. m. Phosph. *Sabad. Staph.*
—, spots, Berb. Dulc. Kal. hdr. Plat. *Rhus.* Sep. *Sulph.*
—, swelling, **Bell.* °*Bry.* Sep.
—, streaks, Sabad.
Hands, eruptions, Bell. Berb. Bov. Bruc. Canth. Carb. an. *Cic.* Cycl. Lyc. *Merc. Ran.* Spig. Spong. **Sulph.* Sulph. ac. Veratr.
—, spots, Alum. Berb. Dros. Electr. Kal. Magn. m. Mang. Natr. Natr. m. *Phos. ac. Plumb. Sabad.* °*Sulph. Tart.* Zinc.
—, scurf, Amm. m.
—, swelling, **Bell.* Electr. Hep. **Lyc. Magn. c. Mur. ac.* Ran. Sulph. *Therid.*
—, callosities, Lach. Phosph.
Lower limbs, eruptions, Electr. Staph.

Lower limbs, pimples, Ant. Chel. Rhod. Staph.
—, spots, Berb. **Calc.* *Cycl.* °Con. Electr. *Graph. Lyc. Petr.* Rhod. Rhus. Sassap. Sil. °*Sulph. Sulph. ac.*
—, herpes, Kreas.
—, rash, Calc. Hyos.
—, swelling, Aur. Bov. °*Bry. Calc. Chin. Lyc. Puls. Sabad.* Zinc.
—, ulcer, N. vom.
—, tubers, *Hep.*
—, callosities, Lach. Phosph.
—, streaks, Calc. Rhus.
Feet, eruption, Bov. Electr.
—, spots, Ant. **Ars. Natr.* Puls. Rhus.
—, chilblains, Kal.
—, spotted swelling, Chin.
—, swelling, Ars. °*Bry.* °*Carb. veg.* Chin. Con. °*Hep. Kal. Mur. ac. Nitr. ac.* **Puls. Raph.* °*Rhus. Sabin.* Sassap. **Sil.* **Stann. Thuj.*

Reddish-yellow, that which is.

Mouth, swelling, Canth.
—, gums, Canth.

Red-marbled.

Spots, Berb. °*Carb. veg.* °*Caust. Crotal. Lyc. Natr. m.* Plat. **Thuj.*

Red-spotted.

Eruption, Dig. Veratr.

Swelling, Chin. Lyc. Rhus v. Sep.

Red Areola, with.

Eruption, Anac.
Blotches, Ant.
Blisters, vesicles, Cann. Crotal. Kal. Kal. chl. Natr. Sil. Sulph. Tab. Vip. torv.
Pimples, Anac. Canth. Cycl. Samb. Tarax.
Pustules, Anac. Borax. Lach. Nitr. ac. Par. Tart. Thuj.
Herpes, °Dulc.
Ulcers, Acon. Ant. Arn. °*Ars.* °*Asa.* Baryt. Bell. °*Calc.* Caust. °*Cham.* Cocc. Corall. Cupr. °*Hep.* Kreas. **Lach.* Lam. °*Lyc.* °*Merc.* Mez. Nitr. ac. N. vom. Petr. Phosph. °*Puls.* Ran. **Rhus.* Sep. °*Sil.* **Staph.* °*Sulph.*
Tubercles, Cocc. Dulc. Phos. ac.

Head, Anac.
Nose, Anac. Natr. Petr. Sil.
Face, Tarax.
Lips, Bell. Samb.
Arms, eruptions, Anac.
Hands, eruption, Anac. Borax. Bov. Canth. Cycl. Natr.
Lower limbs, blotch, Ant.
—, vesicles, Cann. Kal.
Pustules, Lach.

Rhagades.

In general, Aloë. Alum. Ant. Arn. Aur. Baryt.

Bry. **Calc.* Carb. an. Carb. veg. **Cham.* Cyc. Graph. **Hep.* Kal. *Kreas.* Lach. **Lyc.* Magn. c. Mang. *Merc. Natr. Natr. m. Nitr. ac. **Petr.* Phosph. **Puls.* Rhus. Ruta. Sassap. Sep. Sil. *Sulph.* Teucr. Viol. tr. Zinc.

Bleeding, **Merc.* Nicc. **Petr.* Puls. Sassap. **Sulph.*

Burning, Zinc.

Fetid, *Merc.*

Yellow, Merc.

Ulcerated, Bry. **Merc.*

Itching, Merc.

Mercurial, °*Hep.* °*Sulph.*

Humid, Aloës.

After washing, getting wet, Ant. Bry. **Calc.* Cham. Kal. Lyc. Nitr. ac. **Puls.* Rhus. Sassap. *Sep.* **Sulph.* Zinc.

Painful, Graph. Mang. Zinc.

Deep, Mang. Merc.

Head, Ruta.

Nose, **Ant.* Carb. an. Merc.

Face, Sil.

Lips and buccal region, Alum. Amm. Amm. m. *Arn.* °*Ars.* Baryt. Bell. Berb. Bov. **Bry.* *Calc.* Canth. Caps. Carb. an. **Carb. veg.* Cham. *Chin. Colch. Corall. Croc. Dros. Electr. Gins. Graph. Grat. Hep. **Ign.* Kal. Kal. hdr. Kreas. Magn. m. Men. Mez. **Natr. m.* °Nitr. ac. Ol. an. Par. Petr. °*Phosph.* Phos. ac. Puls. Sabad. Selen. °Squill. Staph. Sulph. Tab. Tarax. Tart. °Veratr. **Sulph.* Zinc.

Arms, Sil.

Hands, **Alum.* Graph. Kal. Kreas. **Lach.* °*Magn. c. Merc. Natr. Natr. m.* °*Nitr. ac.* **Petr.* Sil. **Zinc.*
—, fingers. Baryt. Kal. Mang. Merc. **Petr.* Phosph. Zinc.
—, joints, Phosph. **Sulph.*
Feet, °*Hep.*
—, heels, Lyc.
—, soles, Ars.
—, toes, Carb. an. Eugen. **Lach.*

Rheumatic.

Inflammations, °*Acon.* °*Arn.* °*Bell.* °Berb. °Bry. °Calc. ph. °*Cham.* °*Chin.* °*Chinin.?* °Clem. °*Lach.* °*Merc.* °*N. vom.* °*Puls.* °Rhod. °*Rhus.* °Sassap. °Sep. °*Sulph.*
Swelling, °*Acon.* °*Arn.* °*Bell.* °*Bry.* °Calc. ph. °*Cham.* °*Chin.* Cocc. °*Colch.* °Hep. °Kreas. °Lach. °*Merc.* °*N. vom.* °*Puls.* °Rhus. °*Sulph.*

Arms, *Agar.* Ammoniac. **Bell.* **Bry.* **Calc. ph. Grat.* Jod. Meph. Rhus v. Sil. **Thuj.*
—, shoulder and joints, Amm. m. **Calc. ph.* Graph. Grat. Ign. Jod. Lach. Lyc. N. vom. Ol. an. *Phosph.* Phos. ac. Puls. Ran. Rhod. Rhus v. Sabin. *Sulph.* Tart. Teucr.
—, elbow, Grat. Mez. Ran. Rhus v. Tart. Teucr. *Zinc.*
—, upper arm, Coff. N. vom. Phosph. Ran. Stram. *Zinc.*
—, forearm, Gran. Lach.

Hands, Ang. Borax. Lach. *Zing.*
—, wrist-joints, Amb. *Gran.* Grat. *Lach.* Ruta. Zinc.
—, fingers, Ammoniac. Colch. °Lach.
Lower limbs, Amb. °Bry. Chin. Graph. Jod. Meph. Ol. jec. Phos. ac. Poth. Zinc.
—, hips and nates, Cycl. °*Lach.* °*Led.* *Lyc.* Natr. m. Tart.
—, thighs, Agar. Carb. veg. Daph. Gins. Jod. Lach. Sabin. Tart. Veratr. *Zinc.*
—, knee, Crotal. Daph. °*Lach.* Mez. Zinc.
—, legs, calves, &c., Anac. Carb. veg. Gins. Lyc. Mez. Tart. Zinc.
Feet, **Hep.* Ruta. Stram. Zinc.
—, toes, Cinn.

Ridges.

In general, *Ars.* **Bell.* Calc. °*Carb. veg.* Euphorb. **Hep.* Magn. c. Phosph. *Phos. ac. Rhus. Sabad. Stram.*
Brown, *Ars.* °*Carb. veg.*
Burning, Rhus.
Yellow, Stram.
Red, **Bell.* Calc. °*Carb. veg.* Euphorb. **Hep.* Phosph. *Phos. ac.* Rhus. Sabad.
—, redder in the cold, *Sabad.*
Scarlet-red, **Bell.* Euphorb. **Hep.*
White, Magn. c.

Eyes, red, N. vom. Sassap.
Lips, Ars. Stram. Tart. ac.
Abdomen, umbilical region, Phos. ac.
Arms, Euphorb. *Sabad.*

Lower limbs, Calc. *Rhus.*

RING-SHAPED.

Herpes, Clem. Magn. c. °*Natr.* Natr. m. °*Sep.*

ROUGH, WHICH IS.

Eruption, Anac. Phosph. Sep.
Pimples, Alum.
Herpes, °*Bov.* Oleand.
Spots, Baryt. *Merc.* Mur. ac. Nitr. ac. *Sassap.* °*Zinc.*
Nails, Sabad. Sil.

Face, Alum. Anac. Baryt. Bov. Merc. Nitr. ac. Phosph. °Rhus. Sassap. **Sep.* °*Sulph.*
Lower limbs, spots, Mur. ac.

ROUGH SKIN.

In general, °*Bell.* **Calc.* Graph. *Jod.* Kal. Laur. Merc. Natr. Oleand. Phosph. Phos. ac. *Rhus.* Ruta. Sassap. **Sep.* *Sulph.*
Fingers, between the, °*Calc.*

Head, Natr. m. Ruta.
Ears, Phosph.
—, in front of, Oleand.
Lips and mouth, region of, Amb. Anac. Calc. Magn. m. **Merc.* Mur. ac. Natr. m. N. vom. Phos. ac. Plat. Sulph.
Arms, forearm, Mill.
Hands, **Alum.* Baryt. *Hep.* *Kal.* Laur. °*Nitr. ac.* Petr. Phosph. Phos. ac.

Hands, fingers, Laur. °*Petr.*
—, fingers, between the, °*Calc.*
Nails, Sabad. Sil.

Rubeolæ.

In general, °*Acon.* °*Bell.* °*Bry.* Carb. veg.? Coff.? Ign.? °*Merc.* °*N. vom.* Phosph.? °*Puls.* Rhus.? Sulph.?

Round, which is.

Herpes, °Dulc. Hell. Phosph.
Spots, Jod. Led. **Merc.* Natr. Phosph. Zinc.

Saddle-shaped.

Nose, spot, Sep.
—, swelling, Poth.

Salt-rheum.

Ulcers, **Amb.* **Ars.* Calc. Chin. °*Graph.* °*Lyc.* Merc. Petr. Phosph. °*Puls.* °Sep. *Sil.* *Staph.* Sulph.

Sarcomatous, which is.

Eruption, Ars.
Lupia, °Baryt.
Ulcers, Ant. °*Ars.* Cupr. **Hep.* Kreas. **Merc.* *Nitr. ac.* °*Sabin.* Sulph. Thuj.

Face, °Ars.

Buccal cavity, ulcers, °Hep.
Dorsal region, swelling, nape of neck, **Baryt.**

Scaly, Desquamation.

Of the skin generally, Acon. Agar. *Alum.* **Amm.** Amm. m. Ars. Aur. Baryt. Bell. Bov. Calc. Canth. Caps. Carb. an. Caust. Cham. * *Clem.* Coloc. Con. Croton. Dig. Dulc. Euphorb. Ferr. Graph. Hell. Hyos. Jod. Kal. *Laur.* *Magn. c.* Merc. **Mez.* Mosch. Natr. Natr. m. * *Oleand.* Op. Par. Phosph. Phos. ac. Plat. Plumb. **Puls.** Ran. sc. Rhus. Sabad. *Sec.* Selen. Sep. **Sil.** Spig. *Staph.* Stram. Sulph. Sulph. ac. **Tarax.** Tart. *Veratr.*

Lower limbs, knees, Kreas.

Scaly, which is.

Eruption, Agar. *Amm.* Amm. m. Anac. **Ant.** Ars. *Aur.* Bar. m. Bell. Cic. * *Clem.* Cupr. Dulc. *Hep.* Hyos. Kal. *Led.* *Magn. c.* *Merc.* * *Oleand.* **Phosph.* Plumb. Rhus. Sep. Staph. *Sulph.*
Pimples, Dros. Merc.
Herpes, Anac. °Ars. ° *Clem.* Cupr. °*Dulc.* **Kreas.** °Led. °*Lyc.* Magn. c. °*Merc.* Sulph. **Teucr.**
Spots, Kal. Merc.
Scurfs, Croton. ° *Oleand.*

Head, **Alum.* Calc. Crotal. Graph. **Kal. Lach.** °Mez. * *Oleand.* Rhus. Staph.

Ears, pimples, Merc.
—, herpes, Teucr.
Face, Ammon. Anac. °Aur. °Led.
Arms, herpes, Cupr. *Merc.*
Hands, Hep. Laur.
Lower limbs, herpes, °*Clem.* Kreas.

Scarlatina.

In general, °Acon. **Amm.* *Amm. m.* Arn. *Ars.* Baryt. Bar. m. **Bell.* *Bry.* Carb. veg. Caust. Cham. (Coff.) Cop. *Croc.* Dulc. *Euphorb.* Galv. Hep. *Hyos.* Jod. Ipec. **Lach.* °*Merc.* **Phosph.* °*Phos. ac.* Rhus. *Stram.* *Sulph.* Tereb.
Scarlatina, Sydenhamian, **Amm.* **Bell.* Euphorb. Hyos. *Merc.*
—, gangrenous, °Amm. °Ars. °Lach.
—, suppressed, °Phosph.

Abdomen, **Bell.* **Rhus.*

Scarlet-like.

Spots, **Amm.* Amm. m. Arn. °*Ars.* Baryt. **Bell.* Bry. *Carb. veg.* Caust. Cham. °*Croc.* Dulc. *Euphorb.* Galv. °*Hep.* °*Hyos.* Jod. Ipec. Lach. **Merc.* *Phosph.* Phos. ac. Rhus. *Stram.* °*Sulph.*
Rash, °*Acon.* °Amm. ? °Ars. ? °Bell. °*Bry.* ? °Carb. veg. ? °Caust. °*Coff.* °Dulc. ? Galv. °Hyos. °*Ipec.* °Lach. ? °*Merc.* °Phosph. ? °Phos. ac. ? °Rhus. ? °Sulph. ?
Swelling, **Bell.*

Ridges, **Bell.* Euphorb. **Hep.*

———

Face, **Bell.*
Thoracic region, spots, **Bell.* Galv. **Lach.**
Nipples, spots, Lach.
Dorsal region, spots, **Bell.* Galv.
Arms, redness, **Bell.*
—, streaks, Euphorb. *Sabad.*
Hands, swelling, **Bell.*
Lower limbs, redness, Galv.

SCIRRHOUS, WHICH IS.

Indurations, °Bell. Carb. an. ? Carb. veg. ? °*Clem.* Cic.? °*Con.* Jod.?°Lach.? °*Petr.* Phosph.? Ran.? °*Rhus.* °Sep. °*Sil.* °Spong. ? °Sulph.

SCORBUTIC, WHICH IS.

In general, Alum. Amb. Ant. **Ars.* Bell. **Borax.** Bry. Calc. Caps. **Carb. an.* **Carb. veg.* **Caust.** Chin. Cic. Con. Dulc. Hep. Kal. **Kreas.* **Lyc.** **Merc.* **Mur. ac.* **Natr. m.* Nitr. **Nitr. ac.* *N. vom.* Petr. Phosph. Phos. ac. Rhus. **Ruta.** Sabin. Sep. Sil. Stann. **Staph.* Sulph. **Sulph. ac.* Zinc.
Spots, Merc. corr.
Rash, Ars.
Ulcers, *Merc.* **Staph.*

SCROFULOUS, WHICH IS.

In general, °*Alum.* Amm. °*Ant.* °*Ars.* °*Asa.*

°Aur. °*Baryt.* °*Bar. m.* °*Bell.* °*Borax.* °*Bov.* *Bry.*? °*Calc.* °*Carb. an.* °*Carb. veg.* Chinin.? Cin.? °*Cist.* °Con. °Dulc. °*Graph.* °*Hep.* °Jod. °*Kal.* °*Kreas.* °*Lach.* °*Lyc.* °*Magn. c.* °*Magn. m.* °Merc. °*Mez.* °*Mur. ac.* °*Natr.* °*Natr. m.* °Nitr. °*Nitr. ac.* N. mosch.? °*N. vom.* °Ol. jec. °*Petr.* Phell.? °*Phosph.* °*Phos. ac.* °Puls. Ran.? Ran. sc.? Rhab.? °*Rhus.* °*Sep.* °*Sil.* Staph. °*Sulph.* °*Sulph. ac.* Thuj.? °*Zinc.*

Nose, °Aur. °Calc. °Phosph.
Face, °Bov.
Lips, °Ars. °Aur. °Aur. m. °Bell. °Bov. °Calc. °Sil. °Sulph.
Arms, ulcer, °*Lach.*

Herpes, °Aur.
Swelling, Aur. °Bov. Calc. Phosph.
Ulcers, °*Ars.* Aur. °*Bell.* °Bov. °*Calc.* °Carb. an. °*Carb. veg.* °Caust. °*Cist.* °*Graph.* °*Hep.* °*Lach.* °*Lyc.* °N. vom. °*Phosph.* Sep. °*Sil.* °*Sulph.*

Scraping Sensation.

On the skin, in general, *Lyc.* Par. Rhus.

Bones, periosteum, **Asa.* Berb. °*Chin.* Coloc. *Phos. ac.* Puls. **Rhus.* **Sabad.* Spig.

SCRATCHING, AFTER.

Bleeding, bloody exsudations, Chin. Cocc. Kal. Nitr. ac.

Blisters, Amm. Ant. Caust. Chin. Cycl. Hep. Lach. Mang. Natr. Natr. m. Nitr. Phosph. Rhus. Sassap. Spong.

Blotches, Lach. Lyc. Merc. Natr. Nitr. ac. Op. Rhus. Spig. Veratr. Zinc.

Burning, *Amm.* Amm. m. Anac. Arn. *Ars. Bell.* Bov. *Bry.* Calad. Calc. Canth. *Caps. Caust.* Chel. Cic. Cocc. Cycl. Dros. *Dulc. Euphorb.* Guaj. Graph. Grat. *Hep.* Kal. Kreas. *Lach.* Laur. Led. *Lyc.* Magn. art. Magn. arct. Magn. c. Magn. m. *Merc. Mez.* Mosch. N. vom. *Oleand.* Par. *Phosph.* Phos. ac. Plumb. Puls. Ran. Rhod. *Rhus.* Sabad. Sabin. *Samb.* Sassap. *Seneg. Sep. Sil.* Spig. *Squill. Staph. Sulph. Thuj.* Veratr. Zinc.

Ecchymosed, Cycl. Euphorb. Hyos. Kal. Magn. art. Merc. Par. *Sulph.*

Eruption, in general, Alum. *Amm. Ars. Baryt.* Bov. Carb. an. Carb. veg. *Caust.* Kal. Lyc. Magn. c. **Merc.* Natr. Nitr. ac. Phosph. Staph. Zinc.

Herpes, °Dulc.

Itching, relieved by scratching, Alum. *Amb. Amm. Anac.* Ang. Ant. *Arn. Asa.* Berb. Bov. *Bry. Calc.* Camph. Cann. *Canth. Caps.* Caust. Chel. Cic. Cin. *Cycl. Dros. Dulc.* Ferr. magn. Grat. *Guaj. Ign.* Kreas. Laur. Led. Magn. arct. Magn. aust. Magn. c. Magn. m. ***Mang.*** ***Merc.*** Mosch. *Mur. ac. Natr.* Nitr. Oleand. Ol.

an. Phell. *Phosph.* Phos. ac. *Plumb.* Prun. *Rhus. Ruta.* Sabad. *Sabin.* Samb. Sassap. Seneg. *Spig.* Spong. Squill. Stront. *Sulph. Sulph. ac.* Tab. Tarax. Tart. Thuj. Viol. tr. *Zinc.*

Itching, shifting to another place, Anac. Calc. Chel. Con. Cycl. Ign. Magn. art. Magn. c. Magn. m. Mez. Nitr. ac. Spong. Staph. Sulph. ac. Zinc.

—, unchanged, Acon. Agar. Alum. Amb. Amm. Amm. m. Ang. Ant. *Arg. Arn.* Asa. Bism. Bov. Calad. *Cham. Chel.* Cocc. Colch. Croc. *Cupr.* Dros. *Euphorb.* Grat. Hell. *Ipec.* Kal. Laur. *Magn. art. Magn. arct. Magn. aust. Magn. m. Merc.* Mez. Nitr. ac. N. vom. *Puls. Ran. sc.* Rhab. Rhus. Ruta. *Sil. Spig. Spong.* Stront. *Sulph. Sulph. ac.* Tarax. Tart.

—, worse by scratching, *Anac.* Arn. Baryt. *Bism.* Bov. *Calad.* Calc. Cann. Canth. *Caps. Caust.* Cham. Chel. Chin. Cocc. *Con.* Cupr. Dros. Dulc. *Guaj.* Kal. *Led.* Magn. art. Magn. c. Magn. m. Merc. *Mez.* Par. Phosph. Phos. ac. *Puls.* Sassap. Seneg. Sep. *Sil.* Spig. *Spong.* Squill. Staph. Sram. *Stront.* Sulph.

Numbness of the spot scratched, Anac. Oleand. Plumb.

Pain as if ulcerated, Phosph. Staph.

Peeling off of the skin, Dros.

Pimples, Amm. m. Bov. Bry. Chin. Cycl. Graph. Grat. Lach. Laur. Magn. c. Merc. Mosch. Natr. m. Nitr. ac. Phosph. Puls. Rhus. Sabin. Sassap. Sep. Spong. Sulph. Veratr. Zinc.

Pustules, Cycl. Graph. Sassap.

Rash, Amm. Caust. Lach. Merc. Rhus. Selen. Veratr. Sulph.

Red skin, Agar. Arn. Bell. Bov. Graph. Lyc. Merc. Natr. m. N. vom. Oleand. Phos. ac. Puls. Rhus. Spong. Tarax. Teucr.

Red streaks, Euphorb. Phosph.

Smarting, Bry. Carb. an. Hell. *Sulph.* Zinc.

Sore as if raw, Agar. Amb. Ant. Baryt. Bry. Calc. Cann. Caps. Cic. Dros. Hep. Lyc. Magn. art. Magn. aust. Mang. Merc. Mez. Natr. m. Nitr. ac. N. vom. Oleand. Par. Petr. Phosph. Phos. ac. Puls. Rhus. Sabin. Selen. Sep. Sil. Squill. Staph. Sulph. Zinc.

Spots, Ant. Ars. Cocc. Kal. Lach. Mang. Merc. Phosph. Rhus. Sabad. Sep. Sulph. Sulph. ac.

Stinging, Arn. Asa. Baryt. Bry. Canth. Caust. Cycl. Dros. Graph. Merc. Par. Phos. ac. Puls. Rhus. Sabad. Sep. Sil. Spong. Squill. Staph. Sulph. Tarax. Thuj. Viol. tr.

Swelling, Ars. Bry. Caust. Dulc. Lach. Mang. Natr. m. Puls. Ran. Rhus. Sulph. Sulph. ac.

Ulcers, Ang. Ars. Asa. Bell. Caust. Con. Hep. **Lach.* Lyc. Merc. Natr. Nitr. ac. Petr. Puls. Rhus. Sil. Staph. Sulph.

Tension, Caust. Lach. Phos. ac. Stront.

Titillation, Amb. Caps. Chin. Cocc. Merc. Sabad. Sil. Spig.

Tubercles, Agar. Ars. Bov. Bry. Carb. an. Magn. m. Magn. s. Ipec. Natr. m. Nicc. Op. Staph. Sulph. Zinc.

Scurfy.

Eruption, Ars. Electr. Mang. Phos. ac. Sep. (Comp. Scurf.)
Blisters, vesicles, Hell. Natr. *Ran.* Sil. Sulph.
Pimples, Bell. **Calc.* Carb. an. Cham. Hep. Mur. ac. *Oleand. Petr. Sabin. Staph.
Pustules, Ant. Bov. Croton. Dulc. Merc. Tart.
Herpes, °Bov. **Calc.* *Clem.* °*Con.* Graph. °Lach. °Lyc. °Sep. °*Sulph.*
Spots, *Merc.* **Nitr. ac.* Thuj. Zinc.
Swelling, **Merc.*
Ulcers, Ant. **Ars.* Baryt. °*Bell.* Bov. *Bry.* **Calc.* Carb. an. °*Cic.* Clem. **Con.* Electr. **Graph.* Hell. *Hep.* °*Led.* °*Lyc.* **Merc.* Mur. ac. N. vom. Oleand. Par. *Phos. ac.* Plumb. *Puls. Ran.* **Rhus.* *Sabin.* Sassap. °*Sep.* **Sil.* Spong. *Staph.* **Sulph.* Viol. tr.
Tubercles, Sulph.

Ears, eruption, Puls.
Arms, ulcers, Electr. Sabin.
Hands, eruption, Hell. Mur. ac. *Sassap.*
Lower limbs, eruption, Mang.
—, herpes, *Clem.*
—, spots, Zinc.
—, ulcers, Ars. Graph.

Scurfs, Crusts.

In general, **Alum.* Amb. *Amm. Amm. m.* **Ant.* **Ars.* Asa. *Aur. *Aur. m. **Baryt.* **Bell.* °*Bov.*

Bry. ******Calc.* Caps. °*Carb. an.* °*Carb. veg.* Cham. °*Chel.* Chinin. **Cic.* **Clem.* °*Coloc.* Con. Croton. °*Dulc.* Electr. Ferr. magn. **Graph.* **Hell.* **Hep.* Ign. °*Kal.* Kreas. **Lach.* Led. **Lyc.* Magn. c. **Merc.* Mez. Mur. ac. **Natr. m.* Nitr. ac. N. vom. **Oleand.* Par. *Petr. Phosph.* Phos. ac. Plumb. **Puls.* *Ran.* **Rhus.* Ruta. *Sabad.* Sabin. **Sassap.* °*Sep.* **Sil.* Spong. Squill. **Staph.* **Sulph.* Tart. *Thuj. Veratr.* °*Viol. tr.* Vip. torv. Zinc.

—, over the whole body, Dulc.

Black, °*Bell.* Chinin. Vip. torv.

Bleeding, *Merc.* Mez.

Brown, Amm. m. Ant. Berb.

Burning, Amm. m. Calc. Cic. Puls. Sassap.

Crusta lactea, °*Ars.* Baryt.? Bell.? *Calc.?* Carb. veg.? *Cic.?* Dulc.? Lyc.? °*Merc.* Natr. m.? Phosph.? Phosp. ac.? °*Rhus.* Sassap. Sep.? °*Sulph.* Viol. tr.?

Dry, Ars. **Aur.* **Aur. m.* °*Baryt.* °*Calc.* Chinin. Graph. Lach. Led. Merc. °*Sulph.* Thuj.

Fetid, Graph. Lyc. *Merc.* Plumb. Staph. **Sulph.*

Gnawing, Mang.

Gray, Ars. Merc.

Greenish, **Calc.*

Herpetic, °Bov. **Calc.* *Ran.* °*Sep.* Sulph.

Horny, *Graph. Ran.*

Humid, °*Alum.* **Ars.* **Baryt.* **Calc.* Chinin. **Cic.* °*Clem.* **Graph.* **Hell.* °*Hep.* **Lyc.* **Merc.* °*Mez.* °*Oleand.* Plumb. Ran. °*Rhus.* °*Ruta.* Sep. °*Sil.* **Staph.* **Sulph.*

Inflamed, Lyc.

Jerking and painful, Staph.

Itching, Caust. Merc. Phos. ac. *Rhus. Sassap. Sil.
Livid, Chinin.
Painful, Magn. m.
Painful as if sore, Cic. *Sil.*
Raised, Sabin.
Red, redbrown, Amm. m.
Scaly, Croton.
Smarting, Puls.
Suppurating, **Ars.* Plumb. Sil. **Sulph.* (Comp. Humid.)
Tensive, Amm. m.
Yellow, Ant. Aur. Aur. m. **Cic.* Jod. Kreas. Merc. Mez.

Head, °Alum. **Ars.* °Baryt. **Calc.* °*Carb. an.* °Chel. Electr. Ferr. magn. **Graph.* °Hell. °Kal. Magn. c. **Merc.* Mur. ac. **Natr. m.* Nitr. ac. **Oleand.* Paris. Petr. Phosph. **Rhus.* Ruta. Sil. Sulph.
Eyes, Graph. **Merc.* Sep.
Eyelids, Graph. Sep.
Ears, Bov. °*Graph.* °*Hep.* Jod. °*Lach.* °*Lyc.* Mur. ac. °*Puls.* Sassap. Spong.
—, behind the ears, °*Graph.* °*Hep.* °Lyc. °Puls. °*Staph.*
Nose, **Ant.* °Baryt. Bell. Bov. *Carb. an.* Carb. veg. Croton. Natr. m. Nitr. ac. Petr. **Phos. ac.* Ratanh. *Rhus.* Sep. *Staph.* °Sulph.
—, nostrils, **Alum.* Amm. m. **Aur.* Borax. Bov. **Calc.* Carb. an. Cham. °Cic. Ferr. °*Graph.* Hep. Jod. **Kal.* Lach. °Lyc. Magn.

c. **Magn. m.* Merc. Natr. Nitr. ac. Petr. *Phosph. Puls. Sep.* **Sil.* °*Sulph.* **Thuj.*
Nose, at the tip, *Carb. an.* Carb. veg. *Sep.*
Face, °Alum. Ant. **Ars.* **Baryt.* **Bell.* Bry. **Calc.* Carb. veg. **Cic.* °Coloc. °*Dulc.* **Graph.* Hep. Ign. **Lach.* Lyc. °*Merc.* Mur. ac. Nitr. ac. Petr. Phosph. *Phos. ac.* Sassap. **Sep.* Sil. Staph. Sulph. Thuj. Viol. tr. Zinc.
Lips and mouth, region of, **Ars.* Baryt. **Bell.* Berb. °Bry. Calc. °Cann. Cham. Cic. *Ign. Kal. Mur. ac. N. vom. Petr. Phos. ac. Rhus. Sep. *Sil.* Squill. Staph. Sulph.
Chin, Sep.
Buccal cavity, tongue, Chinin.
Sexual parts, Caust. **Nitr. ac.* Thuj.
Nipples, °Lyc.
Dorsal region, Graph. Natr. m.
—, axilla, *Natr. m.*
—, nape of neck, Bell.
Arms, elbows, *Sep.*
—, forearm, °*Alum.*
Hands, Sassap. °Sep.
—, fingers, Anac.
Lower limbs, legs, Ars. Calc. *Sabin.* Staph. Zinc.
Feet, *Sil.*

Sexual Parts.

Aphthæ, labia, Carb. veg.
Balanorrhœa, s. Suppurating.
Black, eruption, Bry.
Blisters, vesicles, Carb. veg. Caust. Graph. *Merc. Nitr. ac. Phos. ac. Rhus.* Staph. Sulph. *Thuj.*

Blisters, glans, Merc. Phos. ac. Rhus. Thuj.
—, labia, Graph. Staph. Sulph.
—, prepuce, Carb. veg. Caust. Graph. Nitr. ac.
Blotches, Arn. Bell. Bov. Sep.
—, glans, Bell.
—, scrotum, Arn.
—, neck of womb, Kreas. Thuj.
—, labia, Calc. Phosph.
—, prepuce, Sep.
Blue-red, swelling, °Arn. Ars.
Brown, spots, Nitr. ac.
Burning, Amb. *Amm.* Anac. Ars. Baryt. *Berb.* Bov. *Calc. Cann. Canth.* **Carb. veg. Caust.* Cham. Euphorb. Hyos. Kal. Kreas. *Laur.* °Lyc. *Magn. arct.* Magn. aust. Merc. acet. Mez. *Nitr. ac.* N. vom. Petr. Puls. Sep. Spong. Stann. **Sulph.* Tereb. Thuj.
—, glans, °Anac. Calc. Stann. Viol. tr.
—, testicles, Baryt. Berb. Nitr. ac. °*Puls.* Tereb.
—, scrotum, Berb. Euphorb. Spong. Sulph. Plat.
—, penis, Caust. Merc. acet. Sep. Spong. Stann.
—, labia, Amm. Calc. Canth. **Carb. veg.* Kal. °*Lyc.* Magn. aust. **Sulph.*
—, vagina, Berb. Cham. Hyos. Lyc. Sulph. Thuj.
Burning, eruptions, Calc. Kal. Nitr. ac. Phosph.
—, ulcers, Hep.
Chancre and chancrous ulcers, Hep. **Merc.* *Nitr. ac. °*Sep.* °Thuj.
After contusion, Con.
Dampness, Calc. *Cann.* Carb. veg. *Hep. Lyc.*

Natr. m. Nitr. ac. **Petr. Sep. Staph.* °Sulph. **Thuj.*

Dampness, glans, dampness, *Cann.* Cinn. *Lyc.* **Merc.* Mez. Natr. m. Nitr. ac. *Sep.* Staph. Thuj.

—, scrotum, Carb. veg. **Petr.* °Sulph.

—, pudendum and thigh, between, Calc. *Hep.*

—, mons veneris, Sulph.

—, prepuce, Nitr. ac.

Eruption, in general, N. vom. Rhus. °*Sep.* Sulph. Tart.

—, glans, Petr. Sep.

—, scrotum, Graph. Rhus.

—, mons veneris, Sil.

—, labia, N. vom. °*Sep.* Tart.

—, vagina, Sulph.

—, prepuce, Merc. Rhus.

Excrescences, °Cinn. °Euphr. °*Lyc.* Magn. aust. °*Nitr. ac.* **Phos. ac. Sabin.* °Staph. °*Thuj.*

—, corona, glandis, Nitr. ac. Phos. ac. Staph. *Thuj.

—, os tincæ, °Thuj.

—, prepuce, *Nitr. ac. Sabin.

Falling off of hairs, Natr. m. Nitr. ac. *Phos. ac. Zinc.*

Fetid, ulcers, Hep. Nitr. ac.

Figwarts, Cinn. °Euphr. Magn. aust. °*Nitr. ac.* °Phos. ac. °Sassap. Sabin. °Staph.? °Thuj.

Fine, eruptions, Kal. Merc.

Flat, ulcers, Corall. **Nitr. ac.* *Thuj.

Gangrene, *Ars. Canth.* Laur. Plumb. °Sec.

—, scrotum, Plumb.

—, penis, Canth. Laur. Plumb.

—, uterus, °Sec.

Gnawing, °Kal. °Lyc. N. vom. Plat.
—, testicles, °Phos. ac.
—, scrotum, Plat.
—, labia, °Kal. °Lyc.
Hard, eruption, Bov. Kreas.
—, swelling, Carb. veg. Merc.
Hæmorrhage, (metrorrhagia), **Acon.* Amm. **Bell.* Bry. *Calc. **Cham.* **Chin.* °Chinin.? *Cin.* °Cinnam.? Cocc. °Coff.? **Croc.* °Diad.? **Ferr.* °Hyos. °Ign.? **Ipec.* Jod. °Kreas. °Led.? Magn. arct. °Magn. aust.? *Merc.* °Natr. Natr. m. N. vom. °*Plat.* °*Puls.* °Rhus. °Ruta.? Sabin. **Sec.* Squill. *Stram.* °Sulph.? °Sulph. ac.
—, urethra, Amm. °Arn. *Ars. °Calc. **Canth.* °Caps. °Caust. °Chin.? °*Con.* °Cop.? Crotal. °Euphorb.? **Ipec.* **Lyc.* **Merc.* Mez. °Mill.? Murex. °N. vom. Op. *Phosph.* °*Puls.* *Sec.* Tereb. Uv. *Zinc.*
Herpes, Croton. °*Dulc.* Natr. m. °*Petr.* *Sassap.*
—, scrotum, Croton. Natr. m.
—, scrotum and thigh, between, °Petr.
—, labia, °Dulc.
—, prepuce, Sassap.
Hydrocele, testicles, Arn. Dig. Graph.? °N. vom.? °*Puls.* °Rhod. °*Sil.* °*Sulph.*
Induration, testicles, °Agn. °Aur. °*Clem.* Cop. N. vom. °Spong.? Sulph.
—, scrotum, Clem. Rhus.
—, prostate glands, Cop. °Jod.
—, neck of womb, Chin. Jod. °Sep.
—, labia, Merc.
—, prepuce, °Lach.
Inflammation, °*Acon.* *Ars.* Calc. Cann. Canth.

Con. Magn. aust. **Merc.* Merc. acet. Mur. ac. Natr. Natr. m. Nitr. ac. N. vom. Phos. ac. Plumb. Puls. Sep. Spong. Staph. Thuj.

Inflammation, glans, Magn. aust. Natr.

—, urethra, **Cann.* **Canth.* Cop. Gran. Sabin.

—, orifice of urethra, Hep. Merc. Sulph. Tab.

—, testicles, °Acon. °Aur. °N. vom. °Spong. ? °Staph.?

—, scrotum, °Ars.? Natr. m. Phos. ac. Plumb.

—, prostate gland, °Puls. °Thuj.

—, penis, Canth. Merc. acet. Plumb. Sep.

—, labia, Calc. Nitr. ac. °N. vom. ? °*Sep.* Sulph.

—, vagina, Nitr. ac.

—, prepuce, Calc. Cann. Con. **Merc.* Mur. ac. Natr. Nitr. ac.

Inflammatory swelling, °Arn. *Merc.* Phos. ac. °*Puls.*

After injuries, °Arn. °Con.

Itching, Acon. Agar. Agn. Alum. *Amb. Amm.* Anac. Ang. Ant. Arn. Ars. Aur. Baryt. *Berb.* Bry. **Calc.* Camph. *Cann. Canth.* Carb. an. **Carb. veg. Caust.* Cham. Chin. Cinn. *Cocc. Coff.* **Con.* Croc. Dig. Dulc. Euphorb. Euphr. Ferr. magn. *Graph. Hep.* Heracl. *Ign.* Ipec. Jod. **Kal. Kreas.* Laur. Led. **Lyc. Magn. art. Magn. arct.* Magn. aust. *Magn.m.* Mang. Meph. **Merc.* Mez. Mur. ac. Natr. **Natr. m.* Natr. s. Nicc. *Nitr. ac. N. vom.* Ol. an. **Petr.* Phos. ac. Prun. *Puls.* Ratanh. Rhod. *Rhus.* Sabin. Sassap. Selen. **Sep.* **Sil.* Spong. Staph. **Sulph. Thuj.* Viol. tr. Zinc.

—, frænulum, Cann. Caust. Hep. Merc.

—, glans, Alum. Amb. Arn. Ars. Calc. Chin. Cinn. Coff. Con. Dig. Hep. Ign. Ipec. Jod.

Kal. Led. Magn. aust. Mang. *Merc.* Mez. *Natr. Natr. m.* Natr. s. *Nitr. ac. N. vom.* Petr. Sabin. *Sep.* Sil. Spong. *Thuj.*

Itching, testicles, Merc.

—, scrotum, Agar. Alum. Amm. Anac. Ang. Ant. Aur. Baryt. *Berb.* Calc. *Carb. veg. Caust.* Cham. Chin. *Cocc.* Coff. Croc. Ferr. magn. *Graph.* Hep. Heracl. Kal. *Lyc.* Magn. aust. Magn. m. Mang. Meph. Mur. ac. Natr. Natr. s. Nicc. *Nitr. ac. N. vom.* **Petr.* Phos. ac. Prun. Puls. Ratanh. Rhod. Selen. Staph. Thuj. Zinc.

—, clitoris, Sulph.

—, penis, Agar. Ant. Ars. Caust. Coff. Con. Hep. Natr. s. *Nitr. ac.* Ol. an. Phos. ac.

—, mons veneris, Agar. Carb. an. Carb. veg. *Kal.* Natr. s. Sulph.

—, labia, Agar. Amb. *Amm.* **Calc.* **Carb. veg.* **Con.* Graph. °*Kal.* Kreas. Lyc. Magn. c. *Merc.* **Natr. m.* Nicc. *Nitr. ac.* **Sep.* **Sil. Staph.* **Sulph.* Thuj.

—, vagina, Canth. **Con.* Kreas. **Sulph.*

—, prepuce, Acon. Agar. Ang. Ars. Bry. Calc. Camph. *Cann. Carb. veg.* Caust. Con. Euphorb. Euphr. Ign. Laur. *Lyc. Magn. arct.* Merc. Natr. *Nitr. ac. N. vom. Puls.* Rhus. Sep. Thuj. Viol. tr.

Itching, eruptions, Amb. Arn. Graph. Lach. *Nitr. ac.* Sep. Sil.

Abuse of mercury, after, °*Thuj.*

Miliary, eruption, Thuj.

Pain as if contused, testicles, Acon. Arg. *Calc.* Dig. Kal. °Lach. Natr. c. Nitr. ac. Rhod. Sabad. Sabin. Thuj.

Redness, Calad. *Calc.* Cann. Carb. veg. Cinn. Corall. Croton. Magn. aust. Merc. Natr. m. Sabin. **Sep.*
—, glans, Calad. Cann. Corall. Croton. Magn. aust. Sabin.
—, scrotum, Merc. Natr. m.
—, pudendum and thigh, between, *Sep.
—, labia, Calc. Carb. veg. Merc. **Sep.*
—, prepuce, Calc. Cann. Cinn. Corall. **Sil.* Sulph.
Painful eruptions, Bov. Con. Nitr. ac. Sil.
—, swelling, °Arn. Ars. Cop. **Merc.* Vip. torv.
Painless, eruptions, Arn. Bell.
—, swelling, Jod.
—, ulcers, Nitr. ac.
Pale-red, eruptions, Cann.
Phimosis, Merc. Sulph.
Pimples, Amb. *Con.* Graph. Kal. *Lach.* Magn. aust. *Merc.* Natr. m. *Nitr. ac.* Phos. ac. Sil. Tart. Thuj. Zinc.
—, glans, Lach. Magn. aust. Nitr. ac.
—, hairy region, Lach.
—, scrotum, Phos. ac. Thuj. Zinc.
—, penis, Phos. ac.
—, mons veneris, Amb. Kal. Sil.
—, labia, Con. Graph. Kal. Natr. m.
—, prepuce, Magn. aust. Nitr. ac. Sil.
Pock-shaped, pimples, Thuj.
Prickling, scrotum, Plat.
Prolapsus, °Bell. Ferr. °Gran.? Kreas. *Merc. °*N. vom.* °Sep. Stann.
—, vagina, Ferr. °Gran.? *Merc. °*Sep.* Stann.
—, uterus, °Bell. °Gran.? Kreas. °*N. vom.* °*Sep.*
Pustules, Bov. Bry.

Rash, Bry. °Dulc. Rhus.
—, glans, Bry.
—, scrotum. Rhus.
—, labia, *Dulc.
Red, eruption, Bov. Kal. Lach. Merc. Petr. Phosph. ac. Sep. **Thuj.* Zinc.
—, spots, Arn. Carb. veg. Caust. Con. Lach. Natr. m. **Nitr. ac.* Petr. Sil. Thuj.
—, swelling, °Arn. Ars. Merc.
—, ulcers, Corall.
Rhagades, glans, Ars.
Scurfs, Caust. **Nitr. ac.* Thuj.
Shining, redness, Merc.
Smooth, excrescences, Thuj.
—, spots, Carb. veg. Petr.
Smarting, Graph. Hep. Heracl. *Magn. art. Puls.* Ran. sc. Staph. Thuj.
—, inguen, Hep.
—, scrotum, Heracl. Ran. sc.
—, labia, Staph.
—, vagina, Graph. Thuj.
—, prepuce, *Magn. art. Puls.*
Smarting, eruption, Graph. Kal. Staph.
Soreness, Alum. Amb. *Amm.* Arn. Calad. Calc. **Carb. veg.* Caust. **Cham.* °*Graph. Hep.* Hyos. *Ign.* °*Lyc.* Meph. **Merc. Natr.* Natr. m. *Nitr. ac.* **N. vom.* Petr. Plumb. **Sep.* **Sulph.* Veratr. ·Zinc.
—, glans, Natr.
—, scrotum, Kal. Natr. m. Petr. Plumb. °Sulph. ·Zinc.
—, pudendum and thigh, between, Caust. *Hep.* Lyc. Merc. *Natr.* **Sep.* °*Sulph.*
—, labia, Amb. Amm. **Carb. veg.* Hep. Natr. **Sep.* Sulph.

Soreness, vagina, Hyos.
Sore, as if excoriated, Amb. Berb. Borax. Cann. Cic. Cinn. Coff. Corall. Ferr. Kal. Kreas. Murex. Phos. ac. Rhod. ***Rhus.*** Sabin. Tab. Teucr. °Zinc.
—, glans, Sabin.
—, scrotum, Berb. Coff. Phos. ac. Teucr.
—, penis, Borax. Cann. Cic.
—, labia, Amb. Berb.
—, vagina, Berb. Ferr. mur. Kal. Kreas. Rhus.
—, prepuce, Cinn. Corall. Sabin.
Sore eruptions, Staph. Zinc.
Ulcers, Hep.
Spots, Arn. Calc. Cann. Carb. veg. Caust. ***Cinn.*** **Lach.* Natr. m. **Nitr. ac.* Petr. Rhus. ***Sil. Thuj.***
—, glans, Arn. Cann. Carb. veg. Cinn. **Lach.* Natr. m. Petr. Thuj.
—, scrotum, Calc. **Sil.*
—, prepuce, Lach. Rhus. Thuj.
Spreading, ulcers, **Merc.*
Stinging, eruption, Calc. Phosph.
—, swelling, Phosph.
—, ulcers, Hep.
Stricture, urethra, Carb. veg. **Clem.* Cop. °Dulc.? °Lach.? °N. vom. °Petr. *Puls.* Rhus.
Suppurating, swelling, Corall. Phosph.
Suppurations, discharge of pus, Caps. Con. Merc. Sassap. Sep.
—, prepuce and glans, between, (balanorrhœa) (Comp. Dampness) Cinn. **Merc.* Mez. *Sep. Cann. Lyc.* Natr. m. Nitr. ac. Staph. **Thuj.*
—, urethra (gonorrhœa), °Agn. *Cann. *Canth. Caps. Chel. Con. °Cop.? Galv. Ipec. Lam.

Merc. Mercurial. °Natr. m.? Nitr. ac. °N. vom.? °*Petr.* Phos. ac. *Puls. Ratanh. Sassap. Sabin. °Tereb.? *Thuj. —Bar. m.? Lach.

Swelling, °Agn. °*Arn.* **Ars.* *Aur. Baryt. Bar. m. Berb. Calad. Cann. *Canth.* **Carb. veg.* °Chin. Cinn. **Clem.* °Con. Cop. Corall. °Dig. Graph. Ign. °Jod. *Kal. *Kreas.* Led. °*Lyc.* Magn. arct. **Merc.* Merc. acet. Natr. c. Nitr. ac. °*N. vom.* Ol. an. Phosph. Phos. ac. Plumb. **Puls.* *Rhod. Rhus. Sabin. °Samb. °*Sep.* Sil. Spig. °Spong. Sulph. *Thuj.* Viol. tr. Vip. torv.

—, frænulum, Cann. Canth. Sabin.

—, glans, Ars. Corall. Natr. Spig.

—, testicles, °*Agn.* °Arn. Ars. **Aur.* Bar. m. °Chin. °*Clem.* °Con. °Dig. °Jod. °Kal. °Lyc. °*Merc.* Nitr. ac. °N. vom. Ol. an. Plumb. **Puls.* **Rhod.* *Spong.

—, scrotum, *Arn. Canth. Carb. veg. Clem. Graph. Ign. Phos. ac. Puls. Rhus. °Samb. °Sep. Vip. torv.

—, epidydimis, Baryt. Magn. arct. Sulph.

—, prostate glans, Cann. °*Puls.* °*Thuj.*

—, penis, °Arn. Cann. Canth. Cinn. Kreas. Led. Merc. acet. Sabin.

—, spermatic cord, Arn. Berb. °Chin. Kal. Phosph. Phos. ac. *Puls.* Spong.

—, neck of uterus, Canth. Sec.

—, labia, Amb. Amm. Bry. Calc. Carb. veg. Kreas. Meph. °*Merc.* Merc. acet. Nitr. ac. °*Sep.* Thuj.

—, vagina, Merc. Nitr. ac. **N. vom.*

—, prepuce, Calad. Cann. Cinn. Corall. **Merc.*

Nitr. ac. Rhus. Sabin. Sil. Sulph. Thuj. Viol. tr.

Ulcers, **Corall.* Graph. Hep. **Merc.* Merc. d. **Nitr. ac.* Phosph. °*Sep.* **Sulph.* **Thuj.*

—, glans, Corall. Nitr. ac. °*Sulph.* *Thuj.

—, labia, Graph. Thuj.

—, pudendum and thigh, between, Graph.

—, prepuce, Hep. *Merc.* *Nitr. ac.* Phosph. °*Sulph.*

Pickling, scrotum, Phos. ac.

Titillation, Acon. Berb. Carb. veg. Chin. Magn. aust. Merc. Natr. m. Phos. ac. Plat. Sil. Spig. Thuj. Val.

—, frænulum, Merc. Phos. ac.

—, glans, Magn. aust. *Natr. m.* Phos. ac. Spig.

—, testicles, Berb. Carb. veg.

—, scrotum, *Berb.* Carb. veg. Chin. Merc. Phos. ac. Sil. Thuj.

—, penis, Val.

—, sexual parts, *Plat.*

Tumors, Natr.

Ulceration, Caust. Merc. Nitr. ac. Thuj.

Urticaria, labia, Tart.

Varices, °Calc. °Lyc. °N. vom.? Zinc.

Wart-shaped, excrescences, Sec. °Thuj.

—, os tincæ, °Sec. °Thuj.

White, ulcers, **Merc.* Thuj.

Yellow, ulcers, Nitr. ac.

Shines, that which.

Swelling, Alum. **Arn.* **Ars.* °*Bry.* **Merc.* Phosph. Ran. *Rhus.* *Sabin.* °*Sulph.* Thuj.

Ulcers, Puls. Staph.

Nose, Borax. Calc. *Canth. Merc.*
—, as if from oil, Calc.
Face, skin of, Plumb. Selen.
Lips, swelling, Staph.
Sexual parts, redness, Merc.
Arms, swelling, **Bry.*
Hands, swelling, *Ran.*
Lower limbs, swelling, °*Bry. Merc.* °*Sulph.*
Feet, swelling, Alum, **Ars. Sabin.* °*Sulph.* Thuj.

SHINES THROUGH, THAT WHICH.

Eruption, Cin. *Merc.* Ran.
Rash, Cin.

SHRIVELLING, WRINKLES.

Wrinkled skin, in general, Amb. Amm. Ant. Bry. **Calc.* Camph. Cham. Cupr. Graph. Hell. Lyc. Merc. Mur. ac. N. vom. Phosph. ac. Plumb. Rhab. Rhod. Rhus. Sabad. **Sassap. Sec.* Sep. Spig. Stram. Sulph. Veratr. Viol. od. Vip. torv.

Nose, Cham.
Hands, fingers, Amb. Cupr. Phos. ac. Sulph.

SMALL, THAT WHICH IS.

Boils, **Arn.* Baryt. Grat. Lyc. Magn. c. Magn. m. Natr. m. *N. vom.* Sulph. Zinc.

Pustules, Evon. Hydroc. Nitr. Tart.
Herpes, °Dulc. °Lach. Magn. Magn. s.
Spots, Bry. Lach. Led. Lyc. Merc. Op. Ratanh. Squill. °*Sulph. ac.* Tart. Vip. torv.
Warts, Baryt. *Calc. *Dulc.* Ferr. magn. Hep. Lach. Rhus. **Sassap.* Sep. *Sulph.*

SMARTING, THAT WHICH SMARTS.

Blotches, Lach. °Sulph.
Eruption, Agn. Alum. Amm. *Amm. m.* Ant. Arn. Ars. Bell. Borax. Bov. Bry. Calc. Camph. Canth. Caps. Carb. an. Carb. veg. Caust. Cham. Chel. Chin. Cocc. *Colch.* Coloc. Con. Dros. *Euphorb.* Hell. *Ipec. Lach. Led. Lyc.* Magn. arct. Magn. aust. Magn. c. Mang. Merc. ***Mez.*** Mur. ac. Natr. Natr. m. N. vom. *Oleand.* Op. Petr. Phosph. Phos. ac. Plat. *Puls.* Ran. Ran. sc. Rhod. Selen. Sil. Spig. *Spong.* Stront. Sulph. Thuj. Veratr. Viol. tr.
Expectoration, Ant. Ars. *Cham.* °*Con.* Ferr. Ipec. °Lach. Merc. °*Phosph.* Sil. *Sulph.*
Herpes, Alum.
Pimples, Agar. *Bell.* Calc. Cham. Coloc. Dig. Kal. Lyc. Merc. Nitr. Teucr. Veratr.
Spots, Puls.
Swelling, N. vom.
Swelling of veins, Grat. Tart.
Vesicles, Graph. Mang. Phos. ac. Plat. Rhod. Rhus. Staph.
Ulcers, Ars. *Bell.* Bry. Calc. Carb. an. Caust. Cham. Chin. *Colch.* Coloc. °*Dig.* Euphorb. °*Graph.* Lach. Lam. °*Led.* °*Lyc.* Mang. ***Merc.*** Mez. Nitr. ac. Petr. Phos. ac. **Puls.* Ran.

Rhus. Ruta. Selen. Sil. Staph. **Sulph.* Sulph. ac. Thuj.
Scurfs, crusts, Puls.

Head, Agn. Bry. Calc. Dros. Grat. Jod. Magn. arct. Merc. Mez. Ran. Rhod. Thuj. Zinc.
—, eruptions and ulcers, Agn. Bry. Coloc. Dros. Jod. Magn. arct. Ran. sc.
Ears, eruptions, Mez. Petr. Puls.
Face, Bell. Bry. Calc. Coloc. Merc. Plat.
Lips and mouth, region of, Bell. Bry. Kal. Merc. Plat. Rhod. Rhus.
Buccal cavity, blisters and ulcers, Merc. Natr. Natr. m. Phos. ac.
Sexual organs, eruptions, Graph. Kal. Staph.
Dorsal region, Ars. Bry.
—, blotches, Lach.
Arms, eruptions, &c., Lyc. Zinc.
Hands, eruptions, Mang.
Lower limbs, pimples, Agar.
Feet, ulcer, Lam.

SMARTING PAIN, AS IF SORE, EXCORIATED.

In general, Acon. Agar. °*Alum.* Amb. Ant. Arg. **Arn.* Ars. °*Aur.* Baryt. Bell. Berb. Borax. **Bry.* **Calc.* Cann. **Canth.* Caps. Carb. an. Carb. veg. **Caust.* Chel. Chin. **Cic.* Coff. Colch. Con. °*Daph.* Dros. Ferr. **Graph.* Hell. ***Hep.** **Ign.* Kal. Laur. Led. **Lyc.* Magn. art. Magn. arct. **Magn. aust.* Magn. c. *Mang.* **Merc.* *Mez.* Mosch. Natr. Natr. m. **Nitr. ac.* **N. vom.* Oleand. Par. **Petr.* *Phosph.* Phos. ac. **Plat.*

******Puls.* Ran. **Rhus.* Rhus v. Ruta. Sabin. Sassap. Selen. **Sep.* Sil. Spig. Spong. *Squill.* *Staph.* **Sulph.* **Sulph. ac.* Tab. Teucr. Val. Veratr. **Zinc.*

Head, *Amb. Anac. Ars. Bry. Calc. *Dros.* Gran. Graph. **Hep.* Jod. Magn. c. **Merc.* **Mez.* Natr. c. *Natr. m.* N. vom. Ol. an. Par. Petr. Phosph. Phos. ac. Ran. Ruta. Staph. Stront. Zinc.

Ears, Borax. Caust. Cic. Galv. Lyc. Magn. c. Phos. ac. Sep.

Nose, Amb. Amm. Ang. *Ant.* Aur. Bov. Camph. Caust. Chin. Cic. Cin. Coff. Colch. Con. Hep. Ign. Lyc. Magn. arct. Magn. c. *Magn. m.* Mang. *Mez.* Natr. m. Nitr. ac. **N. vom.* Phosph. *Rhod.* Rhus. *Sep.* Sil. Spig. Squill. *Staph.* Sulph. Zinc.

Face, Alum. Anac. Borax. Bry. Canth. Con. Dros. Magn. aust. Puls. Sil. Spig.

Lips and mouth, region of, Amm. Ann. Caust. Chin. Euphorb. Graph. Ign. Ipec. Kal. Kreas. Magn. art. Magn. arct. Merc. Phosph. Phos. ac. Plat. Puls. Rhus. Sabad. Sep. Sulph. ac. Teucr.

—, corners of mouth, Bell. Calc. Caust. Graph. Ipec. Magn. arct. Mang. Merc. Natr. m. Sulph. ac.

Chin, Ant. Hep. Magn. aust. Mang. Veratr.

Lower jaw, Bry. Canth. Mang. Veratr.

Buccal cavity, Agar. Alum. Amb. Amm. Ant. Arn. Ars. Aur. Bism. Bry. *Calc.* *Caps.* *Carb. an.* **Carb. veg.* *Cast.* *Caust.* °Cist. Clem. Cocc. Corall. Dig. Electr. **Graph.* Hell. **Ign.* Jod.

Kal. Kreas. **Lach.* Magn. arct. Magn. aust. Magn. c. *Magn. m.* Mang. *Merc.* Mur. ac. Natr. Natr. m. **Nitr. ac.* N. vom. Petr. *Phosph.* Phos. ac. **Puls.* Ratanh. Rhod. Rhus. Ruta. Sabad. Sassap. *Seneg.* **Sep.* Sil. Staph. Stram. Tereb. Teucr. Thuj. **Zinc.*

Buccal cavity, palate, Agar. Alum. *Caust.* Ign. *Mang.* Puls. Thuj.

—, velum palati, Ruta.

—, tonsils, Raph. Rhus.

—, mouth, Agar. Alum. Amm. Electr. Ign. Natr. Phosph. Stram.

—, fauces and throat, Alum. Amm. Aur. Calc. *Caps. Carb. an. Carb. veg. Cast. Caust.* °Cist. Corall. Dig. Hell. **Ign. Kal.* Kreas. **Lach.* Magn. aust. Magn. c. *Magn. m.* **Merc.* **Nitr. ac.* Petr. *Phosph.* Phos. ac. **Puls.* Rhus v. Sabin. *Seneg.* **Sep.* Staph.

—, gums, Alum. Ars. Asa. Aur. Bism. Bry. **Carb. veg.* Clem. Cocc. **Graph.* Jod. Magn. arct. Mur. ac. Natr. m. Nitr. ac. N. vom. Petr. Phosph. Phos. ac. Puls. Ratanh. Rhod. Ruta. Sassap. Sep. Sil. Staph. Tereb. Thuj. *Zinc.

—, uvula, Caust.

—, tongue, Alum. Amb. Amm. Ant. Arn. *Calc. Caust.* Graph. *Ign.* Laur. *Merc.* Natr. Natr. m. *Nitr. ac.* Sabad. Sep. Staph. Teucr. Thuj. Zinc.

Abdomen, Cann. Carb. veg. Croton. Euphorb. °Hyos. Lyc. Phosph.

—, inguinal region, Bry. Calc. Chin. Spig.

Anus, Alum. Amm. Amm. m. Ang. Ant. *Ars.* Aspar. Baryt. Berb. Calc. Cann. Carb. veg. *Caust.* Croton. Euphorb. *Graph.* Grat. Hep.

°*Ign.* Jod. Lal. Lach. Led. Lyc. Magn. art. Magn. c. Magn. m. Mez. Mill. ***Merc. Mur. ac.*** Natr. °*Natr. m.* Natr. s. Nitr. ac. *N. vom.* Petr. Phell. Phosph. Prun. **Puls.* Rhod. Rhus. Sabin. Sassap. Sep. *Spong.* Stann. Staph. *Sulph.* Tab. Veratr. Zinc.

Sexual parts, Amb. Berb. Borax. Cann. Cic. Cinn. Coff. Corall. Ferr. Kal. Kreas. Murex. Phos. ac. Rhod. *Rhus.* Sabin. Tab. Teucr. °Zinc.

—, glans, Sabin.

—, scrotum, Berb. Coff. Phos. ac. Teucr.

—, penis, Borax. Cann. Cic.

—, labia, Amb. Berb.

—, vagina, Berb. Ferr. mur. Kal. Kreas. Rhus.

—, prepuce, Cinn. Corall. Sabin.

Chest, eruption, Rhus.

—, pimples, Calc. Hep. Rhus.

Mammæ and nipples, °*Merc.* °*Sulph.* Tab. Zinc.

— nipples, °*Sulph.* °Zinc.

Dorsal region, neck, Bry.

—, cervical vertebræ, °Con.

—, vertebræ, °Con. Dig. Sep.

—, small of back, Cast. Caust. **Natr.*

—, nape of neck, Bry. Dig. Phos. ac. Sep.

—, back, Cast. Thuj.

—, scapulæ, Coloc. Lach. Plat.

Arms, Bov. Dig. Phosph.

—, shoulders, Arn. Aur. Cic. Con. Magn. arct. Sep.

—, elbow, Carb. an. °*Crotal. Plat.* Stann.

—, upper arm, Graph.

—, forearm, Cupr.

Hands, Berb. Calc. Carb. veg. **Hep.* Lam. Nicc. °*Nitr. ac.* **Rhus.*

—, fingers, Amb. Berb. °*Graph.* *Kal.* Petr. Sulph. ac.

—, thumbs, Magn. art. Mez. Spong.

Lower limbs, nates, Lyc. Magn. aust.

—, hip, Aspar. Berb. Cast. *Cic.* Natr. s. Puls. Sabin.

—, thighs, Arn. Aspar. Bell. Berb. Chel. Coff. Crotal. Kal. Led. Lyc. Mang. Mez. Phosph. Staph. Sulph. Thuj. Zinc.

—, knee, Anac. Asa. Aspar. Berb. *Carb. an.* Caust. Electr. *Led.* Lyc. Val. Veratr.

—, legs, Amb. Aspar. Berb. Chin. Dig. Mang. Plat.

—, tibia, Coff. Mang. Sep.

—, calves, Croc. Crotal.

Feet and joints, Ars. Berb. Chin. Evon. **Hep.* Mur. ac. Natr. Phos. ac. *Plat.* Spig.

—, heel, Borax. Cast. Cycl. Euphorb. *Ign.* Laur. Magn. arct. N. vom. Phos. ac. Sep.

—, toes, Agar. °*Ars.* Berb. Camph. Clem. Cycl. *Lyc. Magn. art.* Magn. aust. Mur. ac. *Natr.* Natr. m. Plat. *Ran.* Sep. Zinc.

Bones, periosteum, °*Con.* Graph. Hep. Ign. Merc. °*Phos. ac.* Sep.

Nails, Alum. Graph. Hep. Kal. Magn. aust. Merc. Mez. Natr. m. N. vom. Puls. Sep. Sulph.

Glands, Alum. Ant. Arn. Bry. Calc. Caust. Cic. Clem. *Con. Graph. Hep. Ign.* Kal. Merc. Mez. Natr. m. *N. vom.* Phosph. Plat. Puls. Rhus. *Sep.* Staph. Sulph. Sulph. ac. Teucr. *Zinc.*

Smarting as if sore.

Blisters, vesicles, Con. Electr. Hell. Magn. c. Natr. Phell. Rhus v. Sil. Staph. Thuj.

Blotches, Ant. Caust. Magn. arct. Phos. ac.

Bloodvessels, swelling of, Amm. Ang. Baryt. *Caust.* *Graph.* Grat. (Hep.) Ign. *Kal.* Magn. arct. Merc. Mur. ac. Natr. m. Nitr. N. vom. ***Phosph.*** ***Puls.*** Rhus. Sil. *Sulph.* Sulph. ac.

Cicatrices of former ulcers and wounds, °N. vom.

Corns, Agar. Amb. Bry. Calc. Caust. Graph. °*Hep.* °*Ign.* Lyc. Magn. art. Magn. arct. Natr. m. Nitr. ac. Phosph.? Rhus. °*Sep.* °*Sil.* °Sulph. Veratr.

Eruption, Acon. Agar. *Alum.* Amb. Ant. ***Arg.*** Ars. *Aur.* Baryt. *Bry.* *Calc.* Cann. Canth. Caps. Carb. an. Caust. Chel. Cin. *Cic.* Coff. ***Colch.*** *Dros.* Ferr. **Graph.* Hell. ****Hep.*** Ign. Kal. Lyc. Magn. art. Magn. aust. Magn. c. Mang. Merc. Mez. Natr. *Natr. m.* *Nitr. ac.* N. vom. Oleand. *Par.* *Petr.* Phosph. ***Phos. ac.*** ***Puls.*** Ran. °***Rhus.*** Rhus v. Ruta. Sabin. Sassap. Selen. *Sep.* Sil. *Spig.* Spong. *Squill.* Staph. *Sulph.* Tab. Teucr. Val. Veratr. Zinc.

Figwarts, Sabin. Thuj.

Nails, on the, Alum. Graph. Hep. Kal. Magn. aust. Merc. Mez. Natr. m. N. vom. Puls. Sep. Sulph.

Pimples, Alum. Arg. Bell. Bov. Bry. Calc. Clem. Guaj. ***Hep.*** Hyos. Lam. Magn. arct. Mez. Phos. ac. ***Rhus.*** *Sabin.* Selen. Spig. Stann. Teucr. Veratr. Zinc.

Pustules, Baryt.
Scurfs, crusts, Cic. ***Sil.***
Spots, Berb. Bry. Electr. °***Ferr. Hep.*** Led. Natr. m. ***Phos. ac.*** Rhod. Sil. ***Veratr.***
Swelling, Aur. Bism. ***Borax. Graph. Hep.*** Natr. Natr. m. °Rhus. Sassap. Sep. ***Sil.*** Thuj. Zinc.
Tumors, Hep.
Ulcers, Alum. Amb. Amm. Ant. Arn. ***Ars.*** Bell. Bov. Bry. ***Calc.*** Caust. Cic. ****Graph.*** ****Hep. Ign.*** Kal. Lam. Lyc. Magn. art. Magn. aust. ***Merc. Mez.*** N. vom. ***Phosph. Phos. ac.*** °***Puls.*** Rhus. °***Sep. Sil.*** Staph. °***Sulph.*** Thuj. Zinc.
Warts, °Hep. °Lach. Natr. m. Nitr. ac. Sabin. Thuj.

Face, Bry. Natr. m. Sil.
Lips, Bry. Con. Natr. m. ***Sil.***
Buccal cavity, eruptions, blisters, Arg. Electr. Lyc. Magn. c. Sil.
—, swollen, which is, Aur. Bism. Graph. Natr. m. Sassap. Sep. Sil. Thuj. Zinc.
—, ulcers, Amm. Bov.
Anus, eruptions, Stann.
Sexual organs, eruptions, Staph. Zinc.
—, ulcers, Hep.
Dorsal region, pocks, Natr.
—, pimples, Bell. Clem. Magn. art. Mez. Spig.
Arms, eruption, Berb. Hyos.
—, swelling, Bov.
Hands, Baryt.
Lower limbs, spots, Electr. Rhod.
Feet, pimples, Bov.
—, swelling, Natr.

Feet, ulcers, Lam.
—, callosities, Lyc.

Smooth, that which is.

Excrescences, **Thuj.*
Herpes, Magn.
Spots, Carb. an. Carb. veg. Corall. Electr. Lach. Magn. c. Petr.
Tubercles, Phos. ac.
Sexual parts, excrescences, Thuj.
—, spots, Carb. veg. Petr.
Thorax, spots, Magn. c.

Soft, which is.

Tumors, Ant. Carb. veg. Daph. Petr. Rhus. Sil.
Swelling, Ars. **Chin. Led.* Petr. Sep. (Comp. Watery.)
Blotches, tubercles, Bell. Crotal. Lach.

Head, °Calc. °Daph.

Soft, getting.

Feet, soles, *Sulph.*
Bones, s. Softening.

Sore, which is.

Pustules, °*Merc.*
Spots, Calc. Carb. veg. Sulph.

Blotches, Sep.

Face, Cic.

Soreness.

In general, Agar. Amb. *Amm.* Amm. m. Ang. Ant. **Arn.* Ars. *Baryt.* **Bell.* Bov. **Calc.* Canth. Carb. an. **Carb. veg.* **Caust.* **Cham.* °*Chin.* Coff. Colch. Dros. Euphr. °*Graph.* Hep. Ign. Kal. Kreas. Lach. **Lyc.* Magn. art. Magn. m. *Mang.* **Merc.* Mez. Natr. *Natr. m.* Nitr. ac. **N. vom.* *Oleand.* *Ol. an.* Op. °*Petr.* *Phosph.* *Phos. ac.* Plumb. **Puls.* Rhus. °*Ruta.* Selen. **Sep.* *Sil.* Spig. *Squill.* **Sulph.* **Sulph. ac.* Vinc. Zinc.

Of children, °*Acon.* Amm. Ant. Baryt. °Bell. °Calc. **Caust.* °*Cham.* °Chin. °*Graph.* °*Hep.* °*Ign.* Kreas. °Lyc. **Merc.* Natr. °*Puls.* °*Ruta.* °*Sep.* Sil. Squill. °*Sulph.*

Head, Bov. °*Calc.*

Ears, behind the, Anac. °*Graph.* Kal. °*Lach.* **Merc.* Nitr. ac. Petr.

Nose, Agar. **Alum.* Caps. Carb. an. °Euphr. Galv. °Graph. **Kal.* Lach. °Magn. m. Mez. *Natr. m.* *Nitr. ac.

Lips, Canth. Caust. Cham. Cupr. Graph. *Ign.* *Kal.* *Lyc.* Magn. c. Merc. Mez. Natr. m. *Phosph.* Sabad. °*Sep.* Zinc.

—, canthi, Ant. Merc. °Phosph. Zinc.

Lower jaw, Mang.

Buccal cavity, Agar. °*Amb.* *Carb. veg.* Chinin. *Dig.* Electr. Ferr. *Graph.* Kal. **Lach.* Lyc. *Merc.* *Mez.* *Mur. ac.* Natr. m. Nitr. ac. Op. Phosph. Phos. ac. **Sabad.* Sep. **Sil.*

—, palate, **Lach.* *Mez.* *Mur. ac.* Nitr. ac. Phos. ac.

—, mouth, Dig. Electr. Kal. **Lach.* Merc. Natr. m. Op. **Phosph.* Sabad.

—, fauces and throat, °*Amb.* *Dig.* Ferr. *Graph.* *Mez.*

—, gums, *Carb. veg.* Chinin. Dig. Kal. °*Lach.* Merc. Nitr. ac. Sep. Sil.

—, tongue, Agar. Carb. veg. Dig. Kal. °*Lach.* Lyc. Mur. ac. Nitr. ac. **Sabad.* **Sil.*

Abdomen, Rhus.

—, inguen, Phos. ac.

Anus, Berb. Calc. *Carb. an.* *Carb. veg.* Ferr. Grat. Kal. Lach. Merc. Natr. m. Nitr. ac. N. vom. Phosph. Sep. Zinc.

—, nates, between the, *Carb. veg.* Natr. m. Nitr. ac. Sep.

—, perineum, Carb. veg.

Sexual parts, Alum. Amb. *Amm.* Arn. Calad. Calc. **Carb. veg.* Caust. **Cham.* °*Graph.* *Hep.* Hyos. *Ign.* °*Lyc.* Meph. **Merc.* *Natr.* Natr. m. *Nitr. ac.* **N. vom.* Petr. Plumb. **Sep.* **Sulph.* Veratr. Zinc.

—, glans, Natr.

—, scrotum, Kal. Natr. m. Petr. Plumb. °Sulph. Zinc.

—, pudendum and thigh, between, Caust. *Hep.* Lyc. Merc. *Natr.* **Sep.* °*Sulph.*

—, labia, Amb. Amm. **Carb. veg.* Hep. Natr. **Sep.* Sulph.

Sexual parts, vagina, Hyos.
Mammæ and nipples, Nitr. ac.
—, nipples, °Arn. °Calc. °Caust. ***Cham.** °***Graph.*** °Lyc. °Merc. °N. vom. °Sep.? °Sil.
Dorsal region, axilla, Ars. Carb. veg. Mez. Teucr. Zinc.
Lower limbs, between the thighs, Ars. Aur. ****Caust.*** Coff. **Graph.* ***Hep.*** Jod. ***Lyc.*** Ol. an. Phosph. ***Rhod. Sulph.***
—, hip, Bov. Mang. ***Petr.*** Sep.
—, nates, Kal. Natr. m. ***Nitr. ac.*** Selen.
Feet, soles, N. vom. Sil.
—, toes, ***Carb. an.*** Coff. ****Graph.*** Mang. Natr. Nitr. ac. Phos ac.

Spongy, which is.

Ulcers, Alum. *Ant.* °*Ars.* Bell. Calc. ****Carb. an.*** ***Carb. veg.*** Caust. Cham. *Clem.* Con. Graph. Jod. Kreas. **Lach.* Lyc. **Merc.* Nitr. ac. N. vom. *Petr.* °*Phosph.* Phos. ac. Rhus. Sabin. °*Sep.* **Sil.* °*Staph.* °*Sulph.* Tart. °***Thuj.***

Ulcers on the lips, Sil.

Spots.

Black, Ars. ***Crotal.*** °***Lach.*** °***Rhus.*** Sec. ***Vip. red.***
Blue, Amm. *Ant.* °*Arn.* Ars. Baryt. Berb. Con. Crotal. **Ferr.* Lach. Led. Merc. Nitr. ac. N. mosch. °***N. vom.*** Op. Phell. Phosph. ***Plat.*** Ruta. ***Sulph.*** ****Sulph. ac.***
Blue-red, Ferr. magn. Lach. Phosph.

Brown, *Ant.* °*Ars.* Aur. Berb. Cann. °***Carb. veg.*** °***Con.*** Crotal. Hyos. Natr. m. °***Nitr. ac.*** °Petr. °***Phosph.*** Plumb. ****Sep.*** °***Sulph.*** Tax. Thuj.

Brown-red, Cann. °*Nitr. ac.*

Burning, Amm. ***Amm. m.*** ****Ars.*** Bell. Berb. Canth. Caust. ***Chel.*** Croc. Cupr. Electr. Ferr. Jod. °*Ipec.* °*Kal.* Lach. Lyc. Magn. c. Magn. m. ***Merc.*** ****Mez.*** Phos. ac. ***Rhus.*** Samb. Squill. Sulph. *Sulph. ac.* Sab. Thuj. Zinc.

As if burnt, Ant. °*Ars.* Carb. veg. °***Caust.*** °*Cycl.* Euphorb. Hyos. Kreas. Lach. Rhus. Sec. Stran.

Chronic, °*Con.*

Claret-coloured, °*Cocc.* **Sep.*

Close together, Calc.

Confluent, °*Bell.* °*Cic.* *Hyos.* Phos. ac. *Val.*

Copper-coloured, Corall. °*Nitr. ac.* Phosph. (Comp. COPPER-COLOURED, that which is.)

Coral-coloured, Corall.

Dark-coloured, Aur. Calc. Corall. Crotal. Phosph. Plumb. Tart.

Death-spots, in old people, Ars. Baryt. °***Con.*** Lach. °Op.? Vip red.

Dirty, Berb. *Sabin.* Sec.

Dry, Baryt. Kal. hdr.

Fiery-red, Ferr. magn.

Like flea-bites, Acon. Bell. Dulc. Graph. Mez. Sec. Stram. Tart.

Freckles, °***Amm.*** °*Ant.* Bry. **Calc.* Carb. veg. ***Con. Dros.*** °***Dulc.*** °*Graph.* Hyos. Jod. ***Kal.*** Lach. Laur. ****Lyc. Merc.*** Mez. Natr. Nitr. ac. ***N. mosch. Petr.*** ****Phosph.*** Plumb. °***Puls.*** °***Sep. Sil.*** Stann. ****Sulph.*** Tart. Thuj.

Gangrenous, Crotal, ***Cycl.*** Hyos.

Gnawing - itching, Phosph.
Gray, Nitr. ac.
Green, Ars. °*Con.* Crotal. Vip. torv.
Hard, Vip. torv.
Hepatic, °*Ant.* Caust. Con. Ferr. Hyos. °***Laur.*** ****Lyc.*** Natr. Nitr. ac. Petr. Phosph. Sep. ****Sulph.*** (Comp. Brown, Yellow, &c.)
Herpetic, Crotal. Graph. *Hyos.* Lyc.****Merc.*** Mur. ac. Natr. m. Phosph. Sabad. Sassap. ****Sep.*** Sil. Zinc.
Humid, Ant. Ars. Carb. veg. *Hell.* Kal. Lach. Selen. **Sil.* °*Sulph.* Tarax.
Inflamed, Ars. Hell.
Irregular, Cocc.
Itching, Agn. Amm. m. Arn. *Berb.* Calc. Carb. veg. Caust. Cinn. °*Con.* Cupr. Dros. Electr. ***Graph.*** Hep. *Jod.* ***Kal.*** °Kal. hdr. *Lach.* ****Led.*** Lyc. Merc. Mur. ac. *Natr. m.* Nitr. ***Nitr. ac.*** Op. Phosph. Par. Ratanh. Sassap. °Sep. **Sil.* Spong. Squill. Sulph. **Sulph. ac.* Tax. ****Zinc.***
Large, Lyc. Phos. ac. Tart.
Leprous, °*Natr.*
Livid, Crotal.
Marbled, *Berb.* °*Carb. veg.* °*Caust.* Crotal. Lyc. ***Natr. m.*** Plat. **Thuj.*
Measle-shaped, Ars.
Miliary, Thuj.
Moles, like, °*Calc. Carb. veg.* ***Graph.*** Nitr. ac. *Petr.* *Phos. ac.* *Sil.* °***Sulph.*** *Sulph. ac.* ****Thuj.***
Nettle-rash, like, Berb.
Painful, as if contused, Berb.
Painful, as if sore, Berb. Bry. Electr. °***Ferr. Hep.*** Led. Natr. m. ***Phos. ac.*** Rhod. Sil. ***Veratr.***

Painful, Alum. Amb. Ars. Berb. Calc. Cann. Caust. °*Con.* Lach. Mosch. Nitr. ac. Petr. Rhod.

Painless, Graph. Led. Phos. ac. Sep. Stann.

Turning pale in the cold, Sabad.

—, under the pressure of the finger, Bry. Ferr. magn.

Pale-red, Cann. Carb. an. Carb. veg. Rhod. Sassap. Teucr. Vip. red.

With peeling off, Amm. Sep.

Petechiæ, Arn. **Ars.* Bell. ***Berb.*** °***Bry.*** Con. ***Hyos.*** ***Lach.*** Led. **N. vom.* Oph. Phell. °***Phosph.*** ****Rhus.*** Ruta. *Sec.* Sil. Stram. Sulph. ac.

—, as if ecchymosed, **Arn.* °*Bry.* °*Calc.* Cham. Chin. °*Con.* Crotal. Dulc. Electr. Euphr. Ferr. °***Hep.*** Lach. Laur. Natr. Natr. m. **N. vom.* Par. Plumb. °***Puls.*** Rhus. °Ruta. Sec. ****Sulph.*** ****Sulph. ac.***

Raised, Calc. Carb. an. Dulc. Kal. Merc. Phosph. Puls. Sassap. Teucr. Thuj.

Rash-like, Mez.

Recurring yearly, Crotal.

Red, Acon. ***Alum.*** ***Amb.*** Amm. ***Ant.*** ****Arn.*** ****Ars.*** ****Bell.*** ***Berb.*** °*Bry.* Calad. **Calc.* Canth. Caps. Carb. an. *Carb. veg.* Caust. Cham. Chin. Cinn. Cist. Cocc. °*Con.* Croc. *Crotal.* *Cycl.* *Dros.* ***Dulc.*** Electr. Ferr. magn. Graph. Hep. Jod. °***Ipec.*** °*Kal.* Kal. hdr. ****Lach.*** ***Led.*** ***Lyc.*** Magn. arct. ***Magn. c.*** ***Magn. m.*** Mang. ****Merc.*** Mez. Mosch. ***Natr.*** ***Natr. m.*** Nitr. ****Nitr. ac.*** Op. Par. ***Petr.*** ****Phosph.*** ***Phos. ac.*** Plat. ***Plumb.*** Poth. Puls. Ratanh. Rhod. ****Rhus.*** **Sabad.* °***Samb.*** ***Sassap.*** ****Sep.*** ***Sil.*** Spong. *Squill.* *Stann.*

Sulph. **Sulph. ac.* *Tab.* Tart. Tax. Teucr. Thuj. Veratr. *Vip. red.* *Vip. torv.* *Zinc.*

Red-checkered, Berb. °*Carb. veg.* °*Caust.* Crotal. Lyc. *Natr. m.* Plat. **Thuj.*

Rough, Baryt. *Merc.* Mur. ac. Nitr. ac. *Sassap.* °*Zinc.*

Round, Jod. Led. **Merc.* Natr. m. Phosph. Zinc.

Scarlet-coloured, **Amm.* Amm. m. Arn. °*Ars.* Baryt. **Bell.* Bry. *Carb. veg.* Caust. Cham. °*Croc.* Dulc. *Euphorb.* Galv. °*Hep.* °*Hyos.* Jod. Ipec. Lach. **Merc.* *Phosph.* Phos. ac. Rhus. *Stram.* °*Sulph.*

Scaly, Kal. Merc.

Scorbutic, Merc. corr. (Comp. Scorbutic.)

Scurfy, *Merc.* **Nitr. ac.* Thuj. Zinc.

Shining through, Phosph.

Small, Bry. Lach. Led. Lyc. Merc. Op. Ratanh. Squill. °*Sulph. ac.* Tart. Vip. torv.

Smarting, Puls.

Smooth, Carb. an. Carb. veg. Corall. Electr. Lach. Magn. c. Petr.

Sore, Calc. Carb. veg. Sulph.

As if from stings of insects, Lyc.

Stinging, Canth. Chel. Lach. Merc. *Nitr. ac.* Puls.

Star-shaped, Stram.

Syphilitic, °*Merc.* °Nitr. ac.

Ulcerated, Hell. *Merc.* Natr. m. *Sabin.* Thuj.

Violet-colored, °*Phosph.* °Veratr.

White, °*Alum.* Amm. °*Ars.* Calc. Carb. an. Electr. *Merc.* *Natr.* Nitr. ac. Phosph. °*Sep.* **Sil.* **Sulph.*

Yellow, Amb. °*Arn.* Ars. Canth. **Con.* Crotal. **Ferr.* Jod. Kal. *Natr.* **Petr.* **Phosph.* *Ruta.* *Sabad.* **Sep.* Stann. °*Sulph.* Tart. Vip. red. Vip. torv.

Head, °*Ars.* Mosch. Kal. Zinc.
Eyes, °Aur. °Bell. °Calc. °Cann. °Con. °*Euphr.* °*Hep.* °*Nitr. ac.* **N. vom.* Puls. °*Ruta.* °Seneg. Sil. °*Sulph.*
Eyelids, Camph. Sil.
Nose, Aur. Calc. Jod. Phos. ac. Rhod. Tax. Veratr.
Face, Acon. Alum. Amb. Amm. Ars. Baryt. Bell. Berb. Bry. °*Calc.* Carb. an. Carb. veg. Croc. °Colch. Ferr. Ferr. magn. Lyc. °*Merc.* °*Natr.* Nitr. ac. Par. Phosph. Samb. Sassap. **Sep.* Sulph. Tab. Vip. red. Zinc.
Lips and mouth, region of, Ars. Berb. Caust. Hep. **Merc.* Mez. °*Natr.* °*Sulph.*
Chin, Natr. m. Sep. °*Sil.*
Abdomen and stomach, region of, Ars. Bell. Canth. *Cal. *Lach.* Led. Lyc. °Natr. m. **Phosph.* *Sabad.* °*Sep.*
—, pit of stomach, Natr. m.
Sexual parts, Arn. Calc. Cann. Carb. veg. Caust. *Cinn.* **Lach.* Natr. m. **Nitr. ac.* Petr. Rhus. *Sil.* *Thuj.*
—, glans, Arn. Cann. Carb. veg. Cinn. **Lach.* Natr. m. Petr. Thuj.
—, scrotum, Calc. **Sil.*
—, prepuce, Lach. Rhus. Thuj.
Thoracic region, Amm. Ars. *Bell.* Carb. veg. Cocc. Crotal. °Ipec. Lach. **Led.* *Magn.* Mez.

Nitr. ac. **Phosph.* °*Sep.* Squill. Sulph. *Vip. torv.*

Nipples, round the, Kal.

Dorsal region, neck, Ars. Bell. Bry. Carb. veg. Cinn. Cocc. Jod. Lyc. Nitr. Phell. Sep. Stann. Vip. torv.

—, axilla, Thuj.

—, hips, Sep.

—, small of back, Sep.

—, nape of neck, Carb. veg. Hyos.

—, back, Lyc. °Sep. Sulph. Zinc.

—, scapulæ, Calc. Cist. Lach.

Arms, Ant. Bry. Crotal. *Cupr.* Lach. Led. *Natr. m.* Petr. *Sabad.* **Sulph.*

—, shoulders, Berb. Sulph. ac.

—, elbows, Calc. *Sep.* Vip. torv.

—, upper arm, Berb. Kal. hdr. *Plat. Rhus.* Tax.

—, forearm, Amm. Berb. Magn. m. *Merc. Sulph. ac. Thuj.*

Hands, Acon. Bell. Berb. Corall. *Dros.* Electr. Ferr. magn. *Jod. Kal. Natr. Natr. m.* °*Nitr. ac. Sabad. Sep.* Squill. Stann. *Tart.* Vip. torv. Zinc.

—, wrist, *Kal. Merc.* °*Petr.*

—, fingers, *Con.* Corall. Ferr. magn. Lyc. Mang. *Natr. m. Phos. ac. Plumb.* Sabad. Squill. Tart.

—, thumb, Lyc.

Lower limbs, Ant. Bry. *Hyos.* °*Natr.* Nitr. °*Sulph.*

—, hips, Rhus.

—, thighs, Amm. Ant. Berb. Cann. Cycl. Electr. *Graph.* Mur. ac. Rhod.

—, legs, **Calc. Chel.* Con. *Lyc.* N. vom. *Phosph. Stann. Zinc.*

Lower limbs, calves, °Con.. Graph. ***Sassap.***
—, shins, Amb. Ant. ***Caust.*** Electr. ***Lach.*** Magn. c. Nitr. ***Phosph. Sil. Sulph. ac.***
—, tendo Achilles, Chel.
Feet, Ant. ****Ars.*** Led. Sec. Squill. ***Sulph. Thuj.***
—, soles, ***Rhus.***
—, toes, Lach. ***Natr.***
Nails, Alum. Ars. Natr. m. **Nitr. ac.* Sep. °***Sil.*** Sulph.

Star-shaped, which is.

Spots, Stram.

Sticking.

In general, ***Agar.*** Agn. Alum. Amm. ****Amm. m.*** Anac. Ant. **Arn. Ars.* **Asa.* **Baryt.* ****Bell.*** Berb. Bov. **Bry.* **Calc.* Cann. **Canth.* Caps. Carb. veg. **Caust.* **Cham.* Chel. Chin. Cin. Clem. **Cocc.* **Colch.* **Con.* Crotal. Cycl. °***Daph. Dig. Dros.*** Dulc. Euphr. **Ferr.* ****Graph.*** Guaj. Hell. Hep. Hyos. **Ign.* Jod. **Kal.* Lach. Lact. Laur. Led. ***Lyc.*** Magn. art. Magn. arct. Magn. aust. Magn. c. Magn. m. ***Men.*** ****Merc. Mez.*** Mosch. Mur. ac. Natr. Natr. m. Natr. s. Nicc. Nitr. **Nitr. ac.* ****N. vom.*** Oleand. Ol. an. Oph. Op. ***Par.*** Petr. Phell. Phosph. ***Phos. ac.*** *Plat.* Plumb. Prun. ****Puls. Ran. Ran.*** *sc.* Rhod. ****Rhus.*** ****Sabad.*** Sabin. ***Sassap. Selen.*** **Sep.* **Sil.* Spig. ****Spong.*** Squill. ****Stann.*** ****Staph.*** Stram. Stront. ****Sulph.*** Sulph ac. Tab. **Tarax.* Tart. Teucr. ****Thuj.*** Veratr. ***Viol. tr.*** Vip. torv. Vip. red. Zinc.

Burning, *Acon.* Alum. *Anac.* Arg. Arn. Ars. *Asa.* Aur. *Baryt.* Bell. Berb. *Bry.* Cann. Caps. Caust. *Cin. Cocc.* Con. *Dig. Hep. Hyos.* Ign. *Lach. Lyc.* Magn. art. Magn. arct. Magn. aust. Magn. c. Men. *Merc. Mez.* Mur. ac. Natr. s. Nicc. *N. vom.* Phell. Phosph. *Phos. ac.* Plat. *Puls. Ran. Ran. sc. Rhus.* Sabad. Selen. *Sep. Sil.* Spig. *Spong.* Squill. *Stann. Staph. Sulph. Sulph. ac. Thuj. Viol. tr.*

Splinters, as if from, *Carb. veg.* Cic. *Colch. Hep.* **Nitr. ac. Petr.* Plat. Ran. **Sil.* Sulph.

Scalp, Agn. Ant. Arn. Asa. *Asar. Berb.* Caust. Chin. Cupr. Cycl. Mez. Petr. Phos. ac. Sulph. Thuj.

Lips and mouth, region of, Agar. Amm. m. Ant. Asa. Bell. Bov. Bry. Caust. Clem. Graph. Grat. Ign. Kal. Magn. arct. Merc. Natr. Natr. m. Nitr. ac. N. vom. Par. Phosph. Phos. ac. Sabad. Sassap. Spong. Stann. Staph. Sulph. Thuj.

Abdomen and stomach, region of, Berb. Mur. ac. Phos. ac.

Mammæ and nipples, Alum. Baryt. Berb. Borax. Carb. an. Cocc. Con. Grat. Kal. Kreas. Laur. Lyc. Magn. aust. Mez. Murex. Natr. m. Ol. an. Phell. Phosph. Plumb. Prun. Rhab. Sabin. Sang. Sep. Zinc.

Bones, periosteum, Aeth. Acon. Agn. Agar. Amm. Anac. Ant. Arg. Ars. Asa. Aur. **Bell.* Berb. Bry. **Calc.* Canth. Carb. veg. **Caust.* Chel. **Chin.* Cocc. Colch. **Con.* Daph. **Dros.* Dulc. Euphorb. Euphr. Graph. **Hell.* Jod. **Lach.* Laur. Lyc. Magn. arct. Magn. c.

Mang. ****Merc.*** Mez. Mur. ac. Natr. Natr. s. Nitr. Nitr. ac. N. vom. Ol. an. Par. Phell. Petr. Phosph. Phos. ac. Prun. ****Puls.*** Raph. ***Ran. sc.*** **Ruta.* Sabin. Samb. ****Sassap.*** °*Sep.* Sil. Spig. Staph. Stront. Sulph. Thuj. Tarax. Tax. ***Val.*** Verb. Viol. tr. Zinc.

Nails, Amm. m. Bell. Carb. veg. Colch. Con. Graph. Hep. ***Kal.*** Lyc. Magn. aust. Natr. s. Nicc. *Nitr. Nitr. ac.* Phos. ac. Sep. *Sil.* ***Sulph.***

Glands, Acon. Agn. Alum. ***Amm. m.*** Ang. Arg. Arn. *Asa.* Baryt. ***Bell.*** Berb. Borax. ***Bry.*** *Calc.* Carb. an. Caust. Chin. *Cocc. Con.* Cupr. Cycl. Euphorb. Electr. Graph. Grat. Hell. Hep. ***Ign.*** Jod. Kal. Lach. Lyc. Magn. art. Magn. arct. **Merc.* Mez. Murex. Mur. ac. Natr. *Natr. m.* Nitr. ac. N. vom. Ol. an. Phell. ***Phosph.*** Phos. ac. Plumb. ***Puls. Ran. sc.*** Raph. Rhab. Rhus. Sabad. Sang. **Sep.* Sil. Spig. *Spong.* Stann. Staph. ***Sulph.*** Sulph. ac. Thuj. Veratr. Zinc.

STINGING, WHICH IS.

Blisters, vesicles, Amm. Calc. Cham. Sil. Spong. Staph.

Blisters, phagedænic, Graph. Magn. c.

Bloodvessels, swelling of, Alum. *Ars.* Baryt. ***Caust.*** Graph. Grat. Kal. ***Merc.*** Natr. m. ***Nitr.*** N. vom. Phosph. Puls. *Sil.* Sulph. Sulph. ac. Tart.

Blotches, ***Petr.*** Sassap. Stram. Zinc.

Chilblains, Magn. aust.

Corns, Agar. ***Alum.*** Ant. Berb. Borax. Bov. **Bry.* °*Calc.* Carb. an. Carb. veg. Caust. Chen. Cocc. Graph. Hep. Ign. Kal. ****Lyc.*** °***Magn. arct.***

Magn. m. *Natr. Natr. m.* Nitr. ac. *Petr.* Phosph. Phos. ac. °*Puls*. Ran. sc. *Rhod.* °*Rhus.* **Sep.* **Sil.* **Sulph.* Sulph. ac. Thuj. Veratr.

Eruption, Acon. Alum. Amm. m. Anac. Ant. Arn. *Ars.* Asa. *Baryt. Bell.* Berb. Bov. Bry. Calc. Camph. Canth. Caps. Carb. veg. Caust. Cham. Chin. *Clem.* Cocc. Con. *Cycl.* Dig. *Dros.* Graph. Guaj. Hell. *Hep.* Ign. Kal. Kreas. *Led.* *Lyc. Magn. art. Magn. arct. Magn. c. *Merc.* Mez. **Mur. ac.* Natr. Natr. m. *Nitr. ac.* N. vom. Petr. Phosph. **Phos. ac. Plat. Puls. Ran.* Ran. sc. *Rhus.* Sabad. *Sabin.* Selen. *Sep.* **Sil.* Spong. Squill. **Staph.* Stront. *Sulph.* Thuj. Verb. *Viol. tr.* Zinc.

Erysipelas, Graph. Phosph. Puls. Rhus. Sulph.

Figwarts, Euphr. Thuj.

Herpes, Anac.

Lupia, Magn. arct.

Nails, on the, Amm. m. Bell. Carb. veg. Colch. Con. Graph. Hep. *Kal.* Lyc. Magn. aust. Natr. s. Nicc. *Nitr. Nitr. ac.* Phos. ac. Sep. *Sil. Sulph.*

Pimples, Alum. Ant. Arn. *Bell.* Calc. ph. *Canth.* Caps. Caust. Cocc. Hell. Kal. Kreas. Magn. art. Magn. arct. Natr. Nitr. Petr. Squill. Staph.

Pustules, Amm. Berb. Dros. Rhus.

Rash, rashlike, Mez. Natr. m. Sulph. Teucr. Viol. tr.

Spots, Canth. Chel. Lach. Merc. *Nitr. ac.* Puls.

Swelling, Acon. Agn. Amm. m. Ant. *Arn.* Ars. Asa. Bell. **Bry.* Calc. *Canth.* Carb. an. °*Carb. veg.* **Caust.* Cham. Chel. *Chin.* °*Cocc. Con. Cycl.* Dig. Electr. °Ferr. **Graph.* Kal. Lach.

Led. Lyc. Magn. c. Mang. *Merc.* Mez. Natr. m. Nitr. **Nitr. ac.* °*N. vom.* Oleand. Petr. **Phosph.* **Puls.* Ran. °*Rhus.* Ruta. *Sabad.* *Sep.* Spong. Stann. **Sulph.* °*Thuj.*

Tubercles, Calc. Caust. Dulc. Cal. hdr. Led. Magn. arct. Magn. c. Phosph. Rhus. Squill. Stram.

Ulcers, Acon. Alum. Ant. Arn. °*Ars.* Asa. Baryt. *Bell.* Bov. °*Bry.* *Calc.* Camph. Canth. *Carb. veg.* Cham. *Chin.* *Clem.* Cocc. Con. *Cycl.* *Graph.* *Hep.* Lam. Led. **Lyc.* Magn. arct. Magn. c. Mang. **Merc.* *Mez.* Mur. ac. *Natr.* *Natr. m.* Nitr. **Nitr. ac.* N. vom. **Petr.* Phosph. °*Puls.* Ran. Rhus. Sabad. Sabin. Sassap. Selen. °*Sep.* **Sil.* Spong. Squill. **Staph.* *Sulph. Thuj.

Warts, Ant. Baryt. °*Calc.* Caust. Euphr. Hep. Lyc. Nitr. ac. Rhus. Sep. Sil. °*Sulph.* Thuj.

Face, Ant. Asa. *Bell.* Bry. Calc. Calc. ph. Caust. Cham. Dros. Kal. Kal. hdr. Kreas. Lach. Led. Magn. arct. Natr. Nitr. ac. Plat. *Rhus.* Sulph. Teucr.

Lips, Bell. Caust. Magn. arct. Mang. Merc. Petr. Phosph. Sil. Squill.

Chin, Bell. Canth. Sil. Stann.

Buccal cavity, blisters, vesicles, Berb. Caps. Cham. Hell. Natr. Natr. s. Spong. Staph.

—, swollen, Laur. Lyc. Merc. Natr. m. N. vom. Petr. Ran.

—, ulcers, Amm. m. Nitr. ac. Staph.

Anus, eruption, Nitr. ac.

—, varices, Alum. *Ars.* Baryt. Caust. Grat. Kal.

Merc. Natr. m. Nitr. N. vom. Phosph. Puls. Sil. Sulph. Sulph. ac.
Sexual parts, eruption, Calc. Phosph.
—, swelling, Phosph.
—, ulcers, Hep.
Dorsal region, blotch, Petr.
—, blisters, Amm.
—, pimples, Arn. Bell. Squill.
—, swelling, Carb. an. Electr. °Merc.
—, tubercles, Squill.
Arms, swelling, **Bry.*
Hands, Arn. Berb. Calc. Canth. Dros. Lyc. Magn. c. Oleand. Puls. Rhus. Sulph.
—, blister, phagedænic, Magn. c.
—, swelling, Oleand.
—, ulcers, Mang. Ran.
Lower limbs, varices, Graph.
—, eruption, Ant. N. vom. Petr. Sabin.
—, spots, Chel.
—, swelling, Graph. **Led.* °*Puls.*
—, ulcers, °Ars. Natr.
Feet, eruption, Calc. Zinc.
—, spots, Lach.
—, chilblains, *Kal.*
—, swelling, °*Carb. veg.* Lyc. Merc. *Phosph.* **Puls.*

Stricture, Contraction.

Anus, Ign. Lyc. Magn. aust. **N. vom.*
Sexual parts, urethra, Carb. veg. **Clem.* Cop. °Dulc.? °Lach. °N. vom. °Petr. *Puls.* Rhus.

Styes.

Eyelids, Alum. °*Amb.* Caust. **Con.* °*Dig.* Ferr. **Graph.* Lyc. °*Merc.* Magn. aust. Men. Phos. ac. **Puls.* Rhus. Seneg. Sep. °Staph. Stann. **Sulph.*
Canthi, Natr. m. Stann. Sulph.

Submaxillary Region.

Blotches, Stann. Staph.
Blisters, Mur. ac.
Bloody, Par.
Bones, swelling of, **Merc.* **Sil.*
Burning, Caust. Par.
Caries, °Cist. *Merc.* °Sil.
Eruption, Canth. °*Graph.* Par. Rhus. Veratr.
Glandular affections, *Amm. Amm. m. Arg. Arn. **Ars.* Aur. **Baryt.* °*Bell.* **Calc.* *Chin.* Cic. Clem. Cocc. *Corall.* Croton. °Dulc. *Graph.* Ign. Jod. Kal. °Kreas. Lact. Led. °*Lyc.* Magn. art. Magn. arct. Magn. aust. Magn. c. °*Merc.* Mez. Natr. **Natr. m.* *Nitr. ac.* *Petr. Phosph. Phos. ac. Puls. Raph. *Rhus.* Sep. **Sil.* Spong. Squill. Stann. **Staph.* **Sulph.* Sulph. ac. Veratr. Zinc.
Itching, Laur. Natr. Oleand. Par. Squill.
Induration, Staph.
Pain as if dislocated, Hep. Ign. Magn. Magn. arct. Rhus. Spig. Spong. Staph.
Pain as if sore, Bry. Canth.
Pain as if ulcerated, Caps. Magn. c. Natr.
Pimples, Par.

Red, Stann.
Smarting as if raw, Mang. Veratr.
Soreness, Mang.
Swelling, °*Acon.* Arn. °Ars. Kal. Lyc. **Merc.* Ol. an. Petr. Phosph. *Sil. Staph. Sulph.
Swelling, sensation of, Sabad.
Tendency to be dislocated, Hep. Ign. Magn. arct. Petr. Rhus. Staph.
Tubercles, Bry. °Graph. Natr. N. vom. Staph. Veratr.

Sun's Heat, as if caused by the.

Blisters in the face, Clem.

Suppressed, which is.

Herpes, °Alum.? Amb. °*Calc.* °*Lach.* °*Lyc.* °Natr.? °Sep.? °*Sulph.*
Itch, °*Amb.* °*Ars.* °*Carb. veg.* °*Caust.* Graph.? Natr. m.? °*Selen.* °*Sep.* °*Sulph.* Zinc.?
Measles, morbilli, °*Phosph.* °*Puls.* °Rhus.
Rash, °*Ipec.*
Scarlatina, Phosph.
Ulcers, °Lach.

Suppurates, that which.

Blisters, phagedænic, Graph.
Blotches, tubercles, Amm. Bov. Nitr. ac.
Eruption, **Ant.* Ars. Bell. **Cic.* Clem. Cocc. Con. Cycl. *Dulc.* Euphr. Hep. Kal. Led. *Lyc.* Magn. art. Magn. c. *Merc.* *Natr.* Natr. m. Petr. Plumb. Puls. **Rhus.* Samb. Sassap. Sec. *Sep.*

Sil. Spig. *Staph.* Sulph. Tarax. Tart. Thuj. Veratr. Viol. od. Viol. tr. Zinc.

Erysipelas, Merc. Phosph.

Figwarts, **Thuj.*

Herpes, Clem. °Dulc. °Lyc. °Merc. Natr. (Comp. Humid.)

Itch, Ant.? °*Caust.* Clem.? Cic.? °*Kreas.* °***Merc.*** Selen.? °*Sep.* Squill.? °*Sulph.*

Lupia, °*Calc.* °*Sulph.*

Nails, Calc. Kal. Phos. ac. Sep.

Pimples, Amm. m. Anthrok. Ant. **Ars.* Aur. Baryt, *Bell.* Berb. Calc. ph. Canth. Caust. Cham. **Cic.* *Clem.* Cocc. Con. Croton. Cycl. **Dulc.* Evon. Graph. Grat. Hep. Hydroc. Hyos. Kal. Kal. chl. Kreas. Lach. Lyc. Magn. art. Magn. arct. Magn. c. Magn. m. ***Merc.** Mez. *Nitr. ac.* Op. °*Petr.* Phos. ac. Plumb. °*Puls.* **Rhus.* Samb. Sassap. Sec. *Sep.* Sil. Spig. **Staph.* Stram. **Sulph.* Tarax. **Tart.* Thuj. Veratr. Zinc.

Pocks, Ars. °*Bell.* °*Merc.* °*Sulph.* Thuj.

Rash, Tart.

Scurfs, crusts, **Ars.* Plumb. Sil. **Sulph.* (Comp. Humid.)

Swelling, *Baryt.* Calc. Carb. veg. Caust. Chin. Corall. Galv. **Lach.* Lyc. °*Mang.* **Merc.* Natr. **Phosph.* **Sulph.* Vip. red. Vip. torv.

Ulcers, **Ars.* °*Asa.* Baryt. Bar. m. Bell. Carb. veg. Chin. °*Chinin.* °Con. Crotal. Dros. *Hep.* °*Lach.* Mang. ***Merc.** Nitr. ac. Paeon. Petr. *Phosph.* °*Phos. ac.* °*Puls.* *Sassap.* **Sil.* **Sulph.* Tart.

Tumors, Ant. °*Ars.* °*Asa.* Bry. **Calc.* Caust. Cic. Cocc. Con. Croc. *Crotal.* Dulc. °*Hep.*

Kal. Lach. Magn. c. °*Mang.* ***Merc.*** Natr. Natr. m. Petr. °*Phosph.* °*Puls.* *Sassap.* Sec. Sep. °*Sil.* Staph. Sulph. Tart.

Vesicles, *Amm. m.* Aur. Bov. Calc. Carb. veg. Magn. c. *Natr.* Petr. Phosph. Puls. Ran. Ran. sc. Rhus. Sassap. Vip. torv. Zinc.

Warts, Ars. Bov. °*Calc.* °*Caust.* °*Hep.* Sil. °*Thuj.*

Head, eruptions, **Ars.* Cic. Nitr. ac. (Comp. Ulcers.)

Canthi, Cham. Cin. Graph. N. vom. Puls. Staph.

Ears, eruption, Cycl. Cal. Sep.

—, lupia, tumor, Merc.

—, pimples, Amm. m.

—, tympanum, °Amm. °Carb. veg.

—, parotid glands, Sassap.

Inguinal glands, °Aur. °*Merc.* **Nitr. ac.* °*Sulph.*

—, ulcerated glands, *Hep.*

Anus, ulcers, Sassap.

Sexual parts, Corall. Phosph.

Dorsal region, swelling, axilla, Petr.

—, neck, Hyos.

Arms, eruption, Lyc.

—, tumor, Crotal.

—, swelling, Galv.

Hands, eruption, Spig.

—, blister, phagedænic, Graph.

—, ulcers, Mang.

Lower limbs, tumors, Sassap.

—, swelling, Chin. Jod.

—, ulcer, °*Sabin.*

Feet, tumor, *Lach.* Sassap.

Feet, blisters, *Con. Graph. Natr. Selen.*
—, chilblains, °*Lach.*
—, ulcers, **Ars.*
—, scurf, *Sil.*

Suppurations and Discharges of Pus.

In general, external and internal, Acon. Amb. Amm. Anac. Ang. Ant. Arg. *Arn. **Ars.* °*Asa.* °*Aur.* Baryt. Bar. m. **Bell.* Bov. Bry. **Calc.* °*Canth.* Caps. Carb. an. **Carb. veg.* Caust. **Cham.* Chel. Chin. Cic. °*Cist.* Clem. Cocc. Con. Croc. Crotal. Dros. **Dulc.* Graph. Hell. **Hep.* Hyos. Ign. Ipec. Kal. Kal. chl. Kreas. **Lach.* **Lyc.* Magn. art. **Mang. Merc.* Mez. Mur. ac. Natr. Natr. m. Nitr. **Nitr. ac.* N. vom. Petr. **Phosph.* Phos. ac. Plumb. **Puls.* Ran. Ran. sc. **Rhus.* Ruta. Sabab. Sabin. Sassap. Sec. Selen. Sep. **Sil.* Spig. Spong. Squill. °Staph. **Sulph.* Sulph. ac. Tart. Thuj. Viol. tr. Vip. torv. Zinc.
Benign, **Calc.* **Cham.* °*Hep.* **Lach.* **Merc.* **Puls.* **Sil.* °Sulph.
Chronic, °*Calc.* °Cham. °*Hep.* °Lach. °Mang. °Merc. °*Phosph.* °*Sil.* °Sulph.
Copious, Acon. Arg. °*Ars.* °*Asa.* Bry. °*Calc.* Canth. Chin. Cin. Graph. Jod. Kal. Kreas. Lyc. Mang. **Merc.* Mez. Natr. *Phosph.* Phos. ac. **Puls.* °*Rhus.* Ruta. Sabin. **Sep.* °*Sil.* Staph. Sulph. Thuj.
Malignant, °Ars. °*Asa.* °*Calc.* °Cham. °*Hep.* °Lach. °Merc. °*Phosph.* °Rhus. °*Sil.* °Sulph. °Vip. torv. (Comp. Unhealthy Skin.)
In membranous parts, °*Sil.*

Suppressed, Acon. Ars. Baryt. *Bell.* Bov. Bry. °*Calc.* Carb. veg. Caust. Chin. Cic. Clem. Coff. *Cupr.* Dros. *Dulc.* Graph. °*Hep.* Hyos. Ign. Ipec. °*Lach.* Led. Lyc. Kreas. Magn. c. °*Merc.* N. vom. Petr. Phosph. *Plat.* Plumb. Puls. Rhus. Sassap. *Sep.* °*Sil.* Spong. Staph. Sulph. *Veratr.*

Eyes, Bell. Bry. **Caust.* °*Euphr.* Graph. Kal. °Kreas. °*Nitr. ac.* Plat. Plumb.

Canthi, Cham. Cin. Graph. N. vom. Puls. Staph.

Ears, Alum. Amm. °*Asa.* °*Aur.* Bell. *Borax.* °*Bov.* °*Calc.* °*Carb. veg.* Caust. °*Cist.* °*Graph.* **Hep.* Kal. Lyc. **Merc.* Petr. **Puls.* °*Rhus.* Sep. **Sulph.* Zinc.

Nose, °Alum. Arg. n. °Asa.? °Aur.? °Aur. m. Cic. Cin. °*Con.* **Lach.* *Merc.* °Petr. *Puls.* Sulph.

Lips, Bry. **Merc.* Phos. ac. Staph.

Chin, Anac.

Buccal cavity, Amm. Baryt. **Bell.* Berb. Canth. °*Caust.* °Gran.? °Ign. °*Lach.* Lyc. **Merc.* °Natr. m. Nicc. Sep. **Sulph.* Sulph. ac.

—, mouth, Canth.

—, tonsils, Baryt, **Bell.* Berb. °Gran.? °Ign. **Lach.* *Merc.* Nicc. °Sep.

—, gums, Canth. °*Caust.* Lach. Lyc. °Natr. m. Sulph. Sulph. ac.

—, tongue, Canth.

Anus, °Lach. Sulph.

Sexual parts, Caps. Con. Merc. Sassap. Sep.

—, glans and prepuce, between (balanorrhoea), Cinn. **Merc.* Mez. *Sep.* *Cann.* *Lyc.* Natr. m. Nitr. ac. Staph. **Thuj.*

Sexual parts, urethra (gonorrhœa), °Agn. °Bar. m.? *Cann. *Canth. Caps. Chel. Con. °Cop.? Galv. Ipec. °Lach. Lam. **Merc.* Mercurial. °Natr. m.? Nitr. ac. °N. vom.? °*Petr.* Phos. ac. *Puls. Ratanh. Sassap. Sabin. °Tereb.? *Thuj.

Mammæ and nipples, °Hep. °*Merc.* °Phosph. °*Sil.*

Dorsal region, axilla, Petr.

—, axillary glands, °Calc. Coloc. *Hep. Sep.* °*Sil.*

—, neck, Hyos. °Ipec.

—, cervical glands, °Cist.

—, lumbar region, °Sil. °Staph.

—, nape of neck, °Sil.

Hand, Eugen.

—, fingers, Borax. **Mang.* N. vom.

—, thumb, N. vom.

Lower limbs, hip-joint, Hep.? Spong.? Staph.?

—, calves, Chin.

Feet, heel, Borax.

—, toes, Lach.

Bones, caries, °*Ang.* Ars.? °*Asa.* °*Aur.* Calc. Caps.? Chin. Con. Cupr. Euphorb.? Graph.? °*Hep.* Jod. °*Lach.* °*Lyc.* **Merc.* °*Mez.* °*Natr. m.* °*Nitr. ac.* Op.? Phosph. Phos. ac. Puls.? Rhus.? °*Ruta.* °*Sabin.* Sec.? Sep.? °*Sil.* Spong.? °*Staph.* °Sulph. Thuj.?

Nails, Calc. Kal. Phos. ac. Sep.

Glands, °*Aur.* Bar. m. **Bell.* **Calc.* Canth. °*Cist.* Coloc. *Dulc.* **Hep.* Hyos. Ign. Kreas. *Lach. Lyc.* **Merc.* **Nitr. ac.* Petr. **Phosph.* Sassap. *Sep.* **Sil.* Squill. **Sulph.*

Swelling of single parts.

In general, *Acon.* Agn. Amb. *Amm.* Anthrok.

**Ant.* **Arn.* **Ars.* **Asa.* Asar. **Aur.* Aur. m. Baryt. **Bar. m.* **Bell.* Borax. **Bov.* °*Bry.* *Calc.* Cann. *Canth.* *Carb. an.* °*Carb. veg.* **Caust.* **Cham.* Chel. **Chin.* Chinin. Cin. Clem. *Cocc.* *Colch.* Coloc. *Con.* Cop. Crotal. Croton. Cupr. °*Daph.* *Dig.* **Dulc.* Electr. *Euphorb.* *Ferr.* Graph. *Hell.* **Hep.* *Hyos.* *Jod.* *Kal.* Kal. hdr. **Lach.* **Led.* **Lyc.* Magn. art. **Magn. arct.* *Magn. c.* Magn. m. Mang. **Merc.* **Merc. corr.* Mez. *Mur. ac.* *Natr.* Natr. m. Nitr. **Nitr. ac.* **N. vom.* Oleand. **Oph.* Op. Petr. **Phosph.* **Phos. ac.* Plat. *Plumb.* **Puls.* Ran. Ran. sc. °Rhod. **Rhus.* **Sabin.* **Samb.* Sassap. *Sec.* **Sep.* **Sil.* *Seneg.* Spig. Spong. Squill. **Stann.* Staph. Stram. Stront. **Sulph.* Sulph. ac. Tereb. *Thuj.* Veratr. Vip. torv.

Aching, Magn. aust. °*Merc.* Mosch. N. vom. Phosph. Seneg. Sep. Stann.

Arthritic, °*Acon.* °*Ant.* °*Arn.* °*Bry.* *Chin.* °*Chinin.* °*Cocc.* °*Colch.* °Hep. °Kreas. °*Merc.* N. vom. °Rhus. °*Sulph.* Thuj.

Arthritic-nodous, °Acon.? °*Agn.* °*Ant.* °Arn. *Asa.* °Aur. °*Calc.* °*Carb. an.* °*Caust.* °*Clem.* °Cic. °Colch.? °Dig. °*Graph.* Hep. Led. °*Lyc.* °*Merc.* Nitr. °Nitr. ac. °*Puls.* Ran. °*Rhod.* °*Rhus.* °*Sabin.* °*Staph.* °*Sulph.*

Black, *Acon.* Aeth. Amm. °*Arn.* **Ars.* Aur. °*Bell.* *Carb. veg.* Con. °*Dig.* Hep. **Lach.* Mang. °*Merc.* N. vom. °*Op.* Oph. *Phosph.* Phos. ac. *Plumb.* **Puls.* *Samb.* Sec. Seneg. *Sil.* *Sulph. ac.* °*Veratr.*

—, black-spotted, N. vom.

—, black-blue, *Acon.* *Amm.* °*Arn.* **Ars.* Aur.

°*Bell.* *Carb. veg.* Con. °*Dig.* Hep. *Lach.* Mang. °*Merc.* N. vom. °*Op.* Oph. *Phosph.* Phos. ac. *Plumb.* **Puls.* *Samb.* Sec. Seneg. *Sil.* *Sulph. ac.* ° *Veratr.*

Bleeding, Canth. °*N. vom.* Ran. sc. Sep. **Sulph.*

Blue, Acon. Aeth. Aur. Lach. Oph. Vip. torv.

—, blue-red, *Ars.* **Arn.* **Bell.* **Cham.* Canth. Con. *Kal.* **Lach.* °*Sil.*

Boring, Bell.

Brown, Lach. Vip.

Burning, Acon. Ant. °*Arn.* **Ars.* Asa. °*Baryt.* **Bell.* **Bry.* *Calc.* *Carb. an.* *Carb. veg.* *Caust.* °*Cham.* *Chin.* *Cocc.* Colch. Coloc. Con. Crotal. *Dulc.* *Euphorb.* Hell. *Hep.* *Hyos.* Jod. *Kal.* *Lach.* *Led.* **Lyc.* Mang. **Merc.* *Mez.* Natr. Natr. m. Nicc. *Nitr. ac.* *N. vom.* *Op.* **Petr.* **Phosph.* *Phos. ac.* °*Puls.* **Rhus.* Samb. Sec. Seneg. **Sep.* °*Sil.* *Spig.* Spong. Stann. **Sulph.* Vip. torv.

Bubbling, N. vom. (Comp. Throbbing.)

Cold, °*Ars.* °*Asa.* Bell. *Cocc.* *Con.* Crotal. *Cycl.* Dulc. Lach. Magn. aust. °Merc. °*Rhod.* °*Puls.* Sec. *Spig.*

Contusion, after, °*Arn.* °*Con.* Sulph.

Corded, Calc. °*Dulc.* Graph. *Hep.* °*Jod.* Lach. Lyc. *Rhus.*

Cracked, broken, Ars.

Cutting, Kal. Stann.

Dirty-looking, Crotal.

Drawing-painful, Amm. m. Cham. Chin. Ferr. Kal. N. vom.

Dropsical, °*Acon.* Anthrok. **Ant.* **Ars.* **Aur.* °*Bar. m.* °Bell. °*Bry.* Canth. Chel. **Chin.* °Chinin.? °*Colch.* Coloc. Con. Crotal. °*Dig.* °*Dulc.*

Euphorb. °*Ferr.* Guaj. **Hell.* Hyos. *Jod.* **Kal.* Lach. °*Led.* **Lyc.* **Merc.* Mez. Mur. ac. Natr. Nitr. Nitr. ac. Oleand. *Op.* Oph. °*Phosph.* *Plumb.* °*Puls.* °*Rhod.* °*Rhus.* °*Ruta.* °*Sabin.* °*Samb.* Sassap. Sec. Seneg. Sep. Sil. **Squill.* °*Stram.* **Sulph.* Tereb. Veratr.

Ecchymosed, **Arn.* **Con.*

Elastic, **Ars.*

Erysipelatous, °*Acon.* *Amm.* *Arn.* *Ars.* **Bell.* *Bry.* *Calc.* Canth. *Carb. veg.* Caust. *Chin.* Euphorb. *Hell.* *Hep.* *Kal.* *Lyc.* Magn. c. °*Merc.* Natr. Natr. m. *Nitr. ac.* Oph. Petr. *Phosph.* Phos. ac. **Puls.* **Rhus.* Ruta. *Samb.* Sassap. *Sep.* Sil. °*Sulph.* Thuj. *Zinc.*

Exuding, **Lyc.* Sep.

Gangrenous, Ars. Euphorb. Vip. torv.

Hard, tight, Acon. Agn. Alum. Amm. Amm. m. *Ant.* **Arn.* **Ars.* *Asa.* Aur. **Bell.* Bov. **Bry.* **Calc.* Canth. **Carb. an.* *Caust.* **Cham.* *Chin.* Cin. *Con.* Dig. *Dulc.* **Graph.* Hell. Hep. *Kal.* Lach. **Led.* **Lyc.* Magn. c. *Merc.* Mez. N. vom. Oph. Par. **Phosph.* Phos. ac. Plumb. **Puls.* **Rhus.* *Sabin.* *Samb.* Sep. **Sil.* Spig. Spong. Squill. **Staph.* *Stront.* **Sulph.* *Thuj.*

Humid, Sulph.

Inflamed, °*Acon.* Agn. Amm. *Ant.* **Arn.* **Ars.* °*Asa.* *Aur.* **Bell.* **Borax.* **Bry.* Calc. *Cann.* Canth. *Carb. veg.* *Caust.* **Chin.* **Cocc.* *Colch.* Con. Crotal. Gran. **Hep.* Hyos. **Jod.* Kal. **Lach.* °Led. **Lyc.* *Magn. c.* °*Mang.* **Merc.* Mez. Mur. ac. Natr. *Natr. m.* Nitr. *Nitr. ac.* **N. vom.* Oph. Petr. **Phosph.* Phos. ac. Plumb. **Puls.* **Rhus.* Sassap. Seneg. **Sep.* **Sil.* Stram. **Sulph.* *Thuj.* Veratr. *Zinc.*

Injuries, after, **Arn.* **Con.* (Comp. INJURIES.)
Itching, Ant. Canth. Caust. Cocc. Lach. Nitr. ac. *Phosph.* Phos. ac. Puls. Rhus. Rhus v. Stram. Sulph.
Knotty, Calc. Dulc. Hep. °*Ign.* Jod. Lyc. Nitr. ac. Phosph. Rhus. Thuj.
Leprous, °Lach.
Livid, Gran.
Lymphatic, *Berb.* °Carb. veg. Oph.
Marbled, spotted, Chin. Gran. Lyc. Rhus v. Sep.
Mercurial, °Staph.
Numb, Sep.
Pain as if dislocated, °Hep.
Pain as from a splinter, Stann.
Painful as if sore, Aur Bism. *Borax. Graph. Hep.* Natr. Natr. m. °Rhus. Sassap. Sep. *Sil.* Thuj. Zinc.
Painful, Amb. *Amm.* **Arn.* **Ars.* *Aur.* Baryt. **Bell.* Bov. °*Bry.* Calc. Canth. Carb. an. Carb. veg. **Caust.* **Cham.* **Chin.* *Con.* Cop. Crotal. Croton. Cupr. °*Daph.* Dig. Dulc. Electr. **Ferr.* **Hep.* Kal. Kal. hdr. **Lach.* **Led.* **Lyc.* Magn. art. **Magn. arct.* *Magn. c.* *Magn. m.* **Merc.* **Merc. corr.* Mez. Mur. ac. Natr. Natr. m. Nitr. **Nitr. ac.* **N. vom.* Oph. **Phosph.* **Phos. ac.* Plat. Plumb. **Puls.* Ran. sc. Rhod. **Rhus.* Sabin. Sassap. Sec. **Sep.* **Sil.* Spig. Spong. Stann. Staph. Stront. **Sulph.* Tereb. **Thuj.* *Vip. torv.*
Painless, Calc. Dros. °*Euphr.* °Lyc. Natr. s. Par. Phosph. Puls. Rhus. *Sep.* Sil. Staph.
Pale, °*Arn.* Ars. **Baryt.* Bell. Bov. **Bry.* *Calc.* Chin. Cocc. Con. Dig. Euphorb. Ferr. Graph.

Hell. °*Jod.* Kal. *Lach.* **Lyc.* *Merc.* Nitr. ac. N. vom. Oph. Plumb. *Puls.* **Rhus.* *Sep.* Spig. Sulph. Vip. torv.

Rheumatic, °*Acon.* °*Arn.* °*Bell.* °*Bry.* °Calc. ph. °*Cham.* °*Chin.* °Cocc. °*Colch.* °Hep. °Kreas. °Lach. °*Merc.* °*N. vom.* °*Puls.* °Rhus. °*Sulph.*

Red, **Acon.* **Ant.* Alum. Amm. Amm. m. **Arn.* **Ars.* **Asa.* Asar. **Aur.* Aur. m. Baryt. **Bell.* *Borax.* Bov. **Bry.* *Carb. an.* °*Carb.veg.* **Cham.* **Chin.* *Con.* Crotal. Electr. **Hep.* *Kal.* Lach. **Lyc.* *Magn. c.* **Merc.* *Mur. ac.* *Natr.* Natr. m. Nicc. Nitr. *Nitr. ac.* **N. vom.* Oleand. °*Oph.* Phell. **Phosph.* Phos. ac. Poth. **Puls.* *Ran.* Ran. sc. *Raph.* °*Rhod.* **Rhus.* Sabin. Sassap. **Sep.* **Sil.* Spong. **Stann.* Stram. **Sulph.* Tab. Therid. *Thuj.*

Red-spotted, Chin. Lyc. Rhus v. Sep.

Sacculated, **Kal.*

Scarlet, **Bell.*

Scrophulous, Aur. °Bov. *Calc. Phosph. (Comp. GLANDS, swelling of.)

Scurfy, **Merc.*

Shining, Alum. **Arn.* **Ars.* °*Bry.* **Merc.* Phosph. Ran. *Rhus.* *Sabin.* °*Sulph.* Thuj.

Smarting, N. vom.

Soft, Ars. **Chin.* *Led.* Petr. Sep. (Comp. Watery.)

Stinging, Acon. Agn. Amm. m. Ant. *Arn.* Ars. Asa. Bell. **Bry.* Calc. *Canth.* Carb. an. °*Carb. veg.* **Caust.* Cham. Chel. *Chin.* °*Cocc.* *Con.* *Cycl.* Dig. Electr. °*Ferr.* **Graph.* Kal. Lach. **Led.* Lyc. Magn. c. Mang. **Merc.* Mez. Natr. m. Nitr. **Nitr. ac.* °*N. vom.* Oleand. Petr. **Phosph.* **Puls.* Ran. °*Rhus.*

Ruta. *Sabad.* *Sep.* Spong. Stann. **Sulph.* °*Thuj.*

Suppurating, *Baryt.* Calc. Carb. veg. Caust. Chin. Corall. Galv. **Lach.* Lyc. °*Mang.* ***Merc.** Natr. **Phosph.* **Sulph.* Vip. red. Vip. torv.

Tearing, °Bry. Euphorb. Kal. Merc. Natr. Puls. °*Rhod.*

Tensive, **Acon.* **Baryt.* Bov. **Bry.* Calc. Cann. Canth. °*Carb. veg.* Chin. Con. Croc. Euphorb. Graph. **Led.* Lyc. Magn. m. Mang. Mur. ac. Par. **Puls.* Rhus. Sep. Sulph. Vip. torv.

Throbbing, **Bell.* Calc. °*Carb. veg.* **Cham.* ***Lach.** Magn. m. N. vom. Sep. **Sulph.*

Titillating, *Acon.* °*Arn.* *Caust.* Chel. *Colch.* *Con.* Lach. °*Merc.* Natr. *N. vom.* Phos. ac. °*Puls.* **Rhus.* Sec. °Sep. Spig. °*Sulph.*

Transparent, *Merc.* Sulph.

Ulcerated, Merc. **Nitr. ac.*

Violet-coloured, Lach.

Watery, œdematous, **Ant.* **Ars.* Aur. °*Bell.* **Bry.* Calc. Canth. Chel. **Chin.* °*Colch.* Coloc. Con. Convolv. °*Dig.* °*Dulc.* Euphorb. Ferr. Guaj. °*Hell.* Hep. **Jod.* **Kal.* Kreas. °*Lach.* °*Led.* **Lyc.* **Merc.* Mez. Mur. ac. Natr. Nitr. *Nitr. ac.* Oleand. *Op.* *Phosph.* *Plumb.* **Puls.* *Rhod.* °*Rhus.* *Ruta.* °*Sabin.* **Samb.* Sassap. Sec. *Seneg.* *Sep.* Sil. **Squill.* Stram. °*Stront.* **Sulph.* *Veratr.* Vip. torv.

White, °*Ant.* °*Ars.* *Bell.* **Bry.* °*Calc.* *Chin.* Dig. Euphorb. Graph. *Hep.* °*Jod.* *Kreas.* °*Lyc.* *Merc.* N. vom. Ol. jec.? °*Puls.* °*Rhod.* °*Rhus.* °*Sabin.* *Sep.* *Sil.* °*Sulph.*

Yellow, Canth.

Head, **Ars.* *Bell.* Cham. Crotal. Cupr. °Daph. Dig. Merc. Op. Phosph. Puls. *Rhus.* Ruta. Sep. Stram. Sulph.

Eyes, Ars. Baryt. **Bry.* Carb. veg. **Guaj.* Hep. Led. **N. vom.* Phosph. Plumb. **Rhus.* Ruta. Stram. **Sulph.*

Eyebrows, *Kal.

Eyelids, **Acon.* Agar. Alum. Ang. Arn. Ars. Asar. Aur. Baryt. **Bell.* **Bry.* **Calc.* Caust. °*Cham.* Cocc. Colch. Cycl. °*Dig.* Euphorb. °*Euphr.* Ferr. °*Graph.* °*Guaj.* Hep. Hyos. °*Ign.* Jod. Kal. °*Kreas.* Lach. Lyc. Magn. aust. Magn. c. Mang. Men. **Merc.* Mosch. Mur. ac. Natr. Natr. m. Nitr. ac. **N. vom.* Op. Phosph. **Puls.* Rhod. **Rhus.* Ruta. Seneg. **Sep.* Sil. Spong. Squill. Stram. **Sulph.* Teucr. *Thuj. Val.

Canthi, Agar. Aur. Bell. Bry. **Calc.* °Chel.? Merc. Petr. Ran. °Ruta.? Sassap. Sil. Stann.

Ear, Alum. °*Anac.* Ant. Baryt. Borax. *Calc.* Caust. Cist. Electr. Graph. *Kal.* Kreas. °*Lyc.* Merc. Natr. m. Nitr. Nitr. ac. Phos. ac. **Puls.* **Rhus.* *Sep.* °*Sil.* Spong. Zinc.

—, behind the ears, Bry. Calc. Caps. Carb. an, Tab.

—, inner ears, *Calc.* Caust. Cist. Electr. Graph. *Kal.* Natr. m. *Sep.*

—, before the ears, Anac. Bry.

—, parotid glands, Amm. Baryt. **Bell.* **Calc.* Carb. an. **Carb. veg.* **Cham.* Cocc. **Con.* Dig. Graph. *Ign.* **Kal.* **Merc.* Nitr. ac. °N. vom.? *Puls.* **Rhus.* Sep. **Sil.* *Sulph.*

Nose, **Alum.* Amm. m. *Arn. Ars. *Aur. **Aur. m.* *Bell. Borax, **Bry.* **Calc.* *Carb. an.* Caust.

Cist. Cocc. Corall. °Graph. *Hep.* °Ign. *Kal.* Lyc. Magn. c. **Magn. m.* *Merc.* *Natr. m.* Nicç. °*Petr.* **Phosph.* Phos. ac. *Rhus.* **Sep.* **Sulph.* Thuj. **Zinc.*

Nose, alæ, Alum. Calc. Carb. an. Magn. m. Merc. Sulph. Thuj. Zinc.

—, nostrils, Bell. Canth. Cocc. Lach. Zinc.

—, dorsum, Phos. ac. Poth.

—, tip, Calc. Kal. Lyc. Merc. Nicc. Sep. Sulph.

—, root, Calc.

Face, Acon. Alum. Amb. Amm. Amm. m. **Arn.* **Ars.* Asa. **Aur.* **Baryt.* **Bell.* Borax. Bov. **Bry.* Calc. Cann. Canth. Carb. an. **Carb. veg.* Caust. Chel. Cic. °Colch. °Coloc. Con. Crotal. Dig. Dulc. Electr. *Euphorb.* Galv. Gran. *Graph.* Guaj. °Hell. *Hep.* *Hyos.* Kal. Kal. hdr. **Lach.* Laur. **Lyc.* Lupul. Magn. c. °Merc. Natr. Natr. m. Nicc. Nitr. ac. **N.vom.* Oleand. Oph. Op. Petr. **Phosph.* Plumb. **Rhus.* Rhus v. Sabin. Sec. **Sep.* Sil. Spig. Spong. *Stann.* **Stram.* **Sulph.* Sulph. ac. Veratr. Vip. red. Vip. torv.

—, cheek, **Arn.* *Aur.* Baryt. **Bell.* Bry. Canth. **Cham.* Chin. Ferr. °Lach. **Magn. arct.* °*Merc.* °*N. vom.* °*Puls.* Spig. Spong. Staph. **Sulph.*

Lips and mouth, region of, Alum. Arg. Arn. **Ars.* Asa. °*Aur.* °Aur. m. Baryt. **Bell.* °Bov. **Bry.* **Calc.* Canth. Caps. Carb. an. Carb. veg. Chin. Dig. Graph. Grat. °Hell. Hep. Kal. Kal. chl. **Lach.* Lyc. Magn. art. Mang. Merc. Merc. corr. Mez. Mosch. Mur. ac. *Natr. **Natr. m.* Nitr. ac. N. mosch. Oleand. Oph. Op. Par,

39

Petr. Phell. Phosph. Puls. *Rhus.* Sep. Sil. °Staph. Stram. **Sulph.* Vip. Vip. torv. Zinc.

—, corners of mouth, Asa. Oleand.

Chin, Carb. veg. Caust. Rhus. Spig. Staph.

Lower jaw, °*Acon.* Arn. °Ars. Kal. Lyc. **Merc.* Ol. an. Petr. Phosph. *Sil. Staph. Sulph.

Buccal cavity, Agar. Alum. Amb. *Amm. Amm. m.* Anac. Aur. **Baryt.* Bar. m. **Bell.* Berb. Bism. Borax. Bov. Bruc. **Calc.* Canth. Carb. an. Carb. veg. Cast. Caust.**Cham. Chin.* **Cist.* Coccin. Cocc. Coff. Con. Crotal. Croton. Dig. Dros. Dulc. Electr. Ferr. **Graph.* Hell. °*Hep.* °*Ign.* Jod. Kal. Kal. hdr. **Lach.* Laur. Lyc. Magn. art. Magn. arct. Magn. c. Magn. m. **Merc. Mercurial. Mur. ac.* Natr. Natr. m. *Natr. s.* Nicc. Nitr. *Nitr. ac.* **N. vom.* Par. Petr. Phell. *Phosph. Phos. ac.* Plat. Plumb. Poth. Puls. Ran. sc. Raph. Sabad. Sabin. Sassap. Sec. **Sep.* Sil. Spig. Spong. **Staph.* Stram. Stront. **Sulph.* Sulph. ac. Tab. *Thuj.* Veratr. Vip. *Zinc.*

—, ranula, °*Thuj.*

—, palate, Bar. m. **Calc. Chin.* **N. vom.* Par.

—, velum palati, °Bell. Coff. °Lach.

—, tonsils, Alum. Amm. **Baryt.* **Bell.* Berb. **Calc.* °Cham. *Graph.* °*Hep.* °Ign. °*Lach.* **Merc.* Natr. Natr. s. Nicc. *Nitr. ac.* N. vom. *Phosph.* Plat. Ran. sc. Sep. **Staph. Sulph.* Tart. *Thuj.* Zinc.

—, mouth, Alum. °Bell. Calc. Canth. Caust. Ferr. °*Merc.* °*N. vom.* Sep.

—, fauces and throat, Ant. Arg. **Bell.* **Calc.* Carb. veg. Caust. *Lach. Nitr. ac.* °Op. Petr. Phos. ac. Poth. Sep. Spig. Sulph. ac. Thuj.

Buccal cavity, salivary glands, Bar. m. *Merc.* Thuj.

—, gums, Agar. *Alum.* Amb. Amm. Amm. m. Anac. Aur. Baryt. **Bell.* Bism. Borax. Bov. **Calc.* Caps. Carb. an. Carb. veg. Cast. **Caust.* **Cham.* Chin. **Cist.* Coccin. Cocc. Con. Croton. Ferr. **Graph.* Hep. Jod. Kal. Kal. hdr. Lach. Lyc. Magn. art. **Magn. arct.* Magn. c. Magn. m. **Merc. Mercurial.* Mur. ac. Natr. Natr. m. Natr. s. Nicc. Nitr. Nitr. ac. **N. vom.* Petr. Phell. Phosph. Phos. ac. Plumb. Puls. Ran. sc. Sabin. Sassap. **Sep.* Sil. Spong. **Staph.* Stront. **Sulph.* Sulph. ac. Thuj. Veratr. Zinc.

—, uvula, °Bell. Berb. Carb. veg. Chin. °Coff. Jod. Lyc. Merc. Natr. s. **N. vom.* *Sabad. Sil.*

—, tongue, Calc. Con. *Crotal.* Dig. °*Dulc.* Electr. Hell. Kal. **Lach.* Laur. Lyc. Merc. Mercurial. Natr. m. Phosph. Phos. ac. Sec. Sil. Stram. Thuj. *Vip. red.* Zinc.

—, lingual glands, *Staph.* Tab.

Abdomen and stomach, region of, Acon. Bell. Canth. Caust. Oph. Puls. Sep.

—, glands, °Ars. °*Aur.* *Calc.* °*Carb. veg.* Clem. **Dulc.* *Graph.* Lyc. **Merc.* Natr. **Nitr. ac.* Phosph. **Staph.* Stann. Stram. **Sulph.* Tereb. °Thuj.

—, umbilical region, Caust. Lach. Lyc.

Anus, Aur. Borax. Croton. Graph. *Hep.* Ign. Lach. Sep. Sulph.

Sexual parts, °Agn. °*Arn.* **Ars.* *Aur. Baryt. Bar. m. Berb. Calad. Cann. *Canth.* **Carb. veg.* °Chin. Cinn. **Clem.* °Con. Cop. Corall. °Dig.

Graph. Ign. °Jod. *Kal. *Kreas.* Led. °Lyc. Magn. arct. **Merc.* Merc. ac. Natr. c. Nitr. ac. °*N. vom.* Ol. an. Phosph. Phos. ac. Plumb. **Puls.* *Rhod. Rhus. Sabin. °Samb. °*Sep.* Sil. Spig. °Spong. Sulph. *Thuj.* Viol. tr. Vip. torv.

Sexual parts, frænulum, Cann. Canth. Sabin.
—, glans, Ars. Corall. Natr. Spig.
—, testicles, °*Agn.* °Arn. Ars. **Aur.* Bar. m. °Chin. °*Clem.* °Con. °Dig. °Jod. °Kal. °Lyc. °*Merc.* Nitr. ac. °N. vom. Ol. an. Plumb. **Puls.* **Rhod.* *Spong.
—, scrotum, °Arn. Canth. Carb. veg. Clem. Graph. Ign. Phos. ac. Puls. Rhus. °Samb. °Sep. Vip. torv.
—, epididymis, Baryt. Magn. arct. Sulph.
—, prostate gland, Cann. °*Puls.* °*Thuj.*
—, penis, °Arn. Cann. Canth. Cinn. Kreas. Led. Merc. ac. Sabin.
—, spermatic cord, Arn. Berb. °Chin. Kal. Phosph. Phos. ac. *Puls.* Spong.
—, labia, Amb. Amm. Bry. Calc. Carb. veg. Kreas. Meph. °*Merc.* Merc. acet. Nitr. ac. °*Sep.* Thuj.
—, vagina, Merc. Nitr. ac. **N. vom.*
—, neck of womb, Canth. Sec.
—, prepuce, Calad. Cann. Cinn. Corall. **Merc.* Nitr. ac. Rhus. Sabin. Sil. Sulph. Thuj. Viol. tr.

Thorax, Bry. Rhus.

Mammæ and nipples, °Bell. Calc. °Graph. **Merc.* Merc. corr. **Puls.* Sabin.
—, nipples, Merc.

Dorsal region, axilla, Baryt.
—, axillary glands, Amm. *Amm. m.* Ars. **Bell.* Clem. Coloc. *Kal.* *Lyc. *Natr. m.* **Nitr. ac.* **Phosph.* Phos. ac. Prun. *Rhus. Sep.* **Sil.* °Staph.? **Sulph.*
—, neck, Ars. **Bell.* Bov. Calc. Canth. Cic. Con. Croc. Crotal. Hyos. °Kal. °Lach. °Lyc. Magn. art. Mang. *Natr.* Nitr. ac. N. vom. Par. Puls. *Sassap.* Sil. Sulph. Tart. Vip. red. Vip. torv.
—, cervical glands, Alum. °Amm. Arn. Bar. m. **Bell.* **Calc.* **Carb. an.* Carb. veg. Caust. Cinn. °Cist. Cupr. °Electr. *Ferr. Graph.* Hell. Ign. *Kal.* °Kreas. °*Lach.* **Lyc. Magn. m.* **Merc. Natr.* **Nitr. ac.* °Phosph. **Sil. Spig. Spong.* °Staph.? Sulph. Tart. Viol. tr.
—, lumbar region, Berb. Lyc. °Sil. °Staph.
—, nape of neck, Baryt. **Bell.* Calc. Puls. Sep.
—, posterior cervical glands, **Baryt.* **Calc.* °*Hell.* °Jod. Mur. ac. °Petr. °Phosph. **Sil.* °Staph.? **Sulph.*
—, back, °Sil. °Staph.
—, vertebræ, °Puls. °Sil.
—, thyroid cartilage, Sil. *Sulph.*
Arms, Alum. °*Ars.* Baryt. **Bell.* Bov. °*Calc. ph.* **Chin.* Crotal. Electr. Oph. °*Puls.* **Rhus.* Sep. °*Sulph.* Vip. torv.
—, shoulders, Acon. **Bry.* °*Calc. ph.*
—, elbow, °*Hep.* °*Lach.* Merc. Puls. °*Veratr.*
—, elbow-joints, Bry. Puls.
—, upper arm, Berb. **Bry.* °*Sep. Sulph.* Vip. torv.
—, forearm, *Berb.* Calc. *Caust.* Dig. Lach. *Lyc. N. vom. Sep.* °*Sulph.* Vip. torv.

Hands, Acon. Amm. m. Ars. Bar. m. **Bell.* °*Bry.* °*Calc.* *Caust.* °*Cham.* Chin. Clem. °*Cocc.* Cupr. *Dig.* *Electr.* *Ferr.* Galv. *Hep.* *Hyos.* °*Lach.* Laur. *Lyc.* *Merc.* *Mez.* *Natr.* *Natr. m.* Nitr. Nitr. ac. N. vom. Phosph. °*Rhod.* *Rhus.* Sec. Sep. Spong. **Stann.* Sulph. Vip. red.

—, wrists, Aur. m. *Carb. veg.* Crotal. °*Euphr.* °*Lach.* Magn. c. Merc. acet. Phosph. Sec. Sep.

—, fingers, Alum. Ammoniac. Amm. Ant. Ars. Berb. Borax. Bry. Calc. Canth. Chin. *Hep.* Jod. °*Lach.* *Led.* Magn. c. °*Mang.* Mur. ac. *Nitr. ac.* Oleand. *Phosph.* Ran. Ran. sc. Rhus. *Sulph.* Thuj. Vinc. Vip. torv.

—, finger-joints, Amb. Berb. Canth. *Carb. veg.* Euphr. Graph. *Hep.* **Lyc.* *Nitr. ac.* Spong. *Sulph.*

—, thumb, Gran. Led. N. vom. *Phosph.*

Lower limbs, *Ars.* *Con.* *Jod.* Lyc.? *Merc.* *Oph.* Sep. °*Sulph.* *Vip. torv.*

—, buttocks, Croton. Vip. red.

—, thighs, Bov. *Chin.* Crotal. Ol. jec.

—, knees, Berb. °*Bry.* **Calc.* **Chin.* °*Cocc.* Ferr. Hep. °*Jod.* Lach. **Led.* **Lyc.* Magn. c. Mur. ac. **N. vom.* Phosph. **Puls.* Rhod. Sassap. Sep. °*Sil.* °*Sulph.*

—, legs, Amb. Ars. *Aur.* Borax. **Bry.* Calc. *Colch.* *Crotal.* Dig. *Dulc.* Graph. °*Kal.* **Lach.* Led. *Lyc.* *Merc.* Natr. °*N. vom.* *Oph.* °*Puls.* Rhod. **Sep.* *Sil.* Stront. *Vip. torv.*

—, tibiæ, Graph. Lach. *Rhus.* Stann. Sulph. ac.

—, calves, Carb. veg. *Chin.* Hyos. Mez. Sulph.

—, tendo Achilles, Berb. Zinc.

Feet, °*Amb.* **Amm.* Arn. **Ars.* °*Asa.* Bar. m. *Bov.* **Bry.* *Calc.* *Carb. an.* Carb. veg. *Caust.* Cham. **Chin.* Chinin. Cocc. Colch. Con. Crotal. °*Dig.* Electr. **Ferr.* **Graph.* Hyos. Indig. Jod. **Kal.* Kreas. **Lach.* *Led.* Lyc. **Natr.* °*Natr. m.* Nitr. ac. N. vom. Op. **Petr.* **Phos.* °*Phos. ac.* Plumb. **Puls.* **Rhus.* Sabad. °*Samb.* Sassap. Sec. **Sep.* **Sil.* **Stann.* °*Stront.* **Sulph.* *Veratr.* Vip. torv. *Zinc.*

—, dorsa of feet, *Calc.* Carb. an. Lyc. *Merc. N. vom.* **Sulph.* Staph. Thuj.

—, joints, *Ferr. Merc.*

—, ankles, Amb. Ars. °*Asa.* Berb. Calc. **Hep.* Kal. *Led.* Lyc. *Mang.* Puls. Sil. *Stann.* Sulph. Zinc.

—, bones; °*Merc. Staph.*

—, heels, *Con. Merc. Raph.*

—, soles, *Cham. Kal.* Kreas. °*Lyc.* Natr. Petr.

—, toes, Amm. Ammoniac. Carb. an. °*Carb. veg.* °*Daph.* Gins. **Graph.* *Merc. Mur. ac. Natr. Nitr. ac.* Oph. *Phos. ac.* Plat. *Sabin.* **Sulph.* *Thuj.* Zinc.

Bones, Amb. Amm. Ant. °*Asa.* °*Aur.* Bell. Bry. °*Calc.* Carb. an. **Clem.* Coloc. Con. °*Daph.* Dig. Dulc. °*Guaj.* Hep. Jod. °*Lach.* Led. °*Lyc.* **Merc.* °*Mez.* Natr. Natr. m. °*Nitr. ac.* Petr. °*Phosph.* °*Phos. ac.* °*Puls.* Rhod. °*Rhus.* °*Ruta.* *Sabin.* Sep. °*Sil.* Spig. **Staph.* °*Sulph.* Thuj. Veratr.

Nails, around the, Natr. m.

Glands, Acon. Agn. Alum. Amb. **Amm.* Amm. m. Ant. Arg. *Arn.* **Ars.* °Asa. °Aur. **Baryt.* Bar. m. **Bell.* Borax. Bov. **Bry.* Calad. **Calc.* Camph. Cann. Canth. Caps. **Carb. an.* **Carb.*

veg. Caust. **Cham.* Chin. Cic. Cinn. °*Cist.* Clem. Cocc. Coloc. **Con.* Corall. Croc. Cupr. Cycl. Dig. **Dulc.* °Electr. Euphorb. *Ferr.* **Graph.* °Hell. **Hep.* Hyos. Ign. **Jod.* *Kal.* °Kreas. °*Lach.* Led. **Lyc.* Magn. c. Magn. m. Mang. **Merc.* *Merc. corr.* Mez. Mur. ac. *Natr.* Natr.m. *Nitr.ac.* °N.vom. Oph. *Petr. **Phosph.* Phos. ac. Plumb. *Puls.* Raph. Ran. Ran. sc. Rhod. **Rhus.* Ruta. Sabad. Sabin. Samb. Sassap. **Sep.* **Sil.* *Spig.* **Spong.* *Squill.* Stann. **Staph.* Stram. Stront. **Sulph.* Sulph. ac. Tart. Tereb. Teucr. °*Thuj.* Veratr. Viol. od. Zinc.

Swelling, sensation of.

In general, Acon. Alum. Amm. Amm. m. Ant. Arn. Ars. Aur. Baryt. **Bell.* *Bry.* °*Calc.* Canth. Caps. Carb. an. Carb. veg. Chin. Cocc. Con. Dig. Dulc. Graph. Guaj. *Hep.* Hyos. *Ign.* **Lach.* Laur. *Merc.* *Nitr.* *Nitr. ac.* N. mosch. **N. vom.* Par. Plat. **Puls.* *Rhus.* *Sabin.* Sassap. Seneg. Sep. Sil. Spig. *Spong.* Stann. Staph. **Sulph.* Sulph. ac. Veratr. *Zinc.*

Lips, Oleand. Rhus.
Lower jaw, Sabad.
Buccal cavity, Alum. Amm. Anac. Baryt. **Bell.* Bry. Chin. Cocc. Daph. *Hep.* Ign. Lach. Lyc. Nitr. N. vom. Plumb. Puls. Rhod. *Sabin.* Sang. Spong. Stront. Sulph. Thuj. *Zinc.*
—, palate, Ign. N. vom. Puls.
—, mouth, Amm. Lyc.

Fauces and throat, Alum. Baryt. **Bell.* Bry. Chin. *Hep.* **Lach. Nitr. ac.* **N. vom.* Plumb. **Puls.* Rhus. *Sabin.* Sang. **Sulph.* Thuj. *Zinc.*

—, gums, Amm. Chin. Daph. Hyos. Nitr. N. vom. Puls. Rhod. Sabin. Spong. Stront.

—, uvula, **Puls.*

—, tongue, Anac. Cocc. Lyc. Magn. aust.

Abdomen, glands, Con. Sil.

Anus, Camph. Graph. Hep. N. mosch. Teucr.

Thorax, Lach. *Merc.*

Arms, shoulders, Kal. hdr. Laur.

Lower limbs, Prun.

—, knee, Alum. Ammoniac. Berb. Canth. Carb. veg. Lach. *Nitr. ac.*

—, legs, Lam. Lyc.

Feet, Plat. Sassap.

—, soles, Bry. °*Calc.*

—, toes, Mur. ac.

Glands, Ant. *Aur. Bell. Bry.* Carb. veg. Chin. Con. Dulc. *Hep. Ign.* Lach. Magn. art. Magn. arct. *Merc.* Natr. m. *Nitr.* Nitr. ac. N. mosch. N. vom. *Puls. Rhus.* Sabin. Spig. *Spong.* Staph. Sulph. Zinc.

Syphilitic, which is.

Herpes, °Nitr. ac. °Thuj.

Spots, °*Merc.* °Nitr. ac.

Ulcers, °*Merc.* °*Nitr. ac.* °*Thuj.*

Nose, °Lach. °Merc. °Nitr. ac. °Thuj.

Buccal cavity, ulcers and eruptions, °Lach. °*Merc.* °Thuj.

Bones, °*Aur.* Carb. veg.? °*Merc.*

Tearing.

Mammæ and nipples, Baryt. Grat. Kal. Ol. an. Phell.

Bones, periosteum, **Agar.* Alum. **Amm. m.* Ang. **Arg.* Arn. Ars. Asa. °*Aur.* **Baryt.* °*Bell.* Berb. Bism. Bov. Bry. Cann. **Carb. veg.* °*Caust.* Cham. Chel. **Chin.* **Cocc.* Coloc. **Cycl.* °*Cupr.* Dig. Dulc. Graph. Hell. Ign. Jod. Kal. Lach. Lact. Laur. °*Lyc.* °*Magn. c.* Magn. m. Mang. Meph. **Merc.* Mur. ac. Natr. Natr. m. Nicc. °*Nitr.* *Nitr. ac.* N. vom. °*Phosph.* °*Phos. ac.* Puls. °*Rhod.* °*Ruta.* Sabad. **Sabin.* Sassap. Sep. **Spig.* Spong. Stann. **Staph.* Stront. *Teucr.* *Thuj.* *Veratr.* Verbasc. Zinc.

Nails, around the, Amb. Baryt. Bism. Camph. *Carb. veg.* Colch. *Coloc.* Jod. Lyc. Nitr. Ol. an. Sulph. ac.

Glands, *Amb.* Amm. *Arn.* Baryt. *Bell.* Bov. *Bry.* *Calc.* Cann. Caps. *Carb. an.* *Carb. veg.* Caust. *Cham.* *Chin.* Cocc. Con. Cycl. *Dulc.* Ferr. Graph. Grat. *Kal.* *Lyc.* **Merc.* Mez. Natr. Nitr. ac. N. vom. Ol. an. Phell. Phosph. **Puls.* *Rhod.* *Rhus.* Selen. Seneg. Sep. *Sil.* *Sulph.* Thuj. *Zinc.*

Tears, that which.

Bloodvessels, swelling of, Sulph. ac.

Blotches, tubercles, Cham. Con.

Corns, °Arn. °Calc. *Cocc.* Ign. °*Lyc.* Magn. m. Rhus. °*Sil.* °*Sulph.* Sulph. ac. Thuj.

Eruption, Kal.
Herpes, Magn. arct.
Nails, around the, Amb. Baryt. Bism. Camph. *Carb. veg.* Colch. *Coloc.* Jod. Lyc. Nitr. Ol. an. Sulph. ac.
Pimples, Dulc.
Swelling, °Bry. Euphorb. Kal. Merc. Natr. Puls. °*Rhod.*
Ulcers, **Ars.* *Bell.* Bry. **Calc.* *Canth.* Clem. Cocc. °*Cycl.* *Graph.* Kal. **Lyc.* Merc. Mez. Nitr. ac. *N. vom.* Phosph. Puls. Rhus. **Sep.* °*Sil.* *Staph.* **Sulph.* Zinc.

Face, Con.
Buccal cavity, Calc. Dulc. **Merc.*
—, eruptions, Dulc.
—, swelling, **Merc.*
—, ulcers, Calc.
Dorsal region, tumor, Petr.
Arms, swelling, **Bry.*
Hands, swelling, **Lyc.*
Lower limbs, varices, Sulph. ac.
—, ulcers, Lyc.
—, swelling, *Puls.* °*Rhod.*
Feet, swelling, Natr.

Tension.

Of the skin, in general, Agn. Alum. Amm. Amm. m. Anac. Ang. °*Ant.* Arg. **Arn.* Asa. Asar. Aur. **Baryt.* **Bell.* Borax. **Bry.* Calc. Canth. **Carb. an.* °*Carb. veg.* **Caust.* Cham. Chin. Colch. *Coloc.* *Con.* Dig. Euphorb. Hell. Hep. Jod. *Kal.* Kreas. *Lach.* Laur. Led. Lyc.

Magn. arct. Magn. c. Magn. m. Mang. Men. Merc. *Mez.* Mosch. Mur. ac. Natr. Natr. m. Nitr. ac. **N. vom.* *Oleand.* *Par.* Petr. *Phosph.* *Phos. ac.* *Plat.* **Puls.* Rhod. **Rhus.* *Ruta.* Sabad. *Sabin.* Sassap. *Sep.* Sil. *Spig.* *Spong.* Stann. *Staph.* *Stront.* *Sulph.* Tarax. *Thuj.* Veratr. Verb. Viol. od. Viol. tr. *Zinc.*

Scalp, Asar. Baryt. Berb. Carb. an. Caust. Lam. Par. Ruta. Sabad. Stront. Spig. Staph.

Bones, periosteum, Arn. Mang. °*Ruta.* Zinc.

Glands, Alum. Amb. Amm. Ang. Arg. Arn. Aur. Baryt. Bell. Bov. Bry. Calc. Carb. an. Caust. Clem. Coloc. Con. Dulc. Graph. Kal. Lyc. Magn. art. Magn. arct. Merc. Mur. ac. N. vom. Phosph. **Puls.* Rhus. Sabad. Sabin. Sep. Sil. Spong. Staph. Stront. Sulph. Thuj.

Tensive, which is.

Bloodvessels, swelling of, Graph.

Eruption, Alum. *Arn.* Baryt. Bell. Canth. Carb. an. **Caust.* Cocc. Con. Hep. Kal. Mez. Oleand. *Phosph.* Puls. **Rhus.* Sabin. Sep. Spong. Staph. *Stront.* Sulph. Tart. Thuj.

Blisters, vesicles, Amm. m. Magn. c. Magn. m. Mur. ac. Natr. Nitr.

Pimples, *Arn.* *Bov.* Con. Mang. Natr. s.

Pustules, Crotal. Magn. s. Nitr. Tart.

Swelling, **Acon.* **Baryt.* Bov. **Bry.* Calc. Cann. Canth. °*Carb. veg.* Chin. Con. Croc. Euphorb. Graph. **Led.* Lyc. Magn. m. Mang. Mur. ac. Par. **Puls.* Rhus. Sep. Sulph. Vip. torv.

Ulcers. °*Asa.* °*Baryt.* Bell. Calc. Carb. an. Carb. veg. °*Caust.* Clem. Cocc. **Con.* Hep. Kal. °*Lach.* Lyc. °*Merc.* Mez. N. vom. °*Phosph.* °*Puls.* °*Rhus.* Sabin. Sep. Sil. **Spong.* Staph. **Stront.* **Sulph.* Thuj. Zinc.
Scurfs, Amm. m.

Tubercles, Caust. Mur. ac.
Erysipelas, Rhus.

Face, **Arn.* Baryt. Bov. Canth. Con. Crotal. Euphorb. Lyc. Magn. s. **Phosph.* Rhus. Staph. Vip.
Lips, Arn. Bov. Magn. c. Magn. m. Mang. Nitr. ac.

Chin, Natr. s. Plat. Verb.

Buccal cavity, vesicles, Magn. c.
Dorsal region, swelling, Bov. Graph. Magn. m. Mang. Mur. ac.
—, tubercles. Caust. Mur. ac.
Anus, swelling, **Bry.* Calc. Sulph.
—, scurf, Amm. m.
Lower limbs, eruption, Nitr. ac.
—, swelling, °Carb. veg. **Led.* Sep.
Feet, swelling, Cann. Chin. **Puls.*

THICKENED, WHICH IS.

Hard skin, Amm. **Ant.* Ars. Borax. Cic. Clem. °*Dulc.* *Graph.* *Lach.* Par. *Ran.* **Rhus.* **Sep.* °*Sil.* Sulph. *Thuj.* Veratr.

Thickening.

Nails, Alum. Calc. **Graph.* Merc. Sabad. Sep. **Sil.* °*Sulph.*
Arm, skin of, Lach.
Feet, soles of, **Ars.*
Bones, s. Swelling.

Thoracic Region.

Blisters, vesicles, Caust.
Blotches, Natr. Sassap.
Blueness, clavicles, Thuj.
Boils, Amm. Chin. Magn. Phosph.
—, small, Amm.
Brownish spots, °Carb. veg. °Sep.
Burning, Baryt. Bov. Caps. Cic. Croc. Graph. Laur. Mez. Mur. ac. Natr. c. Nicc. Phell. Phosph. *Phos. ac.* Ratanh. Sulph. Sulph. ac. Zinc.
—, eruptions, Heracl. Mez.
—, pimples, Staph.
—, herpes, Staph.
—, spots, Amm. m. °Ipec. °Mez.
—, callosities, Rhus v.
Caries, Con.
Creeping, Alum. Coloc. Magn. aust. Magn. m. Mang. Ran. sc.
Dry eruption, Heracl.
Eruptions, which peel off, Led.
Erysipelas, Heracl. Kal. *Led.* °*Lyc.* *Merc.* Mercurial. Mez. *Rhus.* °*Sec.* Tereb. Val.

In the evening, Amm. m. Phos. ac. Ratanh. Nicc.
Formication, Magn. m.
Freckles, Nitr. ac.
Gnawing, Bell. Berb. Phos. ac.
Hard pimples, Bov.
Hepatic spots, °Lyc. *Sulph.*
Herpes, Magn. °*Petr.* Staph.
Itch, Squill.
Itching, Agar. Alum. Anac. Ang. *Ant.* Arn. Baryt. Berb. *Bov.* Calc. Canth. *Carb. veg.* Con. Kal. *Lyc. Natr. m.* Nicc. Phell. *Phosph.* Sabad. *Sep.* Spong. Squill. *Stann. Staph.* Sulph.
—, pimples, Bov. Staph.
—, herpes, Staph.
—, spots, °*Led.* Nitr. ac.
Pain as if ulcerated, °Spig. *Staph.*
Painful, eruption, °Lyc.
—, pimples, Con.
—, swelling, Rhus.
Pimples, Amm. Ant. Bell. Berb. Borax. Bov. Calc. Canth. Chin. Cocc. Con. Dulc. Gins. *Hep.* Jod. *Lach.* Magn. m. Natr. *Plumb. Rhus.* Squill. Staph. *Stront.* Tab. Zinc.
Pocks, Alum. °*Led. Tart.*
Pustules, Aur. Cocc. Evon. Graph. *Hep.* Magn. m. Sil. Stront. Tart.
Pustules, like cowpox, Tart.
Rash, Amm. *Bry.* Calad. Cupr. Galv. Lach. **Led.* Merc. *Sil. Staph.* Stram. Tart.
Red, pimples, Bov. Plumb. Staph. Stront.
—, spots, **Bell.* °Ipec. Magn. c. *Mez.*
—, rash, Amm. **Led.* Staph.

Scarlet-spots, **Bell.* Galv. Lach.
Smarting, Amm. Amm. m. Kal. Natr.
Smooth spots, Magn. c.
Sore, eruption, Rhus.
—, pimples, Calc. Hep. Rhus.
Spots, Amm. Ars. *Bell.* Carb. veg. Cocc. Crotal. °Ipec. Lach. **Led.* *Magn.* Mez. Nitr. ac. °*Phosph.* °*Sep.* Squill. Sulph. *Vip. torv.*
—, like fleabites, Mez.
Swelling, Bry. Rhus.
Swollen, sensation as if, Lach. *Merc.*
Tickling, Kal.
Titillation, Bell. Ran. sc. Spong.
Tubercles, Amm. m. Cann. Caust. Mang. Nicc.
Varicella, °Led.
Yellow spots, Ars. °*Phosph.*

Throbs, that which.

Blisters, phagedænic, Sil.
Swelling, **Bell.* Calc. °*Carb. veg.* **Cham.* **Lach.* Magn. m. N. vom. Sep. **Sulph.*
Ulcers, Acon. Ars. °*Asa.* Bry. °*Calc.* Caust. Cham. Chin. °*Clem.* Con. Hep. Hyos. Ign. °*Kal.* °*Lyc.* °*Merc.* Mez. Mur. ac. Natr. Natr. m. Nitr. ac. Phosph. Puls. Ruta. Sabad. Sep. °*Sil.* **Sulph.* Thuj.
Nails, on the, *Amm. m.* Con. Magn. aust. Sep.
Warts, Calc. Lyc. Nitr. ac. *Petr.* Sep. Sil. Sulph.

Buccal cavity, swelling, Calc. Lach. Magn. m. Sep. **Sulph.*
Arms, swelling, Magn. aust.
Hands, phagedænic blisters, Sil.
Lower limbs, swelling, °Carb. veg.

TICKLES, THAT WHICH.

Bloodvessels, swelling of, Carb. veg.
Pimples, Canth.
Pustules, Mez.
Figwarts, Thuj.
Rash, Bry.
Warts, °*Sulph. Thuj.*

———

Arms, eruptions, Agar.
Hands, eruptions, Agar. Canth.

TICKLING.

Anus, Agar. Bell. Mur. ac. Petr. Phosph. Ran. sc. Tarax. Tereb.
Sexual parts, scrotum, Chin.
Thoracic region, Kal.
Arms, Plat.
—, upper arm, Canth.
Hands, Arg. Ars. Cin. Grat. Lach. Mang. Merc. Mur. ac. Plat. Ruta. *Staph.*
—, fingers, Anac. Ars. Calc. Cocc. Grat. Hell. Merc. Ran. sc. Ratanh. Sep. Verb.
—, thumb, Merc. Ratanh.
Lower limbs, Carb. veg. Coloc. Corall. Ign. Laur. Petr. Sep. Spong.

Feet, Ign. Rhod.
—, heel, Laur. Mur. ac. Ol. an. Ratanh. Rhod.
—, soles, Alum. Euphorb. Graph. Hep. Mang. Ratanh. Ruta. **Sil.*
—, toes, Agar. Amb. Ars. Caust. Euphr. Kal. Sep.
Glands, Kal. Plat.

Titillates, that which.

Bloodvessels, swelling of, Ant. Kal.
Chilblains, Arn. *Colch. Magn. aust.* N. vom. °*Rhus.* Sep.
Erysipelas, Euphorb. **Rhus.*
Pimples, *Bell.* Caust. Magn. m. Veratr.
Rash, Gins.
Swelling, *Acon.* °*Arn. Caust.* Chel. *Colch. Con.* Lach. °*Merc.* Natr. *N. vom.* Phos. ac. °*Puls.* **Rhus.* Sec. °*Sep.* Spig. °*Sulph.*
Ulcers, *Acon.* °*Arn. Bell. Caust. Cham.* °*Clem.* Colch. °*Con.* Croc. Graph. *Hep.* Kal. °*Lach.* Merc. N. vom. *Phosph.* Phos. ac. Plumb. Puls. Ran. **Rhus. Sec.* °*Sep.* Spong. Staph. *Sulph.* Sulph. ac. Tart. Thuj.

Mouth, ulcers, °Lach.
Hands, eruption, Sil.
—, swelling, Caust. Lach.

Titillating.

In general, **Acon. Alum. Amb. Amm.* Amm. m. Ant. *Arg.* **Arn. Ars.* Asa. *Baryt.* **Bell. Bry.*

Calc. Calc. ph. Camph. Canth. Caps. ***Carb. veg.*** *Caust.* **Cham.* *Chel. Chin.* Cin. **Colch. Con. Croc.* Electr.Euphr. Evon. Ferr. magn. *Graph.* Guaj. *Hep. Ign.* **Kal. Lach. Led. Lyc.* Magn. art. **Magn. arct.* Magn. aust. Merc. ***Mur. ac.*** **Natr. Natr. m.* **N. vom.* Par. **Phosph.* **Phos. ac.* **Plat.* Plumb. **Puls.* Ran. Ran. sc. *Rhod.* **Rhus.* **Sabad.* Sabin. *Sec.* Selen. *Sep. Sil. Spig. Spong. Squill. Staph.* **Sulph.* Sulph. ac. **Thuj.* Veratr. *Viol. tr. Zinc.*

Head, Acon. Alum. Amm. Arn. Ars. Baryt. Calc. Carb. veg. Chel. Croton. Lach. Laur. Led. Nitr. ac. *N. vom.* Plat. Ran. Rhod. Rhus. Sabad. Spig. Veratr.

Eyebrows, Croc. Ran.

Ears, Alum. *Amb.* Amm. Ant. Ars. Baryt. Calc. Caps. Carb. veg. Caust. Chin. *Colch.* Coloc. Dros. Kal. Laur. Mill. N. vom. *Plat.* Phell. Ratanh. Rhus. Sabad. *Samb.* Sep. Spig. Sulph. Sulph. ac. Thuj. Tong. Veratr. Zinc.

Face, Acon. Alum. Amb. Anac. Ant. Arn. Bell. Calc. Cann. Colch. Euphorb. Evon. Ferr.magn. Gran. Lact. Merc. N. vom. Ol. an. Paeon. Plat. Ran. Sabad. Sec. Thuj.

Lips, Ant. Arn. Calc. Caust. Lact. Natr. m. Paeon. Phos. ac. Sabad. Stront.

—, of eruptions, Bell. Caust.

Buccal cavity, *Acon.* Alum. Arn. **Baryt.* Carb. veg. Caust. Colch. Ign. Lach. Merc. Natr. m. Petr. Plat. Rhus. Samb. *Sec.* Seneg. Sep. Tab.

—, palate, Caust. Colch. Sabad.

Buccal cavity, mouth, Alum.
—, fauces, throat, Acon. Carb. veg. Colch. Ign. Lach. Petr. Samb. Sec. Sep. Tab.
—, gums, Acon. Arn. **Baryt.* Rhus.
—, tongue, *Acon.* Alum. Merc. Natr. m. Plat. *Sec.* Seneg.
Anus, Agar. Alum. Baryt. Berb. Calc. Carb. veg. Caust. Chin. Cocc. Colch. *Croc.* Ferr. magn. Hep. Ign. Ipec. Kal. Laur. Magn. aust. Mosch. Mur. ac. Natr. *N. vom.* Ol. an. Phosph. Plat. Plumb. Rhus. *Sabad.* Sabin. Sep. Spong. Sulph. Tereb. Teucr. Zinc.
Sexual parts, Acon. Berb. Carb. veg. Chin. Magn. aust. Merc. Natr. m. Phos. ac. Plat. Sil. Spig. Thuj. Val.
—, frænulum, Merc. Phos. ac.
—, glans, Magn. aust. *Nitr. m.* Phosph. ac. Spig.
—, testicles, Berb. Carb. veg.
—, scrotum, *Berb.* Carb. veg. Chin. Merc. Phos. ac. Sil. Thuj.
—, penis, Val.
—, sexual parts, *Plat.*
Chest, Bell. Ran. sc. Spong.
Mammæ, nipples, Sabin.
Dorsal region, axilla, Bry. Mez.
—, neck, °Electr. Sec. Spong.
—, small of back, Lyc. Sassap. Stann.
—, loins, Croton.
—, nape of neck, Lact.
—, back, Acon. Baryt. Caust. Electr. Evon. Graph. Natr. Sec.
—, scapulæ, Anac. Arg. Lact. Magn. arct. Mez. Sil.

Dorsal region, os sacrum, Lyc.
Arms, Amm. Arn. **Bell.* Caps. Cham. Cocc. Croc. Gran. Natr. m. °*Nitr.* Paeon. *Sec.* °*Sulph.*
—, shoulder, Ammoniac. Berb. Cocc.
—, elbow, Berb. Canth. Merc.
—, upper arm, Lach. Sep. Thuj.
—, forearm, Arn. Bry. Con. Plumb.
Hands, Anis. Arn. Ars. *Baryt.* Berb. Bry. Caust. Hyos. Lach. Lam. Mez. Ol. an Op. Par. Phosph. Phos. ac. Plat. °*Ruta.* Sec. Seneg. Spig. *Sulph.* *Veratr.*
—, wrists, Calc.
—, fingers, *Acon.* Agar. *Alum.* *Amm. m.* Baryt. °*Calc.* *Cann.* Cin. Croc. Hep. Kal. Kreas. Lach. Lact. Laur. *Magn. arct.* *Magn. aust.* Magn. m. *Magn. s.* Mur. ac. °*Natr. m.* *Natr. s.* Nitr. ac. *Ol. an.* Op. Paeon. *Ran.* *Rhod.* Rhus. *Sec.* *Sep.* °*Sil.* Staph. *Sulph.* Tab. *Teucr.* Thuj. Veratr. Verbasc.
Hands, finger-joints, Sulph.
—, thumbs, Amm. Cin. Magn. art. *Natr.* *Ol. an.* Plat. Plumb. Sabad. *Teucr.* Zinc.
Lower limbs, Ars. Baryt. Bov. Caps. Caust. Cic. Euphorb. Guaj. Hep. Kal. Magn. art. Magn. c. Nicc. Nitr. ac. Plat. Rhod. *Sec.* Sep. Staph.
—, hips, Baryt. Evon. Kal.
—, thighs, Arg. Chin. Gins. Guaj. Hep. Plumb. Sep. Spig. Sulph. Sulph. ac. Tax.
—, knees, Carb. an. Electr. Gent. Kal. Merc. Rhus. Zinc. oc.
—, legs, calves, Alum. Ant. Baryt. Bell. Calc. Cast. Caust. Graph. *Ign.* Ipec. *Lach.* *N.vom.* *Ol.*

an. Phos. ac. *Plat. Rhod.* Rhus. Sep. Spig. *Sulph. Sulph. ac. Veratr.* Zinc.

Lower limbs, tendo Achilles, Sabin.

Feet, Alum. Amb. Ammoniac. Amm. Arn. Baryt. Bell. Berb. Carb. an. Croc. °*Dulc.* Euphorb. Magn. c. Mang. Mez. Mill. Phosph. Puls. *Rhod.* Rhus. Sassap. °*Sep.* Spong. *Stann.* Tax. Zinc. Zing.

—, soles, Arn. Berb. *Caust.* Clem. Con. Croc. Hep. *Kal.* Laur. Magn. m. Natr. m. Ol. an. Phosph. Plat. Puls. Raph. °*Sep.* Spig. Staph. Sulph. Thuj.

—, heel, Amm. Caust. Ferr. magn. Graph. Natr. Phosph. Stront. Sulph.

—, toes, Alum. Amm. Asa. Berb. Cast. *Caust.* Chin. *Colch.* Euphr. *Hep.* Kal. *Lach.* Lact. Magn. m. Natr. Nicc. Nitr. ac. Plat. *Plumb.* Puls. Ran. sc. *Sec.* Spig. Staph. °*Sulph.* Veratr. Zinc.

Bones, periosteum, Acon. Arn. Cham. Colch. Merc. Plat. Plumb. Puls. Rhus. Sec. Sep. Sulph.

Glands, Acon. Arn. Cann. Canth. Con. Magn. aust. Merc. Natr. Phos. ac. Plat. Puls. Rhod. Rhus. Sabin. Sep. Spong. Sulph. Zinc.

Transparent, Clear, that which is.

Blisters, vesicles, Kal. *Lach. Magn. c.* Magn. m. Mang. Merc. *Ran.*

Pimples, Con.

Spots, Phosph.

Swelling, *Merc.* Sulph.

Mouth, vesicles, Phosph.
Hands, vesicles, Mang. Ran.
Lower limbs, swelling, *Merc.* Sulph.

Tubercles, Blotches.

In general, *Agar. Alum.* Amm. *Amm. m.* Anac. Anthrok. *Ant. Ars.* Aur. *Baryt.* Bell. **Bry.* **Calc.* Cann. Canth. Caps. *Carb. an. Carb. veg.* **Caust.* Chel. Chin. *Cic. Cocc. Con.* Diad. Dig. Dros. *Dulc.* Electr. *Graph. Hell. Hep.* Ign. Jod. Ipec. Kal. Kal. chl. Kal. hdr. Kreas. **Lach.* **Led. Lyc.* Magn. art. Magn. arct. *Magn.c. Magn. m.* Magn. s. *Mang. Merc.* **Mez. Mur. ac.* **Natr. Natr. m. Nitr.* Nitr. ac. *N. vom. Oleand.* Op. *Petr. Phosph.* Phos. ac. *Puls.* **Rhus. Ruta.* Sabin. *Sec. Selen. Sep. Sil. Spig.* Spong. Stann. *Staph.* Stram. *Sulph.* Sulph. ac. *Tarax.* Tart. *Thuj. Val. Veratr.* Verb. Viol. tr. *Zinc.*
Burning, Amm. Amm. m. Calc. Carb. an. Cocc. Dulc. Kal. hdr. Magn. m. Magn. s. Mang. Merc. Mur. ac. Nicc. Nitr. ac. Phosph. Staph.
Suppurating, Amm. Bov. Nitr. ac.
Inflamed, Amm. m. Rhus.
Raised, Oleand. Rhus v. Val.
Gnawing, Rhus.
Yellow, *Ant.* Sulph.
Smooth, Phos. ac.
Scurfy, Sulph.
Hard, Amm. Amm. m. Ant. Bov. **Bry.* Con. *Lach. Magn. c. Magn. s.* Natr. m. Phosph. Rhus. Val.
Miliary, Natr. m.

Itching, Aur. Canth. Carb. an. Cham. Cocc. Dulc. Graph. Kal. Lach. Lyc. Magn. c. Magn. s. Mur. ac. Natr. m. Nitr. Nitr. ac. Op. Rhus. Staph. Stram. Stront. Zinc.
Tuberous, °*Natr.* Phosph. *Sil.*
Leprous, °*Natr.* Phosph. *Sil.*
Humid, Nitr. Selen.
Tearing, Cham. Con.
Erysipelatous, °*Natr.* Phosph. Sil.
Red, *Amm.* Berb. Bov. Carb. an. Carb. veg. Dig. Electr. *Hep.* Kal. chl. Kal. hdr. *Lach.* °*Led.* Magn. c. Magn. m. *Merc.* Mur. ac. Natr. m. Nitr. ac. Op. Phosph. ac. Puls. Sep. Spig. Sulph. Thuj. Veratr.
With red areola, Cocc. Dulc. Phos. ac.
Painful, *Amm.* Ars. Bell. Bov. °*Lach.* Lyc. Phos. ac. Zinc.
Painless, Arn. Bell. Graph. °*Ign.* Led. Oleand. Squill. Veratr.
Tensive, Caust. Mur. ac.
Stinging, Calc. Caust. Dulc. Kal. hdr. Led. Magn. arct. Magn. c. Phos. Rhus. Squill. Stram.
Stab-wound, after, Sep.
Tuberculous, Lach.
Malignant, Ars.
Wart-shaped, Lyc.
Watery, Graph. Magn. c.
Soft, Bell. Crotal. Lach.
White, Dulc. Sulph. Val.
Sore, Sep.
Painful as if sore, Ant. Caust. Magn. arct. Phos. ac.
Drawing-painful, Cham.

Eyes, Aur. Bry. Calc. Ran. sc. Thuj.
Eyelids, Aur. Bry. Calc. Ran. sc. Staph. Thuj.
Ears, Berb. Dros. Lach. Merc. Nicc. Nitr. ac. Phos. ac. Spong. Staph.
Nose, Natr.
Face, °*Alum.* Ant. °*Ars.* Baryt. Bry. Calc. Cann. Canth. Carb. veg. Cham. Chel. Cic. Con. Dig. Dulc. °*Graph.* Hell. Hep. Kal. Kal. hdr. Lach. *Led.* Lyc. Magn. arct. °*Magn. c.* Magn. m. Merc. Natr. Nitr. Nitr. ac. *N. vom.* Oleand. *Puls.* Thuj. Viol. tr. Zinc.
Lips and mouth, region of, Ars. Baryt. Bell. Bry. Caust. Con. Magn. art. Magn. m. Nicc. Sep. Sil. Stront. Sulph.
Chin, Bry. Carb. an. Euphorb. Hep. Magn. m. Oleand.
Lower jaw, Bry. °Graph. Natr. N. vom. Staph. Veratr.
Anus, Carb. veg. Hep. Ign. Stann. Staph. Thuj.
Sexual parts, Arn. Bell. Bov. Sep.
—, glans, Bell.
—, scrotum, Arn.
—, neck of womb, Kreas. Thuj.
—, labia, Calc. Phosph.
—, prepuce, Sep.
Thoracic region, Amm. m. Cann. Caust. Mang. Nicc.
Dorsal region, axilla, Nitr. ac. Phosph.
—, neck, Amm. °Lach. Lyc. Mur. ac. Nicc. Phosph. Phos. ac.
—, small of back, Lyc. Nicc.
—, nape of neck, Ant. Carb. an. Caust. Nicc. Zinc.

Dorsal region, back, Caust.
—, scapulæ, Amm. Squill.
Arms, Ars. Caust. Cocc. Dulc. Mang.
—, shoulder-joint, *Crotal.* Kal. chl. Phosph.
—, elbow, Caust. Magn. c. Mur. ac.
—, forearm, *Agar.* Amm. ***Mur. ac.*** *Nitr.* Phos. aç.
Hands, Ars. Carb. an. *Kal. chl.* *Merc.* ***Rhus v.*** Sep. *Spig.* Stram.
—, wrists, Amm. m.
—, fingers, Berb. Caust. Cocc. *Con.* *Lach.* *Led.* Lyc. Natr. Rhus. Veratr. Zinc.
—, finger-joints, *Zinc.*
Feet, Carb. an.
Glands, °Bry. Calc. **Carb. an.* *Cham. Clem. Dulc. °Graph. °Ign. Lyc. °Nitr. ac. °Phosph. Puls. Rhus.

Tuberous.

Blotches, °*Natr.* Phosph. *Sil.*

Nose, swelling, °Ars. °Merc.

Ulcerated, that which is.

Blisters, vesicles, Calc. Caust. Graph. *Merc.* *Natr.* **Sulph.* *Zinc.*
Blisters, phagedænic, Natr.
Bloodvessels, swelling of, °*Ars.* °*Cham.* Kreas. °*Lach.* °*Lyc.* °*Puls.* °*Sil.* Sulph. Tart.
Eruption, Ars. Caps. Carb. an. Chin. Squill.
Herpes, Zinc.

Nails, °*Alum.* Ant. °*Ars. Baryt.* Bell.? Borax.? Bov. *Calc.* Caust. *Con.* °*Crotal.* Ferr. magn. °*Graph.* **Hep.* Jod. °*Kal.* **Lach. Lyc.* Magn. aust. **Merc.* Natr. m.? °*Nitr. ac.* Petr. Phosph. °*Puls.* °*Rhus.* **Sep.* **Sil.* Squill. **Sulph.* Sulph. ac.

Pimples, **Merc.* Nitr. ac. Sabin. Sep.

Pustules, °*Ars.* °*Dulc.* Magn. m. °*Merc.* Sassap. Sil. Tart.

Rhagades, Bry. **Merc.*

Spots, Hell. *Merc.* Natr. m. *Sabin.* Thuj.

Swelling, Merc. **Nitr. ac.*

Warts, Ars. Calc. **Natr.* Phosph.

Eyes, Amb. Arn. Calc. Caps. Cham. °Clem. **Euphr.* Lyc. Phosph. *Sil.* Staph. **Sulph.*

Eyelids, °*Clem.* Colch. Croc. **Euphr.* Ign. Led. Lyc. Merc. Natr. Natr. m. N. vom. Phosph. Puls. Rhus. *Sil.* **Spig.* Staph. Stram. **Sulph.* Val.

Canthi, Calc. Phosph.

Ears, Alum. **Amm.* Bov. Bry. Camph. Galv. Gran. Graph. Kal. Lyc. **Merc.* °*Puls.* °*Ruta.* Spong. Stann.

Nose, external, *Puls.*

—, nostrils, Alum. Amm. m. **Ant.* *Aur. **Aur. m.* Borax. **Calc.* Caps. Corall. °*Graph.* Hyos. Ign. Kal. °Lyc. **Magn. m.* **Merc.* Natr. *Nitr. Nitr. ac.* Phosph. *Puls.* Ratanh. **Sil. Staph.* Tart. **Thuj.*

Lips and mouth, region of, Amm. m. Arn. **Ars.* °Aur. °Aur. m. Bell. Bry. Caps. Carb. an. Caust. Cham. Chin. Cic. Con. Dulc. Graph.

Ign. Kal. Lyc. Magn. art. Magn. arct. Mang. Merc. Mez. Natr. Natr. m. Nitr. ac. N. vom. Phosph. Phos. ac. Puls. Sep. **Sil.* Staph. Sulph. Zinc.

—, mouth, corners of, °Amm. m. Arn. **Bell.* **Calc.* **Graph.* Hell. Hep. °*Ign.* Mang. **Merc.* °Nitr. ac. N. vom. Phosph. Sil. Zinc.

Chin, Natr. m. Sabin. Sep.

Buccal cavity, Alum. Kal. hdr. Natr. *Natr. m.* Sep.

—, mouth, **Merc.* Natr. *Natr. m.* Rhod.

—, gums, Alum. Kal. hdr. Natr. *Natr. m.* Sep.

—, tongue, Cic. Natr. m.

Sexual parts, Caust. Merc. Nitr. ac. Thuj.

Nails, panaritia, °*Alum.* Ant. °*Ars.* *Baryt.* Bell.? Borax.? Bov. *Calc.* Caust. *Con.* °*Crotal.* Ferr. magn. °*Graph.* **Hep.* Jod. °*Kal.* **Lach.* Lyc. Magn. aust. **Merc.* Natr. m.? °*Nitr. ac.* Petr. *Phosph.* °*Puls.* °*Rhus.* **Sep.* **Sil.* Squill. **Sulph.* Sulph. ac.

Ulcers.

In general, Amm. Ang. °*Ant.* **Ars.* **Asa.* **Aur.* Baryt. Bar. m. **Bell.* Bry. **Calc.* °*Calc. ph.* Canth. **Carb. veg.* Caust. **Cham.* °*Chel.* Chin. °*Chinin.* Cinn. °*Cist.* Clem. Con. Crotal. °*Cupr.* °*Dulc.* °*Euphorb.* Galv. °*Gran.* Graph. Hep. Hyos. Ign. Kal. Lach. **Lyc.* Magn. art. **Merc.* Mercurial. Merc. ac. Merc. d. Mez. Mur. ac. Natr. m. °*Nitr. ac.* °N. mosch.? °*N. vom.* Oph. Petr. °Phell.? °*Phosph.* °*Phos. ac.* Plat. Plumb. **Puls.* Ran. ac. Ran. bulb. Ran. sc. **Rhus.* °*Ruta.* °*Sassap.* Selen. °*Sep.* **Sil.*

°*Staph.* **Sulph.* Sulph. ac. Tart. °*Thuj.* Vip. red. Vip. torv. °*Zinc.*

Aching, Camph. Carb.veg. Chin.**Graph.* Par.**Sil.*

Black, turning, Ant. **Ars.* °*Asa.* Bell. *Carb. veg.* Con. *Euphorb.* °*Ipec.* °*Lach.* *Mur. ac.* Plumb. Rhus. Sassap. *Sec.* °*Sil.* Squill. *Sulph.* Sulph. ac.

Bleeding, Alum. Arn. **Ars.* Asa. Bell. Bov. °*Carb. veg.* Caust. °*Con.* Croc. Dros. **Hep.* Hyos. Jod. **Kal.* Kreas. **Lach.* **Lyc.* Magn. art. *Merc.* Mercurial. Mez. Natr. m. **Nitr. ac.* **Phosph.* **Phos. ac.* **Puls.* Rhus. Ruta. Sabin. Sec. Sep. °*Sil.* °Sulph. Sulph. ac. Thuj. Zinc.

Blisters around, Ars. Bell. Caust. Hep. **Lach.* Magn. art. Merc. Natr. Petr. Phosph. *Rhus.* Sep.

Bloody crust, with, Bell.

Boring, Arg. Aur. *Bell.* Calc. Caust. Chin. Hep. Kal. Natr. Natr. m. Puls. Ran. sc. Sep. **Sil.* °*Sulph.* Thuj.

Bluish, *Ars.* °*Asa.* °*Aur.* Bell. °*Con.* °*Hep.***Lach.* *Mang.* *Merc.* Sec. Seneg. *Sil.* *Veratr.*

Bubbling (throbbing), Mur. ac.

Burning, Amb. **Ars.* Asa. Aur. Baryt. *Bell.* Bov. Bry. Calc. Carb. an. **Carb. veg.* Caust. *Cham.* *Chin.* Clem. Con. Dros. Graph. Hep. Ign. Kal. Lach. °*Lyc.* Mang. **Merc.* **Mez.* Mur. ac. *Natr.* Natr. m. Nitr. ac. N. vom. *Phosph.* Phos. ac. Plumb. **Puls.* *Ran.* **Rhus.* Ruta. Sassap. Sec. Selen. Sep. **Sil.* *Staph.* Stront. °*Sulph.* Sulph. ac. Thuj. Zinc.

Cancerous, °*Amb.* Ant. °*Ars.* °*Aur.* °*Bell.* °*Calc.* *Carb. an.* *Carb. veg.* Caust. °Chel. °Chinin. °*Clem.* *Con.* °*Hep.* Kreas. °*Lach.* °*Merc.* Nitr.

ac. Rhus. °*Sep.* °*Sil.* °*Squill.* Staph. °***Sulph.*** Thuj.

Chronic, malignant, Ars. *Baryt.* Calc. ***Carb. veg.*** Caust. °***Cham.*** °*Chel.* Clem. Con. Croc. °***Graph.*** ****Hep.*** Kal. °*Lach.* °*Lyc.* Magn. c. Mang. °***Merc.*** Mur. ac. Natr. °*Nitr. ac.* °*Petr.* *Phosph.* *Phos. ac.* °***Rhus.*** °*Sep.* °*Sil.* Squill. °***Staph.*** °***Sulph.***

Chronic, old, °*Chel.* Crotal. °*Cupr.* °Euphorb. *Lach.* N. mosch. °*Petr.* °*Phos. ac.* Ran. Ran. sc.

Cold feeling, with, Ars. **Bry.* Merc. ***Rhus.*** °***Sil.***

Confluent, Tart.

Corroded, as if, Merc. Mercurial.

Cutting, **Bell.* °*Calc.* *Dros.* Graph. Ign. *Lyc.* Mur. ac. *Natr.* Phos. ac. Rhus. Sep. *Sil.* Sulph. ac.

Deep, *Ant.* Ars. *Asa.* *Aur.* °*Bell.* *Bov.* °*Calc.* *Carb. veg.* Caust. Chel. Clem. °*Con.* Dros. ***Hep.*** Kreas. **Lach.* °*Lyc.* **Merc.* *Mur. ac.* Natr. Natr. m. **Nitr. ac.* *Petr.* *Phos. ac.* °*Puls.* Rhus. Ruta. Sabin. Selen. °*Sep.* °*Sil.* Staph. °*Sulph.* Thuj.

Digging, Asa. Bell. Bry. Calc. Caust. Chin. Natr. Phosph. Ruta. *Sep.* Stront. Sulph.

Dirty, discoloured, **Lach.* **Merc.* **Nitr. ac.* N. mosch. °*Sabin.* °*Thuj.*

Drawing-painful, Clem. Graph. Mez. Nitr. N. vom. Staph. Sulph.

Fetid, °*Amm.* **Ars.* °*Asa.* Bar. m. Calc. °***Carb. veg.*** Caust. Chin. °*Con.* Graph. °*Hep.* Lach. °*Lyc.* Mang. *Merc.* Mur. ac. Phosph. Plumb. °***Rhus.*** °*Sec.* °*Sep.* **Sil.* **Staph.* Vip. red.

Fistulous, °*Ant.* Ars. °*Asa.* *Aur.* °*Bell.* Bry.

**Calc.* °*Carb. veg.* °*Caust.* Chel. Clem. °*Con. Hep.* Kreas. *Lach.* Led. °*Lyc.* Merc. Natr. Natr. m. °*Nitr. ac.* Petr. °*Phosph.* Phos. ac. °*Puls.* Rhus. °*Ruta.* Sabin. Selen. *Sep.* °*Sil.* Stann. Staph. Stram. °*Sulph.* Thuj.

Flat, Amm. Ang. *Ant.* °*Ars.* °*Asa.* °*Bell.* Carb. an. Carb. veg. *Chin.* Corall. **Lach.* °*Lyc.* **Merc.* Natr, **Nitr. ac. Petr.* Phosph. °*Phos. ac.* °*Puls.* Ran. °*Selen.* °*Sep.* °*Sil.* Staph. Sulph. Tart. **Thuj.*

Gangrenous, Acon. °*Ars.* °*Asa.* Bell. °*Chin.* Con. Mur. ac. Rhus. °*Sabin.* °Sec. Squill. Vip. red.

Gnawed, as if, Lach.

Gnawing-painful, Agn. *Baryt.* Bell. Calc. *Cham.* Cycl. **Dros.* Hyos. *Kal.* Led. *Lyc.* Mang. *Merc.* Mez. Natr. *Phosph.* Phos. ac. °*Plat.* °*Puls.* °*Ran. sc.* Rhus. Ruta. **Staph. Sulph.* Thuj.

Gray, Ars. (Comp. Pus, GRAY.)

Greenish, Staph. (Comp. Pus, GREEN.)

Hard, with hard edges, Arn. °*Ars.* °*Asa.* Bell. Bry. *Calc.* Carb. an. *Carb. veg. Caust.* Cham. Cic. Cin. Clem. Graph. Hep. °Lach. **Lyc.* °*Merc.* Mez. Natr. N. vom. Petr. Phosph. Phos. ac. °*Puls.* Ran. Sep. **Sil.* Staph. **Sulph.* Thuj.

Herpetic, °*Zinc.*

Inflamed, **Acon.* Agn. Ant. Arn. **Ars.* Asa. Baryt. °*Bell.* Borax. Bov. °*Bry. Calc.* Caust. **Cham.* Cin. Cocc. *Colch.* Con. Croc. Cupr. Dig. Galv. *Hep. Hyos. Ign. Kreas. Led.

Lyc. Magn. arct. Mang. **Merc.* *Mez.* *Natr.* *Nitr. ac.* N. vom. Petr. **Phosph.* Plumb. °*Puls.* Ran. °*Rhus.* °*Ruta.* Sassap. Sep. °*Sil.* Staph. *Sulph.* Thuj. Veratr.

Itching, Agn. °*Alum.* °*Amb.* Amm. Anac. *Ant.* Arn. **Ars.* Baryt. *Bell.* °*Bov.* Bry. *Calc.* *Canth.* Carb. veg. °*Caust.* *Cham.* Chel. °*Chin.* *Clem.* Con. Dros. °*Graph.* **Hep.* Ipec. Kreas. Lach. Led. **Lyc.* *Merc.* Mez. Natr. Natr. m. Nitr. *Nitr. ac.* N. vom. Petr. *Phosph.* °*Phos. ac.* **Puls.* *Ran.* **Rhus.* Ruta. Sabad. Sassap. Selen. °*Sep.* **Sil.* Squill. °*Staph.* °*Sulph.* Tart. *Thuj.* Veratr. Viol. tr. Zinc.

Jerking pains, with, Ang. Arn. Cic. *Clem.* Mez. Mur. ac. Plat. *Ruta.* Sulph. ac.

Jerking-painful, °*Asa.* Bell. °*Calc.* °*Caust.* Cham. Chin. Cupr. Lyc. Merc. Natr. °*Natr. m.* Nitr. ac. N. vom. °*Puls.* °*Rhus.* Sep. °*Sil.* Staph. Sulph.

Malignant, Crotal. °*Lach.*

With maw-worms, °*Ars.* Calc. °*Merc.* Sabad.? °*Sil.*

Mercurial, °Alum. °Amm. °Arn. °*Asa.* °*Aur.* °*Bell.* °Calc. °Carb. an. °*Carb. veg.* °Cham. °Chin. °Clem. °Graph. °*Hep.* °*Lach.* °*Lyc.* °Natr. m. °*Nitr. ac.* °Phosph. °*Phos. ac.* °Sassap. °*Sep.* °*Sil.* °Staph. °*Sulph.* °*Thuj.*

Old, torpid, Anac. °Ars. °Calc. Camph. °Carb. an. °*Carb. veg.* °*Con.* Dulc. °*Euphorb.* Jod. Lach. °*Lyc.* Mur. ac. *Nitr. ac.* Oleand. °*Op.* °*Phos. ac.* Plumb. *Sep.* °*Sil.* °*Sulph.*

Painful as if bruised, Ang. Arn. Cham. Chin.

Cocc. Con. Graph. Hep. Hyos. Natr. m. N. vom. Rhus. Ruta. Sulph.

Painful as if burnt, Alum. Ant. °*Ars.* Baryt. **Carb. veg.* Caust. °*Cycl.* Ign. Kreas. Lach. N. vom. Puls. Sabad. Sec. Sep. Stram.

Painful as if sore, Alum. Amb. Amm. Ant. Arn. ***Ars.*** Bell. Bov. Bry. *Calc.* Caust. Cic. ****Graph.*** ****Hep. Ign.*** Kal. Lam. Lyc. Magn. art. Magn. aust. *Merc. Mez.* N. vom. *Phosph.* ***Phos. ac.*** °***Puls.*** Rhus. °*Sep. Sil.* Staph. °*Sulph.* Thuj. Zinc.

Painful as if ulcerated subcutaneously, Arn. Ars. ***Asa.*** Baryt. °Bry. °*Calc.* °*Carb. veg.* °***Con.*** Cycl. °***Graph.*** Hep. Kal. Led. Natr. m. Petr. **Phosph.* ****Puls.*** Ran. Rhus. Sec. ****Sil.*** Staph. ****Sulph.*** Tarax. Val. Zinc.

Painful, Alum. Amm. Anac. Ang. °***Arn.*** ****Ars.*** °***Asa.*** Aur. *Bell.* Carb. an. ****Carb. veg.*** Caust. Cham. Chin. Cic. Cinn. Clem. Cocc. Coff. Con. Croc. Cupr. Dig. Dulc. ****Graph.*** **Hep.* Hyos. Jod. Kreas. °***Lach.*** °***Lyc.*** °*Merc.* ***Mercurial.*** Mez. *Mur. ac. Natr. m. Nitr. ac.* N. vom. ***Petr.*** Phosph. °***Phos. ac.*** °***Puls. Ran.*** Ran. sc. Rhus. ****Sabin.*** Sassap. Selen. °*Sep.* ****Sil.*** Squill. Staph. ***Sulph.*** Thuj. *Veratr. Zinc.*

Painless, *Ars.* Bell. *Carb. veg.* Cocc. Con. Hell. Hyos. Ign. ***Lach.*** Laur. Lyc. Magn. art. Merc. Nitr. ac. Oleand. Op. Phosph. °*Phos.* ***ac.*** Puls. Rhus. Sec. ***Sep.*** Stram. Sulph.

Peeling off of the skin, with, Merc.

Pimples around, Acon. °Ars. °Asa. **Carb. veg.* °*Caust.* Cham. °*Lach.* Magn. art. Merc. Mez. Mur. ac. Natr. Petr. Phosph. °***Puls. Rhus.*** °***Sep.*** Sil. Staph. °*Sulph.*

Proud flesh, with, Alum. Ant. **Ars.* Bell. *Carb. an.* Carb. veg. Caust. °*Cham.* *Graph.* Kreas. °*Lach.* Merc. °*Petr.* Phosph. Sabin. °*Sep.* °*Sil.* Staph. °*Sulph.* Thuj.

Putrid, Amm. **Ars.* *Asa.* Aur. °*Bell.* °*Borax.* Bov. *Bry.* °*Calc.* Carb. veg. Caust. °*Chel.* °*Chin.* Cic. Con. °*Cycl.* *Graph.* °*Hep.* Kreas. *Lyc.* Mang. **Merc.* Mez. **Mur. ac.* Natr. *Nitr. ac.* N. mosch. N. vom. Oph. *Phosph.* °*Phos. ac.* Plumb. **Puls.* °*Rhus.* Ruta. Sabin. Sec. *Sep.* **Sil.* Staph. °*Sulph.* Sulph. ac. Thuj.

Pustulous, Sassap. Tart.

With red areolæ, Acon. Ant. Arn. °*Ars.* °*Asa.* Baryt. Bell. °*Calc.* Caust. °*Cham.* Cocc. Corall. Cupr. °*Hep.* Kreas. **Lach.* Lam. °*Lyc.* °*Merc.* Mez. Nitr. ac. N. vom. Petr. Phosph. °*Puls.* Ran. **Rhus.* Sep. °*Sil.* **Staph.* °*Sulph.*

Salt-rheum, like, **Amb.* °*Ars.* Calc. Chin. °*Graph.* °*Lyc.* Merc. Petr. Phosph. °*Puls.* °Sep. *Sil.* *Staph.* Sulph. (Comp. Blennorrhœa, Salt.)

Sarcomatous, Ant. °*Ars.* Cupr. **Hep.* Kreas. **Merc.* *Nitr. ac.* °*Sabin.* Sulph. Thuj.

Scorbutic, *Merc.* °Staph. (Comp. Scorbutic, that which is.)

Scrophulous, °*Ars.* °Aur. °*Bell.* °Bov. °*Calc.* °Carb. an. °*Carb. veg.* °Caust. °*Cist.* °*Graph.* °*Hep.* °*Lach.* °*Lyc.* °N. vom. °*Phosph.* Sep. *Sil.* °*Sulph.*

Scurfy, crusty, Ant. **Ars.* Baryt. °*Bell.* Bov. *Bry.* **Calc.* Carb. an. °*Cic.* Clem. °*Con.* Electr. °*Graph.* Hell. *Hep.* °*Led.* °*Lyc.* **Merc.* Mur. ac. N. vom. Oleand. Par. *Phos. ac.* Plumb. *Puls.* *Ran.* **Rhus.* *Sabin.* Sassap. °*Sep.* **Sil.* Spong. *Staph.* **Sulph.* Viol. tr.

Shining, Puls. Staph.

Shaggy, Hep. Lach. **Merc.* °*Phos. ac.* Sil. Staph. Sulph. Thuj.

Smarting, Ars. *Bell.* Bry. Calc. Carb. an. Caust. Cham. Chin. *Colch.* Coloc. **Dig.* Euphorb. °*Graph.* Lach. Lam. °*Led.* °*Lyc.* Mang. *Merc.* Mez. Nitr. ac. Petr. Phos. ac. **Puls.* Ran. *Rhus.* Ruta. Selen. Sil. Staph. **Sulph.* Sulph. ac. Thuj.

Sour-smelling, Sulph. (Comp. Pus, Sour-smelling.)

Spongy, Alum. *Ant.* °*Ars.* *Bell.* Calc. **Carb. an.* *Carb. veg.* Caust. Cham. *Clem.* Con. Graph. Jod. Kreas. **Lach.* Lyc. **Merc.* Nitr. ac. N. vom. °*Petr.* °*Phosph.* Phos. ac. Rhus. Sabin. °*Sep.* **Sil.* °*Staph.* °*Sulph.* Tart. °*Thuj.*

Spotted, °*Arn.* Ars. °Con. Ipec. °*Lach.* Sulph. ac.

Spreading-phagedænic, Amm. Anac. **Ars.* *Bell.* Borax, Calc. **Carb. veg.* **Caust.* °*Cham.* °*Chel.* °*Clem.* Con. Cupr. °*Graph.* *Hep.* Ign. Jod. *Kal.* Kreas. °*Lach.* °*Lyc.* Magn. c. **Merc.* *Mercurial.* Mez. °*Natr.* Natr. m. **Nitr. ac.* N. vom. Oph. **Petr.* Phosph. Plumb. *Puls.* **Ran.* **Ran. sc.* °*Rhus.* Ruta. °*Sep.* **Sil.* Spig. °*Squill.* Staph. °*Sulph.* *Sulph. ac.* Zinc.

Stinging, Acon. Alum. Ant. Arn. °*Ars.* Asa. Baryt. *Bell.* Bov. °*Bry.* *Calc.* Camph. Canth. *Carb. veg.* Cham. *Chin.* *Clem.* Cocc. Con. *Cycl.* *Graph.* *Hep.* Lam. Led. **Lyc.* Magn. art. Magn. c. Mang. **Merc.* *Mez.* Mur. ac. *Natr.* *Natr. m.* Nitr. **Nitr. ac.* N. vom. **Petr.* Phosph. **Puls.* Ran. Rhus. Sabad. Sabin. Sassap. Selen. °*Sep.* **Sil.* Spong. Squill. **Staph.* *Sulph. Thuj.

Suppressed, °Lach.

Suppurating, **Ars.* °*Asa.* Baryt. Bar. m. Bell. Carb. veg. Chin. °*Chinin.* °Con. Crotal. Dros. *Hep.* °*Lach.* Mang. **Merc.* Nitr. ac. Paeon. Petr. *Phosph.* °*Phos. ac.* °*Puls. Sassap.* **Sil.* **Sulph.* Tart. (Comp. Pus and Suppuration.)

Swollen, Acon. Agn. Arn. *Ars.* Aur. Baryt. °*Bell.* °*Bry.* Calc. Carb. an. Carb. veg. Caust. Cham. Cic. Cocc. °*Con.* Crotal. Dulc. Graph. °*Hep.* Jod. °*Kal.* Lam. Led. °*Lyc.* Mang. **Merc.* Natr. *Natr. m. Nitr. ac.* N. vom. °*Petr.* *Phosph.* Phos. ac. Plumb. °*Puls.* **Rhus.* Sabin. Samb. °*Sep.* **Sil.* Staph. °*Sulph.* Vip. red. Vip. torv.

Swollen, raised edges, with,°*Ars.* Asa. Bry. Carb. an. Caust. Cic. Cin. °*Hep.* Lyc. **Merc.* °*Petr.* Phosph. Phos. ac. °*Puls.* °*Sep.* °*Sil.* °*Sulph.*

Syphilitic, °*Merc.* °*Nitr. ac.* °*Thuj.*

Tearing, **Ars.* *Bell.* Bry. **Calc.* *Canth.* Clem. Cocc. °*Cycl.* *Graph.* Kal. **Lyc.* Merc. Mez. Nitr. ac. *N. vom.* Phosph. Puls. Rhus. **Sep.* °*Sil.* *Staph.* **Sulph.* Zinc.

Tensive, °*Asa.* °*Baryt.* Bell. Calc. Carb. an. Carb. veg. °*Caust.* Clem. Cocc. **Con.* Hep. Kal. °*Lach.* Lyc. °*Merc.* Mez. N. vom.. °*Phosph.* °*Puls.* °*Rhus.* Sabin. Sep. Sil. **Spong.* Staph. **Stront.* **Sulph.* Thuj. Zinc.

Throbbing, Acon. Ars. °*Asa.* Bry. °*Calc.* Caust. Cham. Chin. °*Clem.* Con. Hep. Hyos. Ign. °*Kal.* °*Lyc.* °*Merc.* Mez. Mur. ac. Natr. Natr. m. Nitr. ac. Phosph. Puls. Ruta. Sabad. Sep. °*Sil.* **Sulph.* Thuj.

Titillating, *Acon.* °*Arn.* *Bell.* *Caust.* *Cham.* °*Clem.* Colch. °*Con.* Croc. Graph. *Hep.* Kal. °*Lach.* Merc. N. vom. *Phosph.* Phos. ac. Plumb. Puls. Ran. **Rhus.* *Sec.* °*Sep.* Spong. Staph. *Sulph.* Sulph. ac. Tart. Thuj.

Wart-shaped, °Ars.

White, white-spotted, °*Ars.* Calc. Con. Dros. Graph. **Lach.* **Merc.* Phosph. Sep.**Sil.* Sulph. Thuj.

Yellow, Calc. Corall. Nitr. ac. Plumb. Zinc. (Comp. Pus, yellow; and YELLOW, THAT WHICH IS.)

Head, **Ars.* Nitr. ac. Ruta.

Eyes, °*Ars.* °Calc. °Clem. °*Euphr.* °Hep. °Lach. °*Merc.* Natr. Ruta. Sil. °*Sulph.*

Ear, Bov. Camph. Kal.

Face, °Ars. °Bry. °Con. Jod. Merc. Natr. Phosph.

Chin, Hep. Merc.

Buccal cavity, Agar. **Agn.* Alum. Amm. °*Aur.* Berb. Borax. Bov. **Calc.* Canth. °*Caust.* Cic. Dig. Dulc. Gran. Graph. °*Hep.* °Jod. Kal. °*Lach.* **Lyc.* **Merc.* **Natr. m.* *Nitr. ac.* **N. vom.* Op. Petr. Phosph. Plumb. Sabin. *Sil.* *Staph.* **Sulph.* Sulph. ac. Thuj. Zinc.

—, palate, °*Aur.* Dulc. °*Lach.* Op. *Sil.*

—, tonsils, Calc. **Lyc.* °Ign.

—, mouth, Agn. Alum. Borax. Canth. °Gran.? °*Hep.* °Jod. **Merc.* *Mercurial.* *Nitr. ac.* °N. vom. Op. Petr. Plumb. Staph. Thuj. *Zinc.*

Buccal cavity, fauces and throat, Jod. °Lach. *Nitr. ac.* N. vom.

—, gums, °*Agn.?* Alum. Aur. Berb. Bov. **Calc.* Hep. °Jod. Kal. Lyc. **Merc. Natr. m.* N. vom. Phosph. Sabin. *Sil. Staph.* Sulph. ac. Zinc.

—, fistula dentalis, Canth. °*Caust.* Lyc. °*Natr. m.* °*Sulph.*

—, tongue, Agar. Amm. Bov. Cic. °Dig. Graph. Lyc. *Merc.* Mur. ac.

Abdomen, region of, °*Ars.* Bar. m. Chin. Cupr. *Hep.* Plumb.

—, inguinal glands, *Hep.*

—, inguinal region, Bar. m. *Hep.*

—, umbilical region, °*Ars.*

Anus, Paeon. Sassap.

—, perineum, Paeon.

Sexual parts, **Corall.* Graph. Hep. **Merc.* Merc. dulc. **Nitr. ac.* Phosph. °*Sep.* **Sulph.* **Thuj.*

—, glans, Corall. Nitr. ac. °*Sulph.* *Thuj.

—, labia, Graph. Thuj.

—, pudendum and thigh, between, Graph.

—, prepuce, Hep. *Merc. Nitr. ac.* Phosph. °*Sulph.*

Mammæ and nipples, °Hep. °*Phosph.* °*Sil.*

Dorsal region, neck, °*Lach.*

Arms, *Electr.* Rhus.

—, upper arm, °*Lach.*

Hands, Dros. °*Sil.*

—, fingers, Alum. Ars. Carb. veg. Kreas. *Lyc.* Mang. Plat. *Ran. Sep.*

—, finger-joints, Sep.

Lower limbs, thigh, Crotal. Kal. Merc. °*Sil.*

Lower limbs, tibia, *Graph.* Lach. *Sabin.* Vip. torv.
—, legs, Ars. Baryt. Bry. Calc. Canth. Carb. veg. Caust. Clem. Ipec. Lach. Lyc. Merc. Mur. ac. Natr. N. mosch. Phosph. Phos. ac. Puls. Ruta. Sabin. Sil. Staph. Sulph. Vip. torv.
—, calves, °*Lach.*
—, nates, Borax.
Feet, *Con.* °*Ipec.* *Phosph.* Puls. Selen. °*Sulph.* *Zinc.*
—, heels, **Ars.* Caust. Lam. °*Natr.* °*Sep.* °*Sil.*
—, soles, **Ars.* **Sep.* Sulph.
—, toes, °*Ars.* Carb. veg. **Graph.* *Nitr. ac.* °*Petr.* Plat.
Glands, °*Bell.* °Clem. °Con. °*Hep.* °*Lach.* °*Merc.* °*Phosph.* °*Sil.* °Sulph.

Unhealthy Skin.

In general, slight injuries or sores heal very slowly, Alum. Amm. *Baryt.* *Borax.* *Calc.* Carb. veg. Caust. **Cham.* Chel. Clem. Con. Croc. **Graph.* Hell. **Hep.* Kal. **Lach.* Lyc. Magn. c. *Mang.* **Merc.* Mur. ac. Natr. °*Nitr. ac.* N. vom. **Petr.* Phosph. Phos. ac. Plumb. *Rhus.* Sep. **Sil.* Squill. °*Staph.* °*Sulph.*

Varicellæ Acuminata.

In general, °*Acon.* **Ant.* Ars. Bell. °*Bry.* °*Carb. veg.* Caust. Cycl. Ipec. Natr. Natr. m. **Puls.* °*Sep.* **Tart.* *Thuj.*

Varicellæ Aquosæ.

In general, Acon. Ant. **Bell.* °*Puls.* °*Rhus.* Sec. °*Sil.* °Sol. n. **Tart.* Thuj.

Vesicles.

In general, Acon. Alum. Amb. Amm. *Amm. m.* Anac. *Ant.* Arg. Arn. **Ars.* Aur. **Baryt.* *Bell.* Borax. Bov. **Bry.* Calad. **Calc.* Camph. Cann. *Canth.* Caps. *Carb. an.* Carb. veg. *Caust.* Cham. Chen. Chin. Cic. **Clem.* Cocc. Coloc. Con. Crotal. Cupr. Cycl. Daph. **Dulc.* Electr. Euphorb. *Graph.* Grat. Guaj. *Hell.* *Hep.* Hyos. *Kal.* Kal. chl. Kreas. **Lach.* Laur. Lob. Lupul. Lyc. Magn. art. Magn. arct. Magn. c. Magn. m. Mang. Merc. Mercurial. Mez. Mur. ac. *Natr.* **Natr. m.* Natr. s. *Nitr.* Nitr. ac. N. vom. Oleand. Ol. an. Op. Oph. Petr. Phosph. Phos. ac. Plat. Plumb. Puls. Ran. Ran. sc. Rhab. Rhod. **Rhus.* Ruta. Sabad. *Sabin.* Sassap. *Sec.* Selen. Seneg. *Sep.* Sil. Spig. Spong. Staph. Stram. Stront. **Sulph.* Sulph. ac. Tab. Tarax. Tart. Thuj. Val. Veratr. Vip. red. Vip. torv. Zinc.
Air, containing, Kal. Vip. torv.
Black, °*Ars.* °Lach. *Natr.* Petr. Vip. torv.
Bleeding, Graph.
Blue, black-blue, **Ars.* Bell. Con. **Lach.* *Ran.* *Rhus.* Vip. torv.
Brown, brownish, Vip. red.
Burning, *Amm.* *Amm. m.* *Aur.* **Baryt.* Bell. Bov. **Bry.* Calc. Canth. Caps. Carb. an.

Caust. Cic. *Graph.* Hep. Lach. Magn. c. Magn. m. Mang. *Merc. Mur. ac. Natr. Natr. m.* Natr. s. Nitr. Nitr. ac. Phell. Phosph. Plat. *Ran.* Ratanh. Sabad. Seneg. Senn. Sep. *Spig.* Spong. Staph. Sulph.
As if from a burn, Amb. Bell. Carb. an. Clem. Lyc. Natr. Phosph. Sep. Sulph.
Close to each other, Ran. Rhus. Veratr.
Confluent, Alum. Phell. Rhus.
Cracked, breaking, **Bry. Crotal. Lach.* Lam. Lupul. Nitr. Phosph. *Vip. torv.*
Cutting, Graph.
Drawing-painful, Clem.
Dry, Rhus.
Erysipelatous, Amm. **Ars.* Baryt. **Bell.* Bry. Carb. an. Chin. Euphorb. **Graph.* **Hep.* *Lach. Petr. Phosph. Ran. **Rhus.* Sabad. **Sep.* °Sol. mamm. Staph. Sulph.
Fistulous, Aur. **Calc.* Petr.
Gangrenous, Acon. Ars. Bell. *Camph.* Carb. veg. Hyos. Lach. Mur. ac. *Ran.* Sabin. *Sec.*
Grape-shaped, *Rhus.*
Grouped, Rhus v. Sulph.
Hard, Lach. Phos. ac. Sil.
As if from heat of sun, Clem.
Herpetic, Nitr. ac.
Humid, Electr. *Hell.* Hep. Lach. Mang. *Merc.* Phosph. Ran. Ran. sc. Raph. *Rhus.* Sulph. Vip. torv.
Inflamed, *Amm. m.* Baryt. Bell. Nitr.
Itching, *Amm. m.* **Bry.* Bruc. * *Calc. Canth.* Carb. veg. *Caust.* Clem. Daph. *Kal.* Kal. chl. Kal. hdr. Kreas. **Lach. Magn. c.* Magn. m. Mang. *Natr.* Natr. m. Nitr. ac. Ol. an. Petr.

Phell. Phosph. Plumb. Ran. Rhus v. Sassap. Seneg. Sep. *Sil.* Spong. *Sulph.*
Itch-like, Lach. Phos. ac. Selen.
Painful as if ulcerated, Mez. Mur. ac.
Painful, Anac. *Bell.* Berb. Borax. Chen. Cic. Graph. *Kal.* Lach. Natr. m. Natr. s. Nitr. ac. N. vom. *Phosph.* Puls. Sulph. Val. Zinc.
Painless, Stront. Sulph.
Pale-red, Rhus.
With peeling off, *Bry. Puls. Rhus.
Pemphigus, °*Bell.* °Dulc.? °*Sep.*
Penetrating deeply, Lach.
Phagedænic, Amm. °*Ars.* Borax. Caust. °*Cham.* °*Clem.* °*Graph.* *Hep.* *Kal.* *Magn. c.* Merc. °Natr. *Nitr. ac.* Oph. Petr. °*Sep.* **Sil.* Sulph.
Putrid, Vip. torv.
Raised, Merc. Selen. Sulph.
Rash, like, Sil.
Red, *Ant.* Cic. Cycl. Crotal. Lach. Mang. Natr. *Natr. m.* Sil. Stront. Val.
With red areolæ, Cann. Crotal. Kal. Kal. chl. Natr. Sil. Sulph. Tab. Vip. torv.
Sac-shaped, **Kal.* Vip. torv.
Sanguineous, *Ars. Aur. Bry. Canth. *Natr. m.* *Sec.* Sulph.
With scarlet-redness, Caust.
Scurfy, Hell. Natr. *Ran.* Sil. Sulph.
Smarting, Graph. Mang. Phos. ac. Plat. Rhod. Rhus. Staph.
Sore and smarting, like a wound, Con. Electr. Hell. Magn. c. Natr. Phell. Rhus v. Sil. Staph. Thuj.
Leaving spots, Caust.
Stinging, Amm. Calc. Cham. Sil. Spong. Staph.

As if from stings of insects, Ant.
Suppurating, *Amm. m.* Aur. Bov. Calc. Carb. veg. Magn. c. *Natr.* Petr. Phosph. Puls. Ran. Ran. sc. Rhus. Sassap. Vip. torv. Zinc.
Tensive, Amm. m. Magn. c. Magn. m. Mur. ac. Natr. Nitr.
Transparent, clear, Kal. Lach. ***Magn. c.*** Magn. m. Mang. Merc. ***Ran.***
Ulcers, around the, *Lach. Rhus.
Ulcerated, Calc. Caust. Graph. ***Merc. Natr.*** **Sulph. Zinc.*
Watery, *Bell. Bov.* Bruc. Clem. Graph. Magn. art. Merc. Natr. Nitr. Plat. Plumb. Rhus. Rhus v. Sec. °*Sulph.* Tab. Vip. red. Zinc.
Whitish, Amm. Berb. Cann. Caust. Clem. Electr. Graph. Hell. Hep. *Lach.* ***Merc.*** Mez. *Natr.* Phosph. Sabad. Sulph. *Thuj.*
Wound, around, **Lach.* Oph. Rhus.
Yellowish, Ant. ****Dulc.*** Crotal. Mur. ac. Ran. Rhus. Vip. torv.

Head, Bov. °Clem. Ol. an.
Eyes, Amm. m. Bell. Croton. °*Euphr.* Magn. arct. Seneg. **Sulph.*
Eyelids, Magn. arct. Rhus. Selen.
Ears, Alum. Chin.
Nose, Amm. Carb. an. Croton. Lach. Magn. m. Natr. *Natr. m.* Nitr. ac. Petr. *Phell.* Phosph. Plumb. **Sil.* Veratr.
Face, Alum. Amm. Amm. m. Ant. Aur. Baryt. Bell. Bov. Bry. Canth. Carb. an. Caust. Cic. Clem. °*Euphorb.* Graph. Lach. Magn. c. Mang. Natr. Nitr. Nitr. ac. Ol. an. Petr.

Phosph. **Rhus.* Sep. *Sil.* Stront. Sulph. Val. Zinc.

Lips and mouth, region of, *Alum.* Amm. Amm. m. °*Ars.* Aur. Bell. Bry. Canth. Carb. an. Carb. veg. Caust. Cic. Clem. Con. Graph. Hell. Hep. Kal. Laur. Magn. c. Magn. m. Mang. Merc. Mez. Mur. ac. Natr. °*Natr. m.* Natr. s. Nitr. Par. Phosph. Plat. Ratanh. Rhod. Rhus. Sassap. Seneg. Senn. Sep. *Sil.* Staph. Sulph. Val. Veratr. Zinc.

—, corners of mouth, Caust. Laur. Mez. Seneg.

Chin, Hep. Natr. Sassap.

Lower jaw. Mur. ac.

Mouth, Amb. *Amm.* *Amm. m.* Anac. Ant. Aur. *Baryt.* Bell. Berb. Borax. Bry. *Calc.* *Canth.* *Carb. an.* Carb. veg. Caps. *Caust.* Cham. Chen. Electr. *Graph.* *Hell. Jod. *Kal.* *Lyc.* Magn. c. Magn. s. Mang. Merc. Mez. Mur. ac. Natr. **Natr. m.* Natr. s. *Nitr. ac.* *N. vom.* Petr. Phell. Phosph. Phos. ac. Sabad. *Sep.* Sil. Spig. *Spong.* Squill. Staph. **Sulph.* Sulph. ac. *Thuj.* *Zinc.*

—, palate, Baryt. Carb. veg. Electr. Natr. s. Phosph. Spig. Sulph.

—, buccal cavity, Amb. Anac. Baryt. Calc. Canth. Caps. Carb. an. °Hell. Jod. Kal. *Merc.* Natr. Natr. m. *Phosph.* Spig. Spong. Staph. **Sulph.* Sulph. ac.

—, fauces, *Calc.* Phos. ac.

—, gums, Aur. Bell. Calc. Canth. Caps. Carb. veg. Kal. Magn. c. Natr. s. Petr. Sep. Sil. Staph.

Tongue, *Amm.* ***Amm. m.*** Ant. ***Baryt.*** Berb. Borax. Bry. Calc. Canth. *Carb. an. Caust.* Cham. Chen. Electr. *Graph.* **Hell.* *Kal. Lyc.* Magn. c. Magn. s. Mang. Mez. Mur. ac. Natr. **Natr. m.* Natr. s. *Nitr. ac. N. vom.* Phell. Phosph. Sabad. *Sep.* Spig. *Spong.* Squill. *Thuj. Zinc.*

Abdomen, Caust. Merc.

Sexual parts, Carb. veg. Caust. Graph. *Merc. Nitr. ac. Phos. ac. Rhus.* Staph. Sulph. *Thuj.*

—, glans, Merc. Phos. ac. Rhus. Thuj.

—, labia, Graph. Staph. Sulph.

—, prepuce, Carb. veg. Caust. Graph. Nitr. ac.

Thorax, Caust.

Nipples, around, °Graph.

Dorsal region, neck, Alum. Magn. c. Vip. red.

—, nape of neck, Caust. Magn. c.

—, back, Caust. Graph. Natr. c.

—, scapulæ, Amm. Ant. Caust. Cic. Lach. Vip. red.

Arms, Amm. m. Ant. Caust. Daph. Kal. chl. Magn. c. Mang. Merc. Natr. ***Natr. m. Puls.*** Sassap. *Sil. Spong. Staph. Sulph. Vip. torv.*

—, shoulder, Amm. m. Magn. c. Mang. Vip. torv.

—, arm, Ant. Caust. Daph. Mang. Merc. ***Natr. m. Puls.*** Vip. torv.

—, elbow, Natr. *Sulph.*

—, forearm, Caust. Sassap. *Sil. Spong. Staph. Sulph.*

Hands, Ant. Bov. *Bruc.* Canth. Caust. °*Clem. Cocc.* Daph. °*Hep. Kal. Kal. chl. Kal. hdr. Lach.* Magn. c. *Merc. Mez. Natr. m.* Phosph. *Rhus. Selen. Spig. Sil. Squill. Sulph.*

Hands, wrists, *Amm. m.* Merc. *Rhus.*

—, finger, Bell. °*Clem.* Cupr. *Cycl.* Electr. *Graph.* Grat. Hell. °*Hep. Kal.* Lach. Laur. Magn. c. Mang. *Natr. Natr. m.* Natr. s. *Nitr. ac.* Phosph. *Phos. ac. Plumb. Ran. Rhus v. Sassap. Sep.*

—, finger-joints, Cycl. Hell. Hep.

—, thumb, *Hep. Lach. Natr.* Natr. s. *Phos. ac. Sep.*

Lower limbs, Ant. Hyos. Vip. torv.

—, hips and nates, Borax. Calc. Oleand. Phos. ac.

—, thigh, Cann. Caust. Sassap.

—, knee, Ant. Carb. veg. Caust. Phosph. Rhus. Sabad.

—, legs, calves, Bell. *Caust. Kal.* Mang.

Feet, °*Ars. Caust. Con. Graph. Lach. Phosph.* Selen. Sep. Tarax. Vip. torv. *Zinc.*

—, soles, Ars. Sulph.

—, heels, Calc. *Caust. Lach.* Lam. *Natr. Petr. Phosph.* Raph. *Sep.*

—, toes, *Graph. Lach.* Natr. Nitr. ac. *Phos. ac. Selen. Sulph.*

Warts.

In general, Amb. °*Amm.* Anac. Ant. Ars. °*Baryt.* Bell. Berb. Borax. Bov. **Calc.* Carb. an. Carb. veg. **Caust.* Chel. Con. Cupr. °*Dulc.* °*Euphorb.* **Euphr.* Ferr. magn. Hep. °*Kal.* Lach. **Lyc.* Magn. aust. **Natr. Natr. m.* **Nitr. ac.* °*Nitr. sp.* Petr. *Phosph.* **Phos. ac.* **Rhus.* °*Ruta.* Sabin. Sassap. °*Sep.* **Sil.* Spig. **Staph.* *Sulph. Sulph. ac. Thuj.

Beating, Calc. Lyc. Nitr. ac. Petr, Sep. Sil. Sulph.
Bleeding, Magn. aust. °*Natr.* Nitr. ac. Thuj.
Burning, Ars. Lyc. °*Petr. Phosph.* °***Rhus.*** Sep. Sulph. Thuj.
Flat, Dulc. Lach.
Hard, Ant. Borax. Dulc. Ran. Sil. °***Sulph.***
Horny, Ant. Borax. Graph.? Ran. °*Sulph.* °***Thuj.***
Indented, Calc. Euphr. Lyc. Nitr. ac. °***Phos. ac.*** °***Rhus.*** Sabin. Staph. °*Thuj.*
Inflamed, Amm. Bov. Calc. *___Caust.___ Hep. Lyc. *_Natr. Nitr. ac._ Rhus. Sep. *_Sil._ Staph. °___Sulph.___
Itching, Euphr. Kal. Nitr. ac. Phosph. Thuj.
Large, °*Caust.* Dulc. °*Natr.* Nitr. ac. Kal. *Sep.*
Old, °*Calc.* °***Caust.*** °*Nitr. ac.* °***Rhus.*** °***Sulph.***
Painful, °*Caust.* Natr. Natr. m. Nitr. ac. Sabin. Sulph. Thuj.
Painful as if sore, °Hep. °Lach. °Natr. m. Nitr. ac. Sabin. Thuj.
Pedunculated, Dulc. °*Lyc.* Phos. ac.? °***Thuj.***
Small, Baryt. *_Calc._ Dulc. Ferr. magn. Hep. Lach. *___Rhus.___ *_Sassap._ °_Sep. Sulph._ *___Thuj.___
Stingings, Ant. Baryt. °*Calc.* Caust. Euphr. Hep. Lyc. Nitr. ac. Rhus. Sep. Sil. °*Sulph.* Thuj.
Suppurating, humid, Ars. Bov. °*Calc.* °***Caust.*** °***Hep.*** Sil. °*Thuj.*
Tickling, °*Sulph.* Thuj.
Ulcerated, Ars. Calc. °*Natr.* Phosph.

Eyes, below the, Sulph.
Eyebrows, *___Caust.___

Eyelids, Nitr. ac.
Canthi, Nitr. ac.
Nose, °Caust.
Face, °***Caust.*** Dulc. °Kal. Nitr. ac. °Sep.
Arms, °*Caust.* Nitr. ac. °*Sep.* °*Sulph.*
—, upper arm, Nitr. ac.
—, forearm, °*Calc.*
Hands, Anac. Berb. °*Calc.* ***Dulc.*** Ferr. magn. ***Lach.*** ***Lyc.*** Natr. m. ***Nitr. ac.*** °*Nitr. sp.* Phosph. °*Rhus.* **Sep.* °*Sulph.* °*Thuj.*
—, fingers, Berb. Ferr. magn. Lach. °*Rhus.* °*Sulph.* Thuj.
—, thumb, *Lach.*

Wart-shaped.

Pimples, Phell.
Ulcers, °Ars.
Blotches, Lyc.

Face, °Ars.
Sexual parts, excrescences, Sec. °Thuj.
—, os tincæ, °Sec. °Thuj.
Dorsal region, pimples, Phell.
Hands, pimples, Lyc.
—, indurations, Borax.

Watery, containing water.

Blisters, vesicles, ***Bell.*** ***Bov.*** Bruc. Clem. Graph. Magn. art. *Merc. Natr. Nitr. Plat. Plumb. Rhus. Rhus v. Sec. °*Sulph.* Tab. Vip. red. Zinc.

Pimples, Coloc. Thuj.
Pustules, Stram.
Blotches, Graph. Magn. c.

Head, tumors, °Daph.
Eyes, Magn. c.
Face, blisters, Bov. Coloc.
Lips, vesicles, Bell. Bov. Clem. Merc. Plat. Rhus. Zinc.
Mouth, blisters, Graph. Natr. Petr.
Dorsal region, vesicles, Vip. red.
Arms, Natr. s. Nitr. Sulph.
Hands, blisters, Bell. *Cocc.* Magn. art. ***Rhus** v.* ***Sassap.***
—, fingers, Cupr. Magn. c. Natr. s. *Plumb. Puls.* ***Rhus** v.*
Lower limbs, œdema, °*Jod.* °***Rhod.***
—, vesicles, *Phos. ac.*
Feet, toes, blister, ***Phos.** ac.*

Weight, Sensation of.

Glands, Bell. Chin. Cupr. Magn. arct. Merc. N. vom. Phosph. Puls. Rhus. Sil. Stann. Staph. Sulph.

White and Whitish, which is.

Blisters, vesicles, Amm. Berb. Cann. Caust. Clem. Electr. Graph. Hell. Hep. ***Lach. Merc.*** Mez. ***Natr.*** Phosph. Sabad. Sulph. ***Thuj.***
Blotches, tubercles, Dulc. Sulph. Val.
Eruption, Agar. Ant. ****Ars.*** Borax. Bov. Bry.

Ipec. Merc. Phosph. *Puls.* Sulph. Tart. Thuj. Val. Zinc.
Herpes, Anac. °Zinc.
Pimples, Ars. Bov. *Carb. veg.* Chel. Coloc. Con. Cycl. Dros. *Kal.* Magn. arct. Magn. m. Mang. Natr. m. Petr. Phos. ac. Staph. Sulph. Zinc.
Pocks, Jod. Lyc.
Pus, Amm. Ars. *Calc.* Carb. veg. Hell. Lyc. Natr. m. Puls. Sep. Sil. Sulph.
Pustules, Cycl.
Rash and rashlike, Agar. **Ars.* Bov. °*Bry. Ipec.* °*N. vom. Phosph. Sulph.* **Val.*
Ridges, Magn. c.
Spots, **Alum.* Amm. °*Ars. Calc.* Carb. an. Electr. *Merc. Natr.* Nitr. ac. Phosph. °*Sep.* **Sil.* **Sulph.*
Swelling, °*Ant.* °*Ars. Bell.* **Bry.* °*Calc. Chin.* Dig. Euphorb. Graph. *Hep.* °*Jod.* Kreas. °*Lyc. Merc.* N. vom. °Ol. jec.? °*Puls.* °*Rhod.* °*Rhus.* °*Sabin. Sep. Sil.* °*Sulph.*
Tumors, Lach. Natr. m.
Ulcers, °*Ars.* Calc. Con. Dros. Graph. **Lach.* **Merc.* Phosph. Sep. **Sil.* Sulph. Thuj.

Head, Ant.
Nose, Carb. veg. Kal. Natr. Natr. m.
Face, Amm. Anac. °Calc. Carb. veg. Clem. Coloc. Dros. Euphorb. Natr. Petr. *Sulph.*
Lips, Hell. Lyc. Magn. c. Magn. m. Mang. Merc. Mez. Natr. Phosph. Zinc.
Mouth, blisters, vesicles, Amm. Berb. Merc. *Thuj.*
—, swelling, Sabin.

Mouth, ulcers, Calc. Dros. Graph. **Merc.*
Sexual parts, ulcers, **Merc.* Thuj.
Arms, eruptions, Agar. Kal. Merc. Natr. m.
Hands, Bov. Cycl. Magn. c. Natr. Nitr. ac. Phos ac.
—, spots, Electr. Nitr. ac.
—, ridges, Magn. c.
Lower limbs, blotches, Ant.
—, blisters, vesicles, Cann. Sabad.
—, pimples, Chel. Staph. Thuj.
—, swelling, Arn.? Ars.? Bell.? °*Calc.*°*Jod.* °*Lyc.* Merc.? N. vom.? Ol. jec. °*Puls.* °*Rhod.* Rhus.? Sil.? °*Sulph.*
Feet, eruption, *Cycl. Graph. Lach.* Sulph.
—, swelling, Kreas.

WITHERING.

Of the skin in general, **Ars.* **Calc.* Camph. Caps. Cham. **Chin.* Clem. Cocc. Croc. **Ferr.* Hyos. **Jod.* Kal. Lyc. Merc. *Phosph.* **Phos. ac.* Rhab. Rhod. Sassap. **Sec.* Seneg. **Sil.* Spong. **Sulph.* * *Veratr.*

YELLOW-SCALED.

Herpes, Cupr.

JAUNDICE, s. Yellow Colour of Skin.

YELLOW COLOUR OF SKIN.

In general, **Acon.* °*Amb.* Ant. *Arn.* **Ars.* Asa.

°*Aur.* °*Bell.* °*Bry. Calc.* Cann. °*Canth.* °*Carb. veg. Caust.* °*Cham. Chel.* **Chin.* Chinin. Cin. Cocc. **Con. Croc. Crotal.* Cupr. Cupr. ac. *Dig.* Dulc. Euphorb. °*Ferr.* Graph. Hell. *Hep.* °*Ign.* **Jod.* Kal. °*Lach. Laur.* °*Lyc. Magn. m.* **Merc.* Natr. Natr. m. *Nitr. ac.* **N. vom.* Oph. °*Op.* Petr. *Phosph.* Phos. ac. °*Plumb.* °*Puls.* °*Ran.?* Rhab. °*Rhus.* Sabad. Sec. **Sep.* Sil. °*Spig.* °*Sulph.* Sulph. ac. *Tarax. Veratr.*

In general, jaundiced, **Acon.* **Ars.* °Bell. **Bry.* °Carb. veg.? °*Cham.?* **Chin.* °Chinin.? *Crotal.* Cupr. Cupr. ac. **Dig.* Hep. **Jod.* °*Lach.* **Merc.* Nitr. ac. °*N. vom.* Oph. Plumb. °*Puls.* °Ran.? °*Rhus.* °Sulph. Sulph. ac.

—, yellow fever, °Crotal. °Acon.

Eye, sclerotica, **Acon.* °Amb. Ant. *Ars.* °*Bell.* °Bry. Calend. Canth. °*Cham.* Chel. °*Chin.* °Cocc. °*Con. Crotal.* **Dig.* Ferr. Ign. Jod. Magn. m. °*N. vom.* °Op. Phosph. Phos. ac. °*Plumb.* Puls. Rhus. Sep. °Sulph. Thuj. Veratr.

Nose, **Aur.* Croton. *Sep.*

Hands, Ign. Spig.

—, fingers, Chel. Phos. ac.

Nails, Amb. Ant. Ars. Aur. Carb. veg. Chel. **Con.* Ign. °*Merc.* °*Nitr. ac.* °*N. vom.* Phos. ac. **Sep.* **Sil.* Spig. °*Sulph.*

Yellow, that which is.

Blisters, vesicles, Ant. **Dulc.* Crotal. Mur. ac. Ran. Rhus. Vip. torv.

Blotches, Tumors, ***Ant.*** Sulph.

Eruption, ***Agar.*** Ant. Ars. Aur. Bar. m. ****Cic.*** Cocc. Cupr. ***Euphorb.*** Hell. Kreas. Led. Lyc. °***Merc.*** *Natr.* ***Nitr.*** *ac.* Par. Phos. ac. ***Sep.*** Val.

Herpes, Cupr. °*Dulc.* Hell. °*Lyc.* °***Sulph.***

Nails, Amb. Ant. Ars. Aur. Carb. veg. Chel. ****Con.*** Ign. °***Merc.*** °*Nitr.* ***ac.*** °*N. vom.* Phos. ac. **Sep.* **Sil.* Spig. °*Sulph.*

Pimples, Ant. Grat. Magn. m. Zinc.

Pus, Acon. Amb. Amm. Anac. Ang. Arg. Ars. Aur. Bov. **Bry.* **Calc.* Caps. ****Carb. veg.*** ****Caust.*** **Cic.* °***Clem.*** Con. Croc. Dulc. Graph. Hep. Jod. °Kreas. Lyc. Magn. c. Mang. ***Merc.*** Natr. Natr. m. Nitr. *Nitr. ac.* N. vom. °***Phosph.*** ****Puls.*** Rhus. °Ruta. Sec. Selen. ****Sep.*** °***Sil.*** Spig. ****Staph.*** Sulph. Sulph. ac. Thuj. Viol. tr.

Pustules, Hyos.

Rhagades, Merc.

Ridges, Stram.

Scurfs, Ant. Aur. Aur. m. **Cic.* Kreas. Merc. Mez.

Spots, Amb. °*Arn.* Ars. Canth. ****Con.*** Crotal. **Ferr.* Jod. Kal. *Natr.* **Petr.* ****Phosph***, ***Ruta. Sabad.*** ****Sep.*** Stann. °*Sulph.* Tart. Vip. red. Vip. torv.

Swelling, Canth.

Ulcers, Calc. Corall. Nitr. ac. Plumb. Zinc. (Comp. Pus, yellow.)

Head, spots, Kal.

Eye, sclerotica, **Acon.* °Amb. Ant. *Ars.* **Bell.* °Bry. Calend. Canth. °*Cham.* Chel. °*Chin.* °Cocc. °*Con.* **Dig.* Ferr. Ign. Jod. Magn. m. °*N. vom.* °Op. Phosph. Phos. ac. °*Plumb.* Puls. Rhus. Sep. °Sulph. Thuj. Veratr.
—, spots, Phos. ac.
Ears, scurfs, Jod.
Face, Amb. Ant. **Cic.* °Colch. °Dulc. Euphorb. °Ferr. Hyos. Kreas. Lyc. °Merc. Magn. m. °*Natr.* **Sep.*
Lips, Merc. Mur. ac. °Natr. Phos. ac. Stram. Zinc.
Mouth, ulcers, Calc. Plumb. Zinc.
Abdomen, spots, Canth. *Phosph.*
Sexual parts, ulcers, Nitr. ac.
Thorax, spots, Ars. °*Phosph.*
Dorsal region, blisters, Ant.
—. spots, Jod.
Arms, eruptions, Hell. Sulph.
—, herpes, Cupr. Hell.
—, spot, Petr.
Hands, eruption, Ran. Sil. Spig.
—, spots, Sabad.
Lower limbs, eruption, Ant. Aur.
—, spots, °Con. Stann.
—, scurf, scald, Mez.

Zone-shaped.

Eruption, Ars. Bry. Cham. °*Graph.* °*Merc.* Natr. °*Puls.* °*Rhus.* Selen. *Sil.* Sulph.
Erysipelas, °*Ars.* °*Graph.* °*Puls.* °*Rhus.*

TABLE OF CONTENTS.

ALPHABETICAL LIST OF THE DIFFERENT PATHOLOGICAL NAMES OF THE MOST IMPORTANT CUTANEOUS DISEASES.

C.

D.

E.

F.

www.ingramcontent.com/pod-product-compliance
Lightning Source LLC
LaVergne TN
LVHW021306110826
845150LV00003B/501

* 9 7 8 1 4 2 5 5 5 9 5 9 5 *